PHARMACEUTICAL LIFECYCLE MANAGEMENT

PHARMACEUTICAL LIFECYCLE MANAGEMENT

MAKING THE MOST OF EACH AND EVERY BRAND

Tony Ellery
Ellery Pharma Consulting
Magden, Switzerland

Neal Hansen
Datamonitor Limited
London, United Kingdom

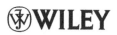

A JOHN WILEY & SONS, INC., PUBLICATION

Published by John Wiley & Sons, Inc., Hoboken, New Jersey
Published simultaneously in Canada

For general information on our other products and services or for technical support, please contact our Customer Care Department within the United States at (800) 762-2974, outside the United States at (317) 572-3993 or fax (317) 572-4002.

Wiley also publishes its books in a variety of electronic formats. Some content that appears in print may not be available in electronic formats. For more information about Wiley products, visit our web site at www.wiley.com.

Library of Congress Cataloging-in-Publication Data:

Ellery, Tony.
   Pharmaceutical lifecycle management : making the most of each and every brand /
Tony Ellery, Neal Hansen.
      p. ; cm.
   Includes index.
   ISBN 978-0-470-48753-2 (cloth)
   I. Hansen, Neal. II. Title.
   [DNLM: 1. Drug Industry–economics.   2. Drug Approval–economics.   3. Economics, Pharmaceutical–legislation & jurisprudence.   4. Marketing–methods.   5. Pharmaceutical Preparations–economics.   QV 736]

   338.4'76153–dc23

                                                                        2011041435

ISBN: 9780470487532

This book is dedicated to
Judith, Glyn, Simon, and David Ellery
and to Nicky, Bethany, and Alex Hansen.

◼◼◼ CONTENTS

ACKNOWLEDGMENTS

Many other experts stand behind the authors in a book of this type, and it is impossible to thank them all. The authors are grateful to Duncan Emerton, Principal Consultant and Head of Biosimilars Practice at Datamonitor Consulting for his insights and expertise that support the chapter on lifecycle management (LCM) for biologics, and to Bruce D. Sunstein of Sunstein Kann Murphy & Timbers in Boston, Massachusetts, USA, for reviewing the chapters on patents and the Hatch–Waxman legislation. Several industry experts also gave invaluable advice, but asked to remain anonymous, an understandable request in view of some of the sensitivities surrounding LCM, and especially late-stage lifecycle management (LCM). The authors are also grateful to Krishna Balakrishnan, Emma Law, and Ruch De Silva of Datamonitor Consulting for support with reviewing the text, completing figures and several of the case studies. Any inaccuracies remain the responsibility of the authors.

ACKNOWLEDGMENTS

The global research-based pharmaceutical industry lies increasingly between the rock of empty pipelines and the hard place of cost containment and more aggressive generic competition. In this environment, it is essential to exploit the whole spectrum of available lifecycle management (LCM) options to maximize the performance of existing brand assets.

This book is intended to pull together all of these potential measures into one reference manual, and to show how different LCM options can be combined to create winning brand strategies. The book contains many real-life case histories, collected in the Appendix, which illustrate specific situations where LCM has been successful, and also instances of attempts to enhance product life cycles that have failed. From each case history we have endeavored to derive lessons which other companies can apply to their projects and brands, or to highlight the mistakes that were made.

Our book will also look ahead to predict which LCM strategies will continue to be effective in the future. Many that have worked well in the past, even the recent past, will not be sustainable as health-care cost containment bites deeper in developed markets, and as generic companies become more expert in challenging brand exclusivities. As Yogi Berra stated, "The future ain't what it used to be."

LCM is highly cross-functional, and the book will evaluate alternative organizational structures and processes, and recommend which of these are optimal to ensure that excellent LCM can be reduced to practice in a company, and how to ensure that best practices are institutionalized and applied by successive project and brand teams, and across different geographies. The effectiveness of the organizational memory is a key aspect of LCM, as LCM strategies frequently do not deliver value until many years after they were initiated, during which time the brand has probably been managed by a succession of three or more project leaders and brand directors.

Included in the book is a practical, hands-on section for project/brand teams on the mechanics of how to actually design and write a convincing LCM Plan. We will also give some advice on how to present the plan to senior management. Having a great LCM strategy is not very helpful if the project or brand team is unable to express clearly and credibly to senior management what can be achieved with the brand, and thus compete successfully with other investment opportunities to get the resources required to implement the LCM strategies included in the plan. In such situations, internal marketing of product ideas is just as important as external marketing of the product itself to regulatory authorities, payers, physicians, and patients. Never, ever, assume that a good LCM Plan will speak for itself.

Finally, the book will show how to link corporate, portfolio, and individual brand LCM strategies, and will address the challenges faced by a branded drug company contemplating creating its own generics division.

Throughout, the book will also sound a note of warning. Effective LCM will not ensure the survival of the large, globally active research-based pharmaceutical companies. The value that can be squeezed out of existing brands can never diminish the need for strongly patented new molecules that address unmet patient needs at an affordable price. Big Pharma has been conspicuously less successful at achieving this goal during the last 20 years than in the 20 years before, and that fact is a prime driver of today's emphasis on LCM, namely the need to make existing brands deliver more profits for longer. But excellent LCM can only ever be a supplementary strategy for such large companies, or serve as a temporary bridge between the current product portfolio and the next crop of NMEs. (Note: We will consistently use the term "NME" = new molecular entity, rather than the almost synonymous "NCE" = new chemical entity.)

Before we go any further, we must first define the scope of our book, and the initial step must be to agree on what we mean when we write "lifecycle management" or LCM.

A good short definition of LCM as it relates to brand management in the branded drug industry is:

> "Optimizing lifetime performance of pharmaceutical prescription brands, every time, within the context of the company's overall business, product, and project portfolio."

Every word in this definition is carefully selected. A company with a portfolio of projects and brands can never hope to maximize the potential of each and every one. Choices have to be made.

This definition is a little broader than the scope of our book, as it covers the processes involved in taking an NME to market in its first indication/first formulation. We will use the term LCM in a narrower sense to cover all of the measures taken to grow, maintain, and defend the sales and profits of a pharmaceutical brand following its development, launch, marketing, and sales in its first formulation and its first indication. There are already plenty of excellent books covering the processes of developing and marketing a new drug, and we do not want to duplicate these efforts here. Moreover, because this book has to cover a vast amount of ground, we will not go into the operational details of how to implement LCM measures. For example, we will not be explaining how to write a patent, how to design a clinical trial, or how to test a new formulation.

But we will also not be making a mistake which is very common in the branded drug industry, and even in Big Pharma, that of using the term LCM to cover only those measures taken to protect brand exclusivity or to capture more of the genericized market once exclusivity has expired. We will certainly include this important aspect of LCM in our deliberations, and we will call it "late-stage LCM," abbreviated to LLCM. LLCM is just one area of LCM, and an excessive focus on LLCM in a company can be very dangerous. Because of the need of companies with weak new product pipelines to lengthen the life cycle of their older brands, LLCM has gained so much in importance in recent years that in some companies LCM is synonymous with LLCM. This is a grave mistake, for at least four reasons:

Focusing on LLCM means that the life cycle of the brand is not optimized during the period when the price is high and the composition of matter patent still provides robust protection.

Many investments are made in LLCM measures which will not provide a financial return as cost containment efforts are making ever more of these measures nonviable. It may well be preferable to invest these resources in building younger brands.

Emphasizing LLCM inevitably leads companies to start considering LCM too late in the brand life cycle for many of the good ideas to be implemented in a timely manner.

Some LLCM measures are cynical and even illegal, and should not be considered if the company wishes to avoid criticism and a deteriorating public image.

From now on we will consistently use the term "branded drug industry" to cover the innovation-based prescription pharmaceutical industry that depends for the bulk of its sales and profits on patented active drug substances. The large multinational branded drug companies we will call "Big Pharma."

As a last remark on definitions, you should note that the term "product lifecycle management" or PLM is widely used in the literature to describe something completely different from the subject of our book. "PLM" is used to describe the process of managing the entire life cycle of an industrial product from its conception, through design and manufacture, to service and disposal. PLM concepts were first introduced where safety was especially important, for example, in the aerospace, medical device, military, and nuclear industries. Since then, manufacturers of other instruments and machinery have also adapted the principles. Books on PLM thus often focus on areas like engineering, cost cutting, and managing product data. Books about PLM are not necessarily going to help you manage the life cycle of a pharmaceutical brand, and you should examine the tables of contents very carefully before investing in such books. If there are chapters on system architecture, database management, and computer-integrated manufacturing, then this is probably not the book you have been looking for!

Finally, you will see that we have not overloaded this book with references. Googling key words will generally provide the reader with a much broader and more up-to-date selection of background reading than we the authors could ever provide. In any case, many of the links that we used to source information will no longer be active by the time the book is published.

TONY ELLERY
Ellery Pharma Consulting

NEAL HANSEN
Datamonitor Limited

LIFECYCLE MANAGEMENT BUSINESS ENVIRONMENT

CHAPTER 1

Challenges Facing the Branded Drug Industry

In 2004, Capgemini conducted an industry-wide survey on pharmaceutical lifecycle management (LCM) ("Increasing the lifetime value of pharmaceutical products," Capgemini Vision & Reality Research, 2004). They held a series of interviews with pharmaceutical industry executives, asking them how important LCM had been for their business in the past 5 years and how they expected its importance to change during the coming 5 years. As can be seen in Figure 1.1, these executives felt that LCM had been important, but 90% predicted that its importance would grow during the 5 years following the publication of the report (2006–2010), with 60% expecting it to become much more important.

Today, just after the time horizon of this prediction, we can look back and state that it has proven to be very accurate, with more and more attention paid to LCM in company statements, conferences, and industry reports.

Why did these executives expect LCM to gain in importance, and why has their prediction proven to be correct?

To set the scene for any discussion of LCM of pharmaceuticals, it is essential that one fully understands the challenges facing the branded drug industry. On the one hand, many of these factors are drivers of the increased interest in LCM; on the other hand, some of the factors actively discourage LCM and put into question the sustainability of certain LCM strategies that were successful in the past.

As we see it, the main challenges are the following:

- Depleted new molecular entity (NME) pipelines/lower R&D efficiency
- Higher development costs
- Safety concerns
- Tougher environment for pricing, reimbursement, and listing

Pharmaceutical Lifecycle Management: Making the Most of Each and Every Brand, First Edition.
Tony Ellery and Neal Hansen.
© 2012 John Wiley & Sons, Inc. Published 2012 by John Wiley & Sons, Inc.

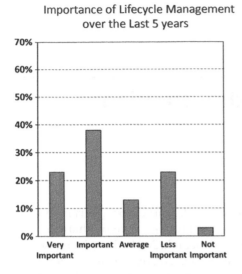
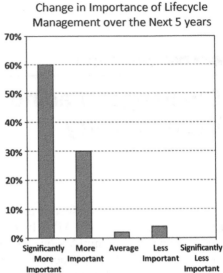

FIGURE 1.1. Increasing importance of lifecycle management. *Source:* Capgemini 2004 Vision & Reality Research, 60 Responses.

- Increased competition
- Earlier genericization
- Faster sales erosion following patent expiry
- Poor image of branded drug industry
- Diversification

1.1   DEPLETED NME PIPELINES/LOWER R&D EFFICIENCY

Since the mid-1990s, the number of NMEs approved by the Food and Drug Administration (FDA) and other health authorities has been declining, as shown in Figures 1.2 and 1.3. In the period from 2006 to 2010, the FDA approved half as many NMEs as in the period 1996–2010.

There is also mounting concern that many of the NMEs that do reach market are not adding significantly to the value of what is already there. In other words, the lack of innovation is not only quantitative in terms of the number of approvals and launches, but also qualitative in terms of the level of innovation as it translates into value for the patient.

A good example of this can be found in the treatment of hypertension. There are two levels at which we can consider "me-too-ism": first, at the level of the drug class, and second, at the level of the disease. Until recently, there were five classes of safe and effective antihypertensives on the U.S. and

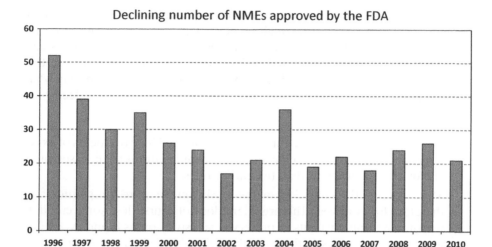

FIGURE 1.2. Reducing R&D productivity—Approvals. *Source:* www.fda.gov.

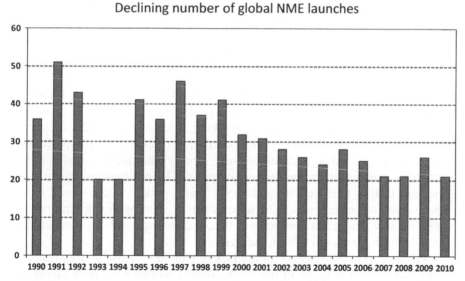

FIGURE 1.3. Reducing R&D productivity—Launches. *Sources:* www.fda.gov & www.pharmatimes.com.

European markets: the beta blockers, ACE-inhibitors, angiotensin receptor blockers (ARBs), Ca-antagonists, and diuretics. Well over a dozen different beta-blockers are available, over a dozen diuretics, and a good half-dozen each of ACE-inhibitors, Ca-antagonists, and ARBs. Some duplication in each class is acceptable from the medical perspective, as different patient groups may respond differently even if there are only tiny variations in the molecular structure of the drugs, but this high level of duplication was not driven by patient need, but by the commercial reality that large companies with a stake in cardiovascular medicine wanted to have their own patented drug in this highly profitable indication. Big Pharma will explain the duplication somewhat differently, particularly emphasizing two aspects which do also indeed play a role:

• Medical breakthroughs are rarer than incremental improvements of existing drugs. The later beta-blockers, for example, are in some cases safer and/or more efficacious than the earlier ones.
• More drugs of the same class on the market mean more competition and therefore lower prices. (This argument does, of course, lose some credibility when a company fights to preserve exclusivity on its brand even after other representatives of the same drug class have already gone generic.)

This, then, is duplication at the drug-class level. Duplication at the disease level is also well illustrated by referring to the hypertension arena. Although all five of the drug classes mentioned above are now available as cheap generics, the first representative of a new class of drug, the renin inhibitors, has already entered the market, and others are bound to follow. In reality, of course, the blood pressure of the vast majority of patients with hypertension can be effectively brought under control using the existing, genericized drugs, either singly or in combination. Companies have continued to invest in hypertension not because it is an unmet need, but because it is a big market, and it is easy to test the drugs. The real solution to the hypertension epidemic does not, of course, lie with better drugs. Stopping smoking, more exercise and less calories and alcohol, better monitoring of the population to ensure that hypertensive patients are identified, and identified early, more aggressive therapy by physicians using existing drugs, and better compliance by patients are vastly more important factors than new drug classes. Clearly, patient needs would be far better served by investing in these aspects rather than by developing me-too NMEs or new drug classes which are barely distinguishable in their clinical effects from the ones already on the market.

Analyzing all of the reasons for the lack of true innovation in drug research would go beyond the scope of this book. Many theories have been advanced, and the truth is likely to lie in a combination of different factors. Here are some of the leading contenders:

• *No More Low-Hanging Fruit*: As already mentioned, there are already safe and effective therapies available for most "easy" diseases, hypertension being a prime example. The diseases which still have a high degree of unmet need, for example, cancer, mental disease, and degenerative diseases of old age, have complex etiologies and are more difficult to treat. One CEO put it like this: "Most of the easy wins have already been made. . . . Now we are into more indirect ways of treating diseases: stopping tumours from growing by preventing their ability to get blood supply. These are much more complicated. This is not to belittle the advances so far, but things are getting difficult" (Lars Rebien Sorenson, CEO of Novo Nordisk, *BusinessWorld*, 2004). Pipeline attrition is of growing concern at both ends of the development process. Early on, better validation of molecular targets for their relevance in man is required to prevent the high rates of efficacy and safety failures. And where projects do fail, the problems must be recognized earlier in the development process. Phase III attrition, and thus the loss of drugs or indication extensions after most of the huge development costs have already been incurred, represents a massive opportunity cost that the branded drug industry can scarcely afford. In 2010—just in cancer—Big Pharma experienced 10 Phase III failures (Pfizer: Sutent® and figitumumab, AstraZeneca: cediranib and zibotentan, Amgen: Vectibix®, Novartis: Zometa® and ASA404, Lilly: Alimta® and tasisulam, Roche: Avastin®).

- *Low Innovation in Big Organizations*: The huge research departments of Big Pharma may not be the ideal breeding ground for innovation, which is more likely to take place in smaller, less structured, and more autonomous groups. This is frequently advanced as an explanation as to why small biotech companies appear to have a better innovation record than the larger companies, and why many Big Pharma companies are closing more and more biotech deals while cutting back on their internal R&D resources. Pfizer, GlaxoSmithKline (GSK), and Novartis are three of many examples of companies that made massive cuts in 2010 and 2011. For years, companies have sought a solution by pursuing megamergers and frequently spoke of "critical mass" in R&D. The trend is now in the opposite direction, with companies breaking their R&D forces into smaller, more autonomous groups, outsourcing and relying increasingly on biotech for innovation. One example of the failure of megamergers to provide the necessary impulse is evident at GSK. The two premerger companies Glaxo Wellcome and Smith Kline Beecham together received 26 NME approvals in the United States in the 6 years prior to their year 2000 merger; in the 6 years following, the merged company, GSK, only managed 15 NME approvals. Another aspect of this problem may relate to executive compensation. In a press release in March 2011, Hay Group consultants stated that biotech and biopharma are innovators not only in the technology and products coming out of their labs, but also in how they measure and reward their executives. Senior executives in Big Pharma are incentivized for the most part to achieve short-term financial results, and this would seem to be inappropriate in an industry with extremely long, multiyear product development cycles.

- *Delayed Peak Sales*: The achievement of peak sales of new introductions is frequently delayed by restrictions of their use to small, high unmet need patient subpopulations until a comprehensive safety database has been accumulated to allow use in broader patient populations. Together with downward pressure on prices, this leads to less funds being available to pump back into R&D.

Whatever the exact contributory effect of these different causes, it is an undisputed fact that less new NMEs are making it to market, and this inevitably means that companies are forced to attempt to squeeze more value out of their existing marketed brand assets.

As we finalize this book, there are early signs that things might be improving. At a Reuters Health Summit in New York in May 2011, the Head of FDA's drugs center, Janet Woodcock, stated that as the FDA had already approved 12 new drugs to date in 2011, she expected last year's total of 21 to be surpassed. She felt this was due to more successful products coming from advancements in science and research investments made a decade or more ago, but added that although she thought that the nadir had been reached, recovery would be gradual. Indeed, by early December, the FDA had approved 30 NMEs, the highest number since 2004. We shall have to wait to see whether this is the start of a new positive trend or the kind of one-off blip that 2004 turned out to be.

1.2   HIGHER DEVELOPMENT COSTS

Although the profit margins of branded drug companies are under increasing pressure, it is important to realize that the reduced number of NMEs reaching market cannot in any way be blamed upon a reduction in R&D budgets, at least up until very recently. Indeed, as can be seen in Figure 1.4, R&D budgets increased steadily during the past quarter century. A simple calculation from Figure 1.4 shows that it cost about US$350 million to put one NME onto the market in 1990, with this figure climbing to US$2.5 billion per NME in 2007. In other words, the efficiency of R&D has dramatically reduced in the last 20 years.

So what are the true costs of developing an NME? Many people were skeptical when, in 2004, the Tufts Center for the Study of Drug Development estimated the costs of bringing a new NME to market as US$800 million (PhRMA, Tufts CSDD Analysis, 2005). This figure included the costs for all of the developmental drugs that did not make it to market, and the direct costs of development were more likely to have been around half of this figure, or US$400 million. And then in 2006, Tufts announced that it had developed the first comprehensive estimate of the average cost of developing a new biotechnology product, and pegged it at US$1.2 billion (PhRMA, Tufts CSDD Analysis, 2006). About half of this sum was needed in preclinical development, the other half for clinical trials. Again, one can discuss whether these are the correct figures. What one cannot dispute is that the costs of development are very high, and still climbing.

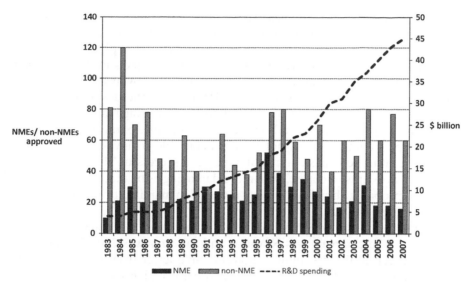

FIGURE 1.4. Increasing R&D spending is not reflective of the number of new NMEs. *Source:* FDA.

Obviously it costs less, and usually a lot less, to develop a line or indication extension of an already marketed NME as part of an LCM strategy. Even in the case of a completely new indication, much of the preclinical work performed for the initial approval can be reused for the new regulatory submission. Added to this, attrition is lower as the molecule is better understood, and there are less likely to be surprises regarding its safety and efficacy. Moreover, the commercial risks following approval are also more manageable because the drug has already been on the market, and its acceptance by health authorities, payers, physicians, and patients is well understood.

1.3 SAFETY CONCERNS

Regulatory requirements for NMEs have increased dramatically in recent years. This means higher development costs per NME and thus, inevitably, less projects and less NMEs. Some of this trend is driven by more stringent health authority demands regarding efficacy and quality, but the overwhelming majority of the increased per-project investment is caused by an increase in safety requirements.

Because of a series of high-profile product withdrawals resulting from safety problems that were not observed or not taken seriously enough during development (e.g., Bextra®, Lipobay®, Vioxx®, and Zelnorm®), more NMEs are being lost in preclinical development as a result of weak or ambiguous safety signals which in the past would not have caused a project to be discontinued.

But late-stage attrition in Phase III trials is increasing as companies some-times do not realize—or do not want to accept—that their NME will not make it to market. This is an inevitable consequence of depleted pipelines, as there are likely to be less short-term alternatives to the projects in Phase III and therefore tremendous financial pressure to make the few available options a success. Once a drug has reached Phase III, most of the development costs have already been incurred or committed, so such late-stage failures are much more damaging than failures early in the project because of the high sunk costs and the opportunity costs of not having been able to invest in alternative profit-generating activities that might have been successful. The rejection of a regulatory dossier is, of course, even more damaging as by that time, significant funds will probably already have been invested in manufacturing capacity and premarketing activities.

Let us look at just one example of how this increased focus on safety can hit a company. The company was Novartis, and the year was 2007. In February, Novartis received the first blow—an approvable letter from the FDA for its DPP-4 inhibitor, Galvus®, where the company had hoped for a straight approval. FDA was concerned about skin lesions seen in monkeys, and also wanted to see additional data regarding use of the drug in Type 2 diabetes patients with severe renal problems. Analysts assumed that the failure to get an approval letter would delay the market entry of Galvus by at least a year, and that this would allow Merck's DPP-4 inhibitor Januvia® to build a dominant market leadership position, but by the end of the year, things looked even worse for Galvus, and Novartis was admitting that the drug might never reach the U.S. market. That prophecy turned out to be correct, although the drug did get approval in Europe and many other countries and generated sales of close to US$400 million in 2010, more than doubling the previous year's result. The second blow in 2007 came in March, when the FDA requested that Novartis withdraw from the U.S. market its irritable bowel drug, Zelnorm, after analysis of clinical trial data had revealed a higher incidence of cardiovascular side effects in patients receiving Zelnorm than in patients receiving placebo. Still Novartis's miserable year was not finished, and in September, the company received a nonapprovable letter from FDA for its COX-2 inhibitor, Prexige®. Again the issue was safety, with the FDA concerned about the death of two patients in Australia suffering from liver disease, and in any case sensitized to the whole COX-2 inhibitor drug class following the withdrawal of Vioxx. All three of these 2007 decisions to withdraw or not to approve Novartis drugs were based on safety data which were far from black and white. Although these things are hard to prove in retrospect, a few years earlier—prior to the with-drawal of Vioxx—it is very likely that these data would not have been inter-preted as strictly, and that all three drugs might well now be on the U.S. market. Moreover, during the same period, three other Novartis products were also labeled with black-box warnings (Elidel®, Myfortic®, and Tasigna®). The neg-ative decisions by the FDA must have cost Novartis many billions of U.S. dollars in cumulative sales, and the value of Novartis shares dropped by 18% in 2007.

More recent examples of the increasing focus on safety issues can also be cited. The sales of GSK's Avandia® in Europe were suspended in 2011, and its use in the United States restricted to Type 2 diabetes patients who have both failed on every other diabetes medicine and have been made aware of the drug's substantial risks to the heart, which include stroke and heart attacks. Avandia's main class rival, Takeda/Lilly's Actos®, did not escape the crackdown on safety either, with concerns over a potential higher incidence of bladder cancer leading to withdrawals in Germany and France, and an eventual strong warning across the rest of Europe. And it was not only the older drugs that felt the impact of caution on safety of antidiabetic agents. In June 2011, an FDA advisory committee voted against AstraZeneca/BMS (Bristol-Myers Squibb)'s first-in-class SGLT2 inhibitor dapagliflozin on the evidence of potential increased cancer risks with the new agent.

Indeed, older, established brands are frequently perceived as safer than newer drugs, although this judgment should in reality be considered suspect and frequently does not stand up to close scrutiny. After all, the older drugs were not subjected to the same level of safety testing during development as is today the case. It is indeed interesting to speculate whether companies today would have persisted with the development of such therapeutic mainstays as penicillin and aspirin. Penicillin is associated with a 5% rate of hypersensitivity reactions and a 1% likelihood of anaphylaxis, and aspirin can cause gastric bleeding and intracranial hemorrhage. Recently, a meta-analysis was performed of 31 clinical trials involving more than 116,000 people taking either naproxen, ibuprofen, diclofenac, Pfizer's Celebrex®, Merck's Arcoxia® or Vioxx, Novartis's Prexige, or a placebo. All of the drugs were associated with a higher risk of stroke, heart attack, or cardiovascular death. While Vioxx showed the highest risk of heart attack (2.12 times compared with placebo), it was Arcoxia (4.07) and diclofenac (3.98) that posed the highest risk of cardiovascular death (Trelle, S., Reichenbach, S., Wandel, S., et al. 2011. "Cardiovascular safety of non-steroidal anti-inflammatory drugs: Network meta-analysis." *BMJ*). While Vioxx was withdrawn from the U.S. market in 2004 and Arcoxia received a nonapprovable letter from the FDA in 2007, diclofenac remains on the market after over 30 years as one of the most successful drugs in history, with the original brand, Novartis's Voltaren®, topping US$700 million in annual prescription sales in 2010.

Health authorities have been heavily criticized for allowing "dangerous" drugs to reach market in recent years, and there can be little doubt that they see less potential for criticism if they allow older drugs to continue to be sold than if they allow new ones with potentially serious side effects to reach the market. Thomas Paine explained the phenomenon rather elegantly in his 1776 book, *Common Sense*, when he stated that "A long habit of not thinking a thing wrong gives it a superficial appearance of being right. Time makes more converts than reason."

But companies must still be cautious of what they claim for their older drugs; Pfizer was warned by the FDA in June 2010 for failing to promptly

Health economics studies are essential for getting pricing and reimbursement

Regulatory	Pricing and reimbursement	Purchase
• Safety • Efficacy • Quality	• Effectiveness in the real world • Cost-effectiveness (value for money)	• Budget impact

FIGURE 1.5. Importance of health economic studies. *Source:* Ellery Pharma Consulting.

Figure 1.5 summarizes the different levels of studies that are required before a new drug will actually get used.

As mentioned in the OECD extract cited earlier, currently in the United States, there are no government price controls over private sector purchases. However, federal law does require pharmaceutical manufacturers to pay rebates on certain drugs to be eligible for reimbursement under several state and federal health-care programs.

While the United States relies mainly on competition to keep downward pressure on the price of drugs, all other major OECD countries practice price control in one form or another. The mechanisms employed vary considerably between countries, but the aim is always to achieve a reduction of drug budgets. It goes beyond the scope of this book to conduct a comprehensive global analysis of drug pricing and reimbursement, but we will spend some time looking at this important area as the measures can also impact LCM strategies like new formulations and fixed-dose combinations. Depending upon the market, the methods used include company profit control, price cuts and price freezes, reference pricing, prescription restrictions, physician budgets, patient co-pays, or self-pays, health economics analyses, parallel trade, tendering, generic substitution, and over-the-counter (OTC) switching. Price controls can be applied at the manufacturing or at the retailing level.

The most direct control is to set a fixed sales price and not allow sales at any other price. In other cases, governments will set very low reimbursement prices so that the patient has to pay the excess to the real price; this encourages the patient to look for a cheaper alternative, and this would be a generic if one is available. Some governments, including Japan and Canada, regularly reduce the reimbursement prices of marketed drugs.

Reference pricing is the preferred method for keeping prices down in some countries, where the government sets the level of reimbursement based on that in another country or basket of countries. Or the government may set reimbursement at the level of the average or lowest price of other drugs in the same therapeutic class. This last practice has been strongly criticized by the branded drug industry because it undervalues the properties of new market entries in existing classes, although these in some cases have efficacy or safety advantages, or may be more suitable than existing brands for treating certain patient subgroups. This form of reference pricing often penalizes new formulations, setting their prices at the same level as the generic of the original formulation.

Another method used to restrict usage of expensive new drugs is to limit the quantity that can be sold. Alternatively, a higher price may be allowed if low volumes are sold, but the price is cut if the sales volume rises above a predetermined level.

Actually limiting the amount of profit that a company is allowed to make on a product is an effective indirect way of controlling price and volume. This is practiced, for example, in the United Kingdom.

These measures all affect pricing and reimbursement. But as stated earlier, getting a price and reimbursement is not the last problem that a drug must overcome to be commercially successful.

The next hurdle is actually getting onto the formulary, that is the list of drugs that the government, hospital, or insurer is willing to purchase and/or reimburse. A drug which is not included in the formulary will not get prescribed or dispensed unless an exception is granted, and this is hard to achieve. Even in situations where drugs not included in the formulary can be legally prescribed, the fact that they are not reimbursed will severely limit usage.

NMEs and LCM measures such as new indications and new formulations will be subjected to exactly the same kind of cost containment pressure at the price, reimbursement, and listing levels. Getting significant usage of line extensions at a premium price over the original product is becoming increasingly difficult, and in many cases, health economics studies are likely to be required which are so expensive, and so uncertain in their outcome, that the line extension does not offer an attractive commercial opportunity. However, line extensions can benefit to some extent from the experience already gained with the molecule on the market. The concerns of payers will be known and understood, and in some cases, arguments may already have been found or data already generated to address these concerns. In addition, if positioned and designed correctly, as we will see in later chapters, such line extensions can improve the value proposition and thus the formulary status of a whole franchise. The risk of failing to get a return on investment in developing a line extension may thus still be less than for an NME.

Pricing and reimbursement pressure is not going to go away. Indeed, it shows every sign of increasing in every developed market. Let us look at Europe first. Even as we finalize this book, it is uncertain whether the main European currency, the Euro, will survive, or whether countries with weaker economies such as Greece will have to revert to their old currencies, with enormous financial implications of doing so. The problems started in Greece, Ireland, and Portugal but have now spread to Italy and Spain, with the rating agencies even casting a critical eye on the situation in France and Germany.

It is indeed staggering to look at the levels of debt that most western countries have accumulated. Within the Eurozone, Spain, France, and Italy each have total debts (government, nonfinancial business, household, and financial institutions) of between 300% and 400% of GDP. This compares with figures of 400% for the United Kingdom (which is not in the Eurozone, having retained the pound sterling as currency), 300% for the United States, and nearly 500% for Japan. The healthiest European Union (EU) economy is Germany, but even here debt is at the same level as in the United States. The ratings agencies Standard and Poor's and Fitch have responded by downgrading or placing on credit watch all of the Eurozone economies. Eurozone economies which have already lost the top AAA Standard and Poor's rating include Belgium, Greece, Ireland, Italy, Portugal, and Spain, while it is worth remembering that both Japan and the United States are also not rated AAA.

Moreover, Japan, the second biggest drug market in the world behind the United States, is currently coping with the aftermath of the catastrophic March 2011 earthquake and the ensuing nuclear plant problems in Fukushima, and facing rebuilding costs estimated to be in excess of US$300 billion.

As we write, it is not clear how these various crises will play out, but—looked at from the narrow perspective of our book—they are bound to both increase price pressure on pharmaceuticals as countries all over the world fight to contain public spending and increase the pressure on funding in new product development. This latter factor will particularly impact biotech and other R&D-focused organizations as previous sources of funding become more difficult to find.

1.5 INCREASED COMPETITION

It is helpful to consider competition at three different levels:

Molecule. The company must compete with other companies offering the same molecule once the patent has expired, been invalidated, or been infringed "at risk" by a generic company. This form of competition has grown much stronger in recent years and will continue to do so, as we shall see in later sections of our book.

Drug Class. The company must compete with other companies offering different molecules in the same drug class. The dearth of innovative new classes of drug has driven ever more companies to develop "me-too" drugs, in other words, drugs that are in the same class but are claimed to offer some advantage regarding efficacy, safety, or convenience. This is not a new phenomenon, as the period of time that the first drug of a new class will have the market to itself before the next entry in the same class arrives has been growing shorter for decades; this trend is shown in Figure 1.6.

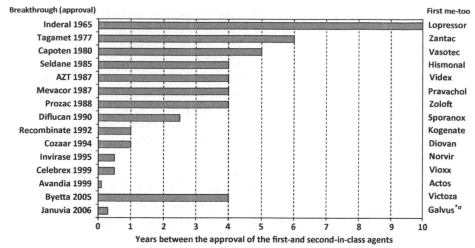

FIGURE 1.6. Delays getting shorter to second-in-class entries. *Source:* Adapted from Wilkerson Group, 2000.

Disease. The company must compete with other companies offering solutions for the disease which lie outside of the drug class. This can be a very broad competitive arena and can be divided into two sublevels:

· Competition with other prescription drug classes
· Competition with therapies other than prescription drugs (including, e.g., OTC medications, vaccines, surgical procedures, alternative medicine, even changed lifestyles)

Increased competition is a strong driver of LCM. New indications and more differentiated formulations may help to differentiate a drug from other offerings in the same drug class or for the same disease, and can be employed proactively and/or reactively to attain or maintain competitive advantage. And after patent expiry, patented line extensions may enable a brand to retain a higher share of the genericized market when facing intramolecular competition.

1.6 EARLIER GENERICIZATION

There are several different causes of earlier genericization, but the net result is the same: brands lose their exclusivity earlier in the life cycle.

The main reason for earlier genericization is that generic companies are now large, rich, confident, and experienced enough to enter into patent litigation with branded drug companies, or even to launch their generic product at risk, when they believe a patent to be invalid.

In the United States, the Hatch–Waxman legislation actually offers generic companies an incentive to invalidate drug patents, by providing 180-day marketing coexclusivity with the brand to the generic company that files the first Abbreviated New Drug Application (ANDA).

We will be looking at the Hatch–Waxman legislation in the United States later in the book, but another of its immediate effects when it was first passed back in 1985 was to establish the so-called safe harbor which allowed generic companies to conduct bioequivalence studies with patented drugs before patent expiry, thus enabling them to launch their generics on the very day that the patent expired instead of some months afterward.

A more recent event that may dramatically weaken some patents and thus further encourage earlier generic entry to the market is the 2007 ruling in the KSR versus Teleflex case. We will look at this landmark decision in depth later, but the bottom line is that the ruling has raised the bar on what can be considered a "nonobvious" invention. Some new formulations and fixed-dose combinations that were considered innovative and therefore granted a patent in the past will find it more difficult to obtain and maintain patent protection in the future.

There is no excuse for companies that do not prepare their brands for basic patent expiry. After all, on the day the patent is granted, a company knows exactly when the patent will expire two decades into the future. Planning for patent invalidation or at-risk generic launches is much more difficult, as the time point of the generic entry is not known in advance.

LCM strategies for maximizing the period of exclusivity, or at least limiting the impact of early genericization, include the construction of complex combinations of patents which are hard to invalidate and slight modifications of the drug substance which effectively create a new brand franchise. Again, we will be looking at this in considerable detail later in the book.

In practice, it is getting more difficult to obtain secondary patents, and many that are granted are very vulnerable to circumnavigation or challenge by generic companies. There is thus a large question mark against the sustainability of many LCM strategies which are based on the robustness of secondary patents.

1.7 FASTER SALES EROSION FOLLOWING PATENT EXPIRY

A separate but related issue is the rate at which generics gain market share from the brand once the patent has expired or has been invalidated. Clearly, generic substitution is an effective means of reducing health-care spending on drugs, as in many markets, generics cost only a tiny fraction of the brand price.

As was the case with pricing and reimbursement, different countries have chosen different mechanisms to promote generic substitution. As an example, in the United Kingdom and Spain, pharmacists are allowed to substitute

Country	Pro-Generic reforms
United States	• ANDA reviews to continue in parallel with the processing of Citizen's Petition to minimize the delay of Gx marketing approval
United Kingdom	• The Department of Health is considering imposing mandatory generic substitution by pharmacists
Germany	• Although not a reform, a precedent set in the approval of a near generic version of Plavix indicates opportunity for the future approval of other near generics with minor differences in composition compared to the originator • Germany is the largest Gx market in the EU and has had a range of pro-Gx legislature
France	• Price cuts for both branded and Gx drugs
Spain	• Price cuts of up to 25% on Gx drugs in July 2011 • Changes to reference pricing system as soon as the first Gx in a therapeutic group is added to the reimbursement list • Plans to make mandatory prescribing by active ingredient instead of brand name • A new Medicines Bill was passed that gave pharmacists the authority to carry out Gx substitution in 2006
Italy	• Price cuts of 12.5% on generic and off-patent drugs from June 2011 • Pharmacists were incentivized to dispense Gx by receiving 8% of the margin on the generic drug in 2009
Japan	• Incentives for physicians prescribing Gx drugs • Implementation of guidance for biosimilars' approval in March 2009

FIGURE 1.7. Health-care reforms in the 7MM aimed at increasing the use of generics. *Sources:* www.scripintelligence.com; Datamonitor pharmaceutical market overview reports.

brands prescribed by the physician with a generic. In the United Kingdom, substitution is encouraged by requiring physicians to prescribe drugs by the International Nonproprietary Name (INN) instead of by brand name, and pharmacists are incentivized to dispense generics. In Spain, physicians receive a lump sum payment if they reach annual generic subscribing targets. Figure 1.7 shows an overview of some of the methods used to encourage generic approvals and generic usage in seven top pharmaceutical markets.

The introduction of an improved formulation of the original brand, protected by a secondary patent, has historically been one of the most successful strategies for maintaining postpatent sales, and we will look at several examples of this strategy later in the book. The new formulation is introduced a year or two before the basic patent expires, the sales force persuades physicians to prescribe the new formulation, and by the time the generic arrives in the old formulation, the market has moved on to the new formulation so that there are few sales remaining for the generic to cannibalize.

But here as well the LCM environment is getting tougher. The new formulation must overcome a whole series of barriers before it can be commercially successful, and we will be looking at this later in the book. The barriers include:

- As mentioned earlier, will the secondary patent be granted, or is it too "obvious"?
- Is it robust? Can it withstand challenge?
- Can it be circumvented, that is, can another formulation with the same advantages be made without infringing the patent?
- Is the new formulation differentiated enough to get a premium price?
- After basic patent expiry, will it be reimbursed, listed, prescribed, and dispensed at that price, or will prescription sales move to the generics?

The combined effect of less new drug approvals and faster sales erosion by generics is demonstrated by the following figures. Murray Aitken, an IMS vice president, was quoted by *Forbes* in May 2010 as stating that 81% of U.S. drug sales in 2009 were for medicines where a generic was already available, compared to 61% in 2003; in 2003, 84% of patients prescribed a drug where a generic was available would get the generic, compared with 91% in 2009—put another way, in 2009 the brand was only retaining 9% of sales following genericization in 2009 compared with 16% in 2003, a drop in market share of 44%. With the one exception of Lipitor (which was due to go generic in 2011), the most prescribed drugs in the United States were now all generics (*Forbes*, "The death of the blockbuster," May 28, 2010).

1.8   POOR IMAGE OF BRANDED DRUG INDUSTRY

This is a controversial area, but as it is a key aspect of the problems that the branded drug industry are facing, and has a considerable impact on LCM strategies, it does need addressing here.

Once upon a time, around 25 years ago, branded drugs were regarded as one of the most innovative, socially aware, and ethical of all industries. This started to change as the profitability of branded drug companies rose to levels that were far above the average for other manufacturing industries, while at the same time innovation started to flag. Gradually, the perception gained strength that branded companies, and especially "Big Pharma," were not only exploiting sick people to line their own pockets, but were failing to even provide worthwhile new drugs that might at least partly justify this behavior. A Harris Interactive poll in 2010 showed the extent of the problem, comparing how much trust consumers have in different industries, highlighted in Figure 1.8. The results of these Harris polls are always rather depressing, but at least drug companies have improved by 1% since the last report in 2008. Looked at from the other side, however, it still means that nearly 90% of the U.S. public consider the pharmaceutical industry to be untrustworthy and dishonest.

What on earth are the reasons for this change in perception? Most of us in the industry are still proud of our contribution to the reduction of human pain

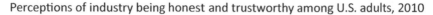

Perceptions of industry being honest and trustworthy among U.S. adults, 2010

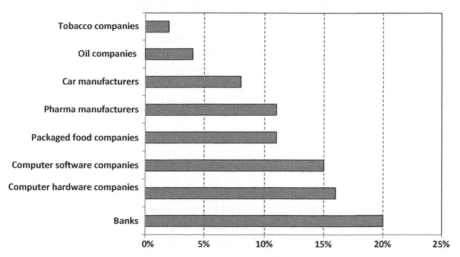

FIGURE 1.8. Public image of the pharmaceutical industry. *Source:* www. harrisinteractive.com.

and suffering, but that is not the way we look from outside of the industry. There are several reasons, and we have already touched on some of them.

1.8.1 Prosperity of the Branded Drug Industry

In many countries, society has the perception that good health—and therefore also health care—are basic human rights almost on the same level as clean drinking water and free oxygen to breathe. While society accepts that richer members of society are likely to enjoy better food, bigger houses, faster cars, and more elegant clothing, it seems wrong that they should also have better disease prevention, more effective therapies when they are ill, and consequently, less disability and a longer life expectancy. As long as poorer countries and weaker members of society do not enjoy the same benefits of good health care as the better-off citizens of the developed countries, it therefore seems to many to be vaguely indecent that pharmaceutical companies should reap huge profits in creating and selling drugs that are unaffordable for a large portion of the population.

And the branded drug industry is indeed very profitable. According to *Fortune* magazine, the profits of the U.S. pharmaceutical industry as a percentage of sales stood at 19% in 2008. Manufacturers of network and communications equipment were slightly more profitable at 20%, and medical equipment manufacturers not far behind at 16%, but all other manufacturing industries stood at 10% or less (*Fortune*, May 4, 2009). In this context, it is worth remembering that the profitability of retail pharmacies, pharmacy benefit managers

(PBMs), and payers is less than 5%. Executive compensation, which has been strongly criticized for the financial sector during the recent downturn, seems to be less of an issue for the drug industry in most countries. But there is sometimes criticism of chief executive compensation, for example, recently in the cases of Bill Weldon at J&J and Dan Vasella at Novartis.

The pharmaceutical industry is in a particularly vulnerable position when it comes to defending what is sometimes seen as its financial excesses, as it is in continual negotiation with governments and third-party payers regarding prices and reimbursement.

1.8.2   Lack of Innovation

We have already looked at this issue. In the 10 years from 1987–1997, the branded drug industry introduced important new classes of medicine to world markets. Examples include serotonin-specific reuptake inhibitors (SSRIs) for depression, statins for lowering cholesterol, proton pump inhibitors (PPIs) for gastric ulcers, ARBs for hypertension, and highly active antiretroviral treatment (HAART) therapy for AIDS. Since then, apart from Gleevec®, which is effective in a number of rare cancers, very few major new drug classes have launched, with one of these being the COX-2 inhibitors, which have since had to be withdrawn for safety reasons. As long as the branded drug industry was producing important new drugs, there was a broad acceptance that the companies should be allowed to earn good profits. Once innovation flags, but profits remain high, the potential for criticism obviously rises.

1.8.3   Marketing Spend and Tactics

While Big Pharma has repeatedly stated that it needs high profit margins to finance its expensive and high risk research efforts to find new drugs, critics have been quick to point out that the R&D spend of these companies is less than half of their sales and marketing spend. Indeed, a report by two University of York researchers in 2008 revealed that the U.S. pharmaceutical industry spent 24.4% of its sales dollars just on promotion compared with 13.4% on R&D (Gagnon and Lexchin. 2008. "The cost of pushing pills: A new estimate of pharmaceutical promotion expenditures in the United States," *PLos Medicine*). Some specific marketing practices have also come under heavy fire. In 2009, following a 4-year investigation, Pfizer was fined a total of US$2.3 billion for illegally promoting Bextra and other brands. The illegal marketing practices included paying physicians, resort trips, and kickbacks for prescribing Pfizer drugs for off-label indications; Pfizer had already been fined a total of US$500 million over illegal marketing since 2002 even before the 2009 judgment.

Industry critics point out that the affordability of even large fines is a problem regulators face in deterring such activity. In the case of drugs generating billions of dollars in sales every year, even fines of US$1 or US$2 billion do not offset the money to be made from off-label marketing.

Some controversial direct-to-consumer advertising campaigns have also come under fire, and lawsuits have targeted questionable pricing to state Medicaid programs. In just one recent year, the U.S. Justice Department had 150 cases on its docket of alleged fraud by pharmaceutical companies (*FORC Journal*, 2007, Vol. 18, Edition 3, Fall).

The less brands a company has on the market, and the less differentiated these brands are, the more necessary it becomes to utilize all possible marketing strategies to stimulate sales.

1.8.4 Safety Issues

Again, we have already considered this. But from the public image perspective, the main issue has not always been the safety issues per se, but rather how the pharmaceutical industry is perceived to have handled them. The popular press abounds with articles stating that pharmaceutical companies hide negative results from the public and continue to sell drugs that they know to be dangerous. One recent example in the *New York Times* of June 13, 2010 related to Avandia.

However, the most prominent recent example of concealment of negative results related to Merck's Vioxx. Hailed initially as a breakthrough pain therapy, Vioxx was withdrawn from the market in late 2004 after results from a clinical trial indicated an increased risk of heart attacks in patients taking the drug. Shortly afterward, *The Lancet* published a meta-analysis of available studies which indicated that "the unacceptable cardiovascular risks of Vioxx were evident as early as 2000" (*The Lancet*, 2004, Vol. 364, No. 9450, pp. 1995–1996).

In May, 2008, Merck was found guilty of using deceptive marketing tactics to promote Vioxx, and 30 states will split the resulting US$58 million settlement. At that time, the amount was the largest multistate settlement against a pharmaceutical company.

Legal cases involving the families of patients who were prescribed Vioxx and who died of heart attacks continued to appear in the press, and in 2007 Merck announced that it would fund a US$4.85 billion settlement expected to resolve roughly 50,000 lawsuits (Merck Press Statement, November 9, 2007).

Still the controversy continued, and in 2009, the U.S. Circuit Court of Appeals agreed to allow a class-action securities lawsuit connected to what Associated Press has described as "tens of billions of dollars in shareholder value" that plummeted when Vioxx was withdrawn from the market (reported in *WSJ*, April 27, 2010). Investors are accusing Merck of omission of critical information and releasing misleading information on Vioxx's risks.

Merck's defense was that its investors should have been aware, based on information in the public domain, that problems could have been existing with Vioxx, citing a U.S. FDA warning issued to the company regarding Vioxx in late 2001.

Merck was also relying on a 2000 study, the Vigor trial, which compared Vioxx to naproxen. In this trial, Vioxx patients had a fivefold increased risk for heart attacks (*New England Journal of Medicine*, 2000; 343:1520–1528). Merck maintained in a press statement that this should have provided investors with adequate warning of potential problems with Vioxx. But Merck had long argued in the opposite direction, against the interpretation that Vioxx was causing the heart attacks. Merck had maintained that naproxen was in fact preventing them. The investors' lawyer, David C. Frederick, stated that "It would be the height of irony that for Merck's success in concealing its fraud through the scientific uncertainty that was occurring with the naproxen hypothesis, that it would have this suit thrown out on statute of limitations grounds and never face the day in court that the investors here expect and deserve" (reported in *Washington Times*, December 1, 2009).

And to add to Merck's woes, in 2009, Scott S. Reuben, former chief of acute pain at Baystate Medical Center, admitted that data for 21 studies he had authored had been fabricated in order to enhance the analgesic effects of the drugs. It was pointed out that Dr. Reuben was also a former paid spokesperson for Pfizer, which owns the original Vioxx patent (*WSJ*, March 11, 2009).

Perhaps Merck could not have done more to avoid the Vioxx safety issue and subsequent withdrawal; after all, it is logical and acceptable that side effects with a low incidence will only appear after a drug has been approved for usage in broad patient populations. But, in retrospect, Merck would no doubt have liked to handle certain aspects of the case differently.

One key learning from the Vioxx case is how ready public opinion is to believe the worst of a large pharmaceutical company, even that the company is knowingly selling a drug which kills patients. As such, the Vioxx case is a prime example of just how far trust in the pharmaceutical industry has deteriorated.

1.8.5   Keeping Generics Off the Market

Some of the measures that branded drug companies employ to maintain exclusivity and keep generics off the market have met with considerable public and official criticism in recent years. There is growing concern that the majority of patents taken out by the pharmaceutical industry protect minor and often obvious "improvements" in existing drugs, and that they only serve to delay or prevent cheaper generic medicines reaching the market rather than providing any tangible benefit for patients.

On July 8, 2009, announcing the adoption of the European Commission Final Report on its competition inquiry into the pharmaceutical sector, Neelie Kroes, the European Commissioner for Competition, stated that "The inquiry has told us what is wrong with the sector, and now it is time to act. When it comes to generic entry, every week and month of delay costs money to patients and taxpayers. We will not hesitate to apply the antitrust rules where such delays result from anticompetitive practices. The first antitrust investigations are already under way, and regulatory adjustments are expected to follow dealing with a range of problems in the sector." The Final Report stated that "The inquiry concentrates on those practices which companies may use to block or delay generic competition as well as to block or delay the development of competing originator products."

In February 2009, the U.S. Federal Trade Commission (FTC) sued the branded drug company Solvay and the two generic companies Watson and Par Pharmaceuticals for attempting to delay generic competition to Solvay's branded testosterone-replacement drug AndroGel®, a prescription pharmaceutical with annual sales of more than US$400 million (FTC press release, February 2, 2009). According to the Commission's complaint, Watson and Par each sought regulatory approval from the FDA to market generic versions of AndroGel. In their FDA filings, both companies certified that their products did not infringe the only patent Solvay had relating to AndroGel, and also that the patent was invalid. The complaint charged that Solvay subsequently agreed to pay the generic companies to abandon their patent challenges and agree not to bring a generic AndroGel product to market until 2015.

"At a time of escalating health care costs, these unlawful agreements deny patients the benefit of competition between branded and generic pharmaceuticals and ultimately cost consumers hundreds of millions of dollars a year," said Acting FTC Bureau of Competition Director David P. Wales.

In his separate statement, FTC Commissioner Leibowitz stated, "This is yet another example of pharmaceutical companies turning competition on its head. . . . Congress enacted the landmark 1984 Hatch–Waxman Act to encourage early generic entry and save consumers money, but these anticompetitive deals threaten to destroy that benefit and make crucial portions of the Hatch–Waxman Act extinct in all but name."

The main focus of LLCM (late-stage lifecycle management) in branded drug companies is, indeed, to utilize all available measures to maintain brand exclusivity for as long as is legally possible. Every loophole in the pertinent legislation will be taken advantage of as the financial benefits of blocking generic entry are so gigantic.

Among our case histories in this book, we will be looking more closely at a pivotal case of LLCM, that of AstraZeneca's Nexium®. This was commercially very successful, but also encapsulated several controversial elements of how a major branded drug company with a poor pipeline managed to rejuvenate an old brand to compensate for a lack of NMEs. It prompted the former editor of the influential *New England Journal of Medicine*, Marcia Angell, to make the much-quoted statement in 2004 that the story of Nexium and drugs like it is proof that the pharmaceutical industry is "now primarily a marketing machine to sell drugs of dubious benefit" (Marcia Angell. 2005. *The Truth About the Drug Companies: How They Deceive Us and What to Do About It*, Random House).

Summarizing all that we have written so far in this first chapter, it can be categorically stated that the branded drug industry is facing more challenges

Top 10 pharma sales growth forecast 2013–2014

Rank	Company	% growth
1	Pfizer	−1.7
2	Novartis	2.9
3	GSK	6.2
4	Merck & Co.	−0.6
5	Roche	1.9
6	Sanofi	2.5
7	AstraZeneca	1.4
8	Johnson & Johnson	−0.5
9	Abbott	−3.1
10	Eli Lilly	−9.4

FIGURE 1.9. Growth forecasts. *Source:* Datamonitor PharmaVitae Explorer.

today than at any time in its recent history. Empty pipelines, higher development costs, lower prices, increased competition, and shorter brand life cycles constitute such a powerful combination of threats that many industry observers are asking whether we are currently seeing the beginning of the end of Big Pharma as we know it. In January 2010, on a single day, AstraZeneca announced it will cut 8,000 jobs worldwide, and GSK announced that 12,000 positions will be eliminated by 2014. And then in July 2010, Merck announced following its merger with Schering Plough in the previous year that 15% of its workforce, or 15,000 persons, would be put out of work over the following 2 years. It is in this environment that interest in LCM blooms, as desperate companies try to squeeze more sales and profits out of their diminishing portfolio of brand assets.

Industry analysts are almost united in their projections that that the branded drug industry will be unable to maintain the growth and profit levels that it has taken for granted for the last quarter century. As an illustration of what is expected, Figure 1.9 shows recent estimates for top-line growth for the leading companies from 2013–2014.

1.9 DIVERSIFICATION

As the discovery of new drugs becomes increasingly difficult, some branded drug companies are looking to spread risk by diversifying their businesses away from an overdependence on prescription drugs. Whether to follow this trend, and how widely to diversify away from the core business, is a quandary faced by many large and mid-sized brand companies, and there is no consensus yet on what the best approach might be. The very broadly diversified chemical/ pharmaceutical company seems to be a thing of the past. Historically, the drug industry grew out of the chemical industry in many cases, and was just one part of a widely diversified business portfolio based on chemistry. Just to take one of many examples, before its merger with Sandoz to form Novartis in the late 1990s, Ciba Geigy's business portfolio consisted of industrial chemicals (dyes for textiles, paper and leather, pigments for paints and plastics), precision balances, contact lenses, contact lens disinfectant solutions, plastics, health-care products (pharmaceuticals, OTC, and diagnostics), and agricultural chemicals (herbicides and pesticides). Later, companies tended to narrow their focus, with major players like Pfizer, Merck, and Roche concentrating their efforts on prescription drugs. Companies like Johnson & Johnson (J&J), with a broad business portfolio within what could loosely be defined as "health care," were rather unfashionable. Today, J&J looks almost like a role model as Big Pharma prescription drug companies spread out into adjacent areas like OTC, generics, diagnostics, medical devices, and eye care.

In the context of our book it is worth bearing in mind that this diversification of business interests can open up new in-house opportunities for LCM, both for increasing and defending prescription brand revenues.

The most obvious example of diversification supporting LCM is where a brand company sets up its own generics division, working on the time-honored principle of if you can't beat 'em, join 'em. The best industry example of diversification into generics is Novartis. Novartis's generics arm, Sandoz, is the second biggest generics company in the world behind Teva. Generics have a long history at Novartis, as both of the predecessor companies had generic businesses even before their 1996 merger. Ciba Geigy had sold generics under the Servipharm, Geneva, and Multipharma brands starting in the 1970s, and Sandoz had had a generics division, Biochemie, since the 1960s, adding the Azupharma acquisition shortly before the merger with Ciba Geigy. Within Novartis, all of these generic companies were grouped together under the resurrected Sandoz company name in 2003, and the subsequent acquisitions of BASF Generics, Lek, Hexal, and Eon enabled Sandoz to climb to its current position among the industry leaders.

Novartis is, of course, not alone in its endeavors to diversify into generics. In its 2009 Annual Report, Pfizer wrote "Pfizer is a growing force in the rapidly expanding but highly contested generics marketplace. While we have a huge generics catalog of our own, we recently entered into major licensing agreements with three India-based pharmaceutical companies, Claris Lifesciences, Aurobindo Pharma, and Strides Arcolab. These agreements will bring hundreds of high quality generic medicines to underserved populations around the world and add numerous products to Pfizer's portfolio of established brands in key markets." Pfizer tried to buy Germany's Ratiopharm in early 2010 but was outbid by Teva. Speculation through 2010 suggested that Pfizer's next target for strengthening its generics interests might be Stada, but that deal never materialized. Instead, in its Q4/2010 earnings call, Pfizer had to announce that the sales of its Greenstone generics unit had slumped by 14%.

Other Big Pharmas were also actively building up their stakes in generics. In 2009, Sanofi-Aventis acquired Zentiva, a branded generics group with products tailored to the Eastern and Central European markets, as well as Kendrick, one of Mexico's leading generics manufacturers, and Medley, a leading generics company in Brazil. Then in May 2010, Sanofi-Aventis strengthened its position in the emerging Japanese generics market by launching a joint venture with Nichi-Iko K.K., the leader and fastest growing generics company in Japan. The joint venture is 51% owned by Sanofi-Aventis.

GSK increased its shareholding in Aspen during 2009; Aspen is a major supplier of generics and branded generics in South Africa and also exports to some markets. GSK also acquired BMS's mature products business in Egypt during 2009 and, in 2010, added Argentina's Laboratorios Phoenix.

AstraZeneca, one of the Big Pharmas which has suffered most from patent expiries of its leading drugs in recent years, stated in its 2009 Annual Report that it intends to selectively supplement its Emerging Markets portfolio with branded generic products sourced externally and marketed under the AstraZeneca brand, and in 2010 announced three generics pacts with Aurobindo, Torrent, and Intas.

Will this recent interest of Big Pharma in the generics industry prove to be successful? It is something of a credibility tightrope walk for a company active in both the branded and generic industries to on the one hand aggressively defend its own intellectual property while at the same time trying to find loopholes in the intellectual property of its competitors. Also, it is difficult to house the two different mind-sets, business models and company structures under one corporate umbrella, as we will be discussing later in the book. Not all Big Pharmas have jumped onto the bandwagon. Large companies that have, so far at least, distanced themselves from building their own generic businesses include Roche and BMS.

Once exclusivity has been lost, most large branded drug companies have to continue to invest in their old brands by managing them in units with names like "established medicines" or "mature products." The situation might be different if industry pipelines were full, but in the current situation, companies cannot afford to give up on their patent-expired brands even after exclusivity has been lost. Again, we will be looking at the options for LCM of genericized brands in more detail later.

Another common diversification strategy for Big Pharma, and one that is much older than the current trend to move into generics, is the maintenance of an OTC business unit. There are several reasons why a brand company in the prescription drugs sector would wish to be involved in the OTC sector as well:

• Shifting prescription brands to OTC status as part of brand LCM, either as an expansion strategy in mid-life cycle or as a way of escaping from generic competition following patent expiry. We will be looking at this in detail later in the book.

· Benefiting from the trend for third-party health-care cost containment by moving more medicines to OTC status.
· Gaining better understanding of the self-pay prescription/OTC hybrid model prevalent in many emerging markets.
· Cycling prescription drug marketers through the OTC business to give them a better understanding of direct-to-consumer (DTC) advertising and marketing.
· Getting more public recognition for the company name.

Other business diversification strategies which can provide brand LCM opportunities and are therefore relevant to the subject of this book include moves into animal health, medical devices, diagnostics, and drug delivery. Gaining access to proprietary medical devices and drug delivery systems can be a valuable strategy for both expansion and defense of a brand.

Two common diversification strategies that do not directly benefit pharmaceutical brand LCM are medical nutrition and vaccines.

The world champion at diversification is, and have been for many years, J&J. Their business portfolio includes such brand names as Johnson's Baby Care®, Piz Buin®, Band Aid®, Listerine®, Carefree®, o.b.®, Tylenol®, Pepcid®, Benecol®, Acuvue® Contact Lenses, DePuy, Cordis, Lifescan, Ortho®, Ethicon®, Duragesic®, Risperdal®, Remicade®, Janssen, Centocor, and McNeil. In April 2011, J&J announced that they were acquiring for US$21 billion Synthes, a leading manufacturer of instruments, implants and biomaterials for the surgical fixation, correction, and regeneration of the human skeleton and its soft tissues.

Another diversification dimension which is very relevant for brand LCM is geographical. Most brand companies are intensifying their efforts in emerging markets, especially the BRICT countries (Brazil, Russia, India, China, and Turkey) where intellectual property, pricing, and reimbursement are treated differently compared to the traditional top-priority markets in North America, Western Europe, and Japan. In one recent example, in May 2010, Abbott announced it had bought India's Piramal for nearly US$4 billion to gain the number 1 position in the Indian pharmaceutical market.

The key question for diversification, however, remains—is the goal to de-risk the business through spreading bets across a number of different sectors or to create synergies that allow each different operation to increase the value of its neighbors? For many companies, diversification is now simply a necessity to cope with a blended reality of the future of the pharmaceutical industry. As growth markets such as India and China become more important, the boundaries between prescription drugs, generics, and consumer health care will become even more blurred, and it will be those companies that can adapt to the needs of different markets that will succeed.

CHAPTER 2

The Life Cycle of Industries, Technologies, and Brands

In this chapter we will examine the typical life cycle of industries, technologies, brands, and services outside of the pharmaceutical industry, and then in the next chapter we will look at the rather special situation confronting branded pharmaceuticals. It is essential to understand both. On the one hand, the branded drug industry can learn a lot by observing industries that had been practicing lifecycle management (LCM) for decades before it became a priority for branded drugs. On the other hand, many LCM strategies employed in other industries just will not work in the case of drugs. Understanding these additional opportunities and the inherent limitations will help drug LCM managers to design effective strategies that optimize brand performance over the whole lifetime, from cradle to grave.

Before looking at product life cycles from the perspective of the company selling the product, it will be helpful to take the opposite view, that of the customer. In the drug industry this can mean the physician, the pharmacist, the patient, and the payer, and it is critical to understand how different customer groups react to innovation, as a brand will target different categories of customer during its life cycle.

2.1 DIFFUSION OF INNOVATIONS

In the 1950s, Beal, Rogers, and Bohlen at Iowa State College first published their seminal research on technology adoption by consumers (Beal, G.M., Rogers, E.M., and Bohlen, J.M. 1957. "Validity of the concept of stages in the adoption process." *Rural Sociology* 22(2): 166–168). Their work was built on early papers by Ryan and Gross, dating from the early 1940s (Ryan, B. and Gross, N.C. 1943. "The diffusion of hybrid seed corn in two Iowa communities." *Rural Sociology* (8): 15–24). Iowa State is not the first address that comes

Pharmaceutical Lifecycle Management: Making the Most of Each and Every Brand, First Edition. Tony Ellery and Neal Hansen.

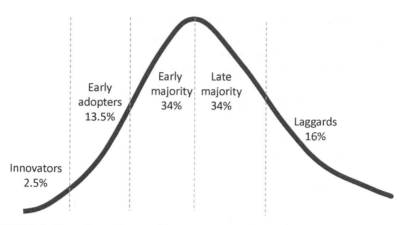

FIGURE 2.1. Roger's psychographic customer profiles. Adapted from Rogers (2003), *Diffusion of Innovators.*

to mind when one thinks of breakthrough marketing research, and indeed the authors' original purpose had been to understand purchasing patterns of hybrid seed corn by farmers. The fifth edition of Rogers's standard work on the subject is still in print as we write (Everett M. Rogers. 2003. *Diffusion of Innovations*, 5th Edition, Free Press).

The main finding of this whole body of work was that customers can be generally divided into five groups regarding their willingness to adopt new technologies. These groups are usually labeled "innovators," "early adopters," "early majority," "late majority," and "laggards."

The distribution of customers in each group takes the form of a bell curve, as shown in Figure 2.1, whereby the percentages used by Rogers are approximate and illustrative rather than absolute.

How are these five different groups characterized?

Innovators. These are the first individuals to adopt an innovation. They are adventurous and ready to take risks, and tend to be young and well-off. They are very sociable and closely follow the latest scientific and technological developments. They associate closely with other innovators and are often part of peer networks. In the case of physicians, they are unlikely to be the key opinion leaders yet, as they would have too much to lose if they pinned their names onto a fad that proved unsuccessful, but rather those physicians who bet on the right innovations will in all probability evolve to become the opinion leaders of the future. Innovators do not have the credibility and track record to motivate the majority of customers to move to the new technology, and the innovation will not be a success unless the next group, the early adopters, latches onto it.

Early Adopters. This is the second category of customers to adopt an innovation. Their profile is similar to that of innovators, except that they are more established and are therefore somewhat less willing to risk their status until the innovators have shown the new idea to be potentially viable. In the case of drugs, established medical opinion leaders would fall into this group. They are more integrated into social systems, whereas the innovators are often considered to be too "weird" or "geeky" for their recommendations to be taken seriously. Added to which, the innovators do not usually care whether others follow their lead or not, while the early adopters do. The early adopters are the change agents, with the weight and credibility to act as role models for the customer categories that follow. They are the "go to" people that a company will check with before considering investing in a new idea or technology.

Early Majority. The next category to adopt the innovation is the early majority. These individuals will follow the lead of the opinion leaders after a varying degree of time, once the level of uncertainty and risk has proven to be limited. In his book, *Crossing the Chasm*, Geoffrey Moore refers to a gap—a chasm—between the first two groups and the early majority (Geoffrey A. Moore. 1999 *Crossing the Chasm: Marketing and Selling High-Tech Products to Mainstream Customers*, HarperBusiness). A product that fails to cross this gap will not achieve widespread acceptance, and it will either fail or be niched.

Late Majority. These individuals will adopt an innovation after the average member of the society. They are skeptical of new developments, and are unwilling to take risks so they want to stand back and watch until enough experience has been gained to convince them that the innovation is generally accepted and commonplace.

Laggards. This is the last category to adopt an innovation. These individuals are typically suspicious of change and resistant to it. They tend to be traditionalists, and not very socially active. They are usually older. Often they will only adopt an innovation once earlier alternatives—the ones they grew up with—are no longer available.

2.2 THE LIFECYCLE CURVE

The lifecycle curve of a typical industrial product or service, which is shown in Figure 2.2, will largely mirror the innovation diffusion curve shown in Figure 2.1.

It is important to understand that the curve shown in Figure 2.2 is only one of many possible shapes, although the phases of development, introduction, growth, maintenance, and decline are almost invariable. Furthermore, the timescale varies enormously. And the lifecycle curve is not only applicable to single products and services—brands, product families, categories, and even industries go through the same phases.

Let us look at some examples of how the length and form of life cycles can vary.

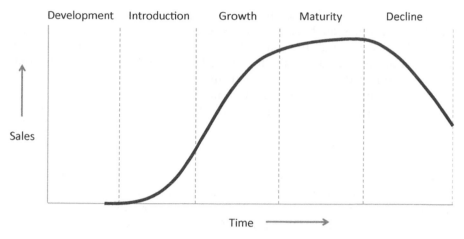

FIGURE 2.2. Typical life cycle of an industrial product/service. *Source*: Ellery Pharma Consulting.

Money, in the form of coins or paper notes, has enjoyed a very long life cycle. The first stamped coins that are known to have been used as currency date from around 650 B.C., and coins are still in general use today. However, the gradual fall in popularity of cash began with credit cards, and the spread of "virtual money" in the form of online purchasing and online banking looks set to drive what will surely be an extremely prolonged Decline Phase.

The first automobile powered by an internal combustion engine running on petrol was introduced to the market by Karl Benz in 1888, and by 1893, he had sold about 25 vehicles. The Introduction Phase was prolonged, until Henry Ford's first mass-produced motor car, the Model T, allowed the industry to enter its Growth Phase starting in 1914. Today, nearly a century later, this petrol-based internal combustion engine technology may be considered to have reached the interface between its Maturity and Decline Phases, as concerns about global oil reserves and rising carbon dioxide levels in the atmosphere drive the search for viable new power sources.

The toy known as the Hula Hoop was created in 1958, and quickly evolved to become the biggest toy fad that America and Europe had ever witnessed. Worldwide in 1958, over 100 million Hula Hoops were sold, 25 million within 4 months in the United States alone, and at the peak of its popularity, the company Wham-O (which later had a second huge success with the Frisbee) was manufacturing 20,000 Hula Hoops per day. Clever marketing tactics, including giving away Hula Hoops free to kids at playgrounds, meant that the Introduction Phase was kept very short before almost exponential growth followed. But within just 1 year, Hula Hoop sales declined precipitously and in the early 1960s ground to a complete halt. There was no true Maturity Phase, just steep Growth followed by steep Decline. The lifecycle curve looks like a tall, thin pyramid!

As stated earlier, industries, technologies, product categories, brands, and individual products all have life cycles. Generally speaking, the life cycle will be longest for industries, and shortest for individual products, though this is not always the case as the following two examples illustrate. The commercial airship industry only lasted from about 1920 until 1937; the rapid evolution of airplanes was already threatening the future of airships in the 1920s, and the Hindenburg disaster in May 1937 effectively put an end to the industry after less than 20 years. Compare this with the branded soft drink, Coca-Cola, which was first marketed under this name in 1888 and is still going strong today.

Before we look at the specifics of branded pharmaceutical life cycles, it is important to understand the characteristics of the different lifecycle phases, and therefore why different technologies, different product categories, and different brands can have such vastly different life cycles.

2.3 LIFECYCLE PHASES

2.3.1 Development Phase

In this phase, the company invests money to develop a product from the initial idea through to introduction onto the market. There are no sales revenues from the product during the Development Phase.

The impact of failure of a development project upon a company depends on a number of factors:

1. *The Size of the Project.* This can vary immensely. At one end of the spectrum, the software for a simple new PC game can be developed very cheaply. At the other end, new product development in the commercial aircraft industry can be extremely expensive, some estimates putting the development costs of Boeing's new Dreamliner to be as much as US$8–10 billion.

2. *The Size of the Company.* Obviously, a larger company with many development projects can withstand the loss of one project better than a small company with just one or two projects.

3. *The Timing of the Failure.* "Make your mistakes early" is a good principle in product development. If a project must be redirected, or even discontinued for technical or commercial reasons, the damage to the company is much less if this attrition occurs early in the development process. At this stage the sunk costs are still low, and resources can be freed up for company ventures with a higher chance of success. Failures later in development mean writing off higher investment costs, and the opportunity cost may be very significant. The most damaging failures of all are always the ones that happen after market entry, as marketing expenses are also wasted and the failure can even damage the company's reputation. New Coke, the Ford Edsel, and Betamax are examples of such postlaunch failures.

4. *The Reason for the Failure.* There are several aspects of this. If multiple projects are based on the same technology, then the failure of one project may signal the imminent failure of others as well. A similar situation may be encountered when a company uses the same third party for key aspects of multiple projects, or when they are depending on the expertise of the same in-house expert for several projects.

2.3.2 Introduction Phase

Once the initial development has been completed and the product introduced to the market, sales start off low until customer awareness has been built and the benefits of the product over existing offerings have been recognized. In most industries, the Introduction Phase can be shortened by premarketing the product during the Development Phase, especially to the early adopters. The costs associated with product introduction, distribution, marketing, training, and so on, mean that the product will usually not become profitable during the Introduction Phase. The cost of goods is also likely to be high, as sales volumes are low and economies of scale cannot yet be realized. Investments in additional plant and equipment to increase production capacities may be necessary, and amortization of these investments further depresses profitability.

Premium prices are usually charged during the Introduction Phase, however, as early adopters tend to be financially well-off and are willing and able to pay for something that they perceive as new and exclusive. Occasionally, the opposite introduction strategy is selected, offering the product at a low price initially to gain market share and realize economies of scale.

Depending on the industry and the product, some companies will give away product samples initially, especially to early adopters, again with the intention of building sales quickly and shortening the Introduction Phase. We have already mentioned how Hula Hoops were given away to children on playgrounds; needless to say, this tactic will have been most successful when the "thought leaders" among the children were chosen for these gifts.

2.3.3 Growth Phase

This is the period of rapid sales growth. The early adopters have fulfilled their function, and awareness of the product and a desire to own it are penetrating into the early majority. Customers are asking for the product, and this will increase distribution as more and more retailers want to carry it. If an initial high-price strategy has been selected, prices can be kept high during the Growth Phase, especially if demand exceeds supply. As it becomes clear to the company that they have a success on their hands, new product features and packaging can be introduced both to expand sales and to build higher entry barriers to competitors who have noticed the success and are moving their new products toward market. Marketing costs remain high, and the number of sales staff may be increased. As the Growth Phase progresses and the product becomes established, the late majority also starts dipping into its pockets.

2.3.4 Maturity Phase

Sales growth starts to flatten and reaches a plateau. The early adopters have moved on to the next generation of products, and the early majority is starting to follow them. Most sales are going to the late majority, with even the laggards finally starting to take an interest. This is the most profitable phase for the product. Marketing expenditure has been reduced because the product is now widely known. Economies of scale have been realized in production. Competitors have appeared, and modifications may be made to the product and features added to differentiate the brand and to defend the brand franchise. Other tactics may be tried to improve the aging brand's competitiveness— sales promotions, price cuts, and so on. The major effort will be in preventing existing customers switching to the new competitors rather than in gaining new customers.

2.3.5 Decline Phase

Different factors can cause sales to dip at the end of the Maturity Phase. It may be that the market is saturated, that everybody has already bought the product in the case of nonperishable goods. An example would be the decline in sales of CDs of classical music; once you have bought one or two versions of the Beethoven symphonies on CD, you probably will not be buying any more, and the CDs you already have will last for decades.

It may be that new, incrementally better competitive products have entered the market—digital single lens reflex (SLR) cameras would be a good example, where 10-megapixel models replaced 8-megapixel models, and then were themselves replaced by 12-megapixel models, all within the space of a couple of years.

Rather than just an incremental change, a disruptive change in technology may make the previous generation of products obsolete. Thus, audio CDs sent vinyl LP sales into a sharp decline in the early 1980s.

Customer tastes may change, and this is what often happens to fads and fashions. The Hula Hoop, the Yo-Yo, and Cabbage Patch dolls are good examples of the former. And it is fascinating to watch the evolution of spectacle frames, how they vary in thickness, color, and size on an almost annual basis. Obsolescence here is all about customer taste, and the power of advertising in persuading customers to buy the latest fashion when their existing spectacles are still working fine.

During the Decline Phase, a company has a limited number of options:

1. *Concentrate on Selling to Laggards.* There is still a niche market for vinyl LPs, and it is not very price sensitive so that premium prices can be

set to compensate for higher production costs as economies of scale are lost. Long after most major recording companies had fully converted to the production of CDs, United Record Pressing of Nashville, Tennessee, continued—and continues to this day—to manufacture only vinyl records. In some industries, laggards can remain loyal customers for decades.

2. *Harvest the Product.* Reduce marketing support and other costs (e.g., by moving production to a third-party low-cost country and/or by reducing the number of product variants).

3. *Find New Uses for the Product.* Also known as "repurposing," this strategy has been used as a late-stage lifecycle management (LLCM) strategy for drugs, though in other industries it is usually used as a way of gaining commercial success for products which failed to fulfill their original purpose. A famous example was provided by 3M, where researchers trying to find a strong new adhesive in 1970 only succeeded in developing a weak, pressure-sensitive adhesive which did not meet the requirements. The inventor, Spencer Silver, tried to ignite interest for the product within 3M but was not successful in doing so until, 4 years later, another 3M scientist, Arthur Fry, found a new use for the product. Fry was a member of his church choir, and used markers in his hymnal to keep his place. But they kept falling out. So he tried Silver's weak glue to stick them to the pages. It was not until 10 years after Silver's original invention that 3M started marketing Post-it Notes, which today are still one of the most widely used of all office products. Stepping away from industrial products for a moment, the city of London, England, provides a fine example of repurposing as an LLCM strategy! London Docks had been the main point of entry for goods destined for the capital city of the United Kingdom since the 17th century. But between 1960 and 1970, the shipping industry adopted the container system for transporting cargo. This meant much larger vessels, and the River Thames in London was not deep enough to accommodate them. Around 83,000 jobs were lost during the 1960s, and by 1980, the last commercial dock had closed. In 1981, the London Docklands Development Corporation (LDDC) was set up; the LDDC led a gigantic redevelopment program between 1981 and 1990 to convert the docklands into a combined residential, commercial, and light industrial district. Warehouses were converted into luxury apartments and offices, docks were converted to accommodate pleasure craft, and London City airport was built. The Canary Wharf project included Britain's tallest building, and created a major financial center. The decline of London Docks had been turned into a very successful commercial venture by repurposing the entire area.

4. *Discontinue the Product.* This may mean withdrawing the product from the market, or in certain cases, selling the brand to a smaller company which can still make a success of it.

CHAPTER 3

The Life Cycle of a Pharmaceutical Brand

As we have seen, the characteristics of product life cycles vary considerably between industries. Let us now concentrate on the class of product that is the subject of this book, the branded prescription pharmaceutical.

There are a number of specific features of the pharmaceutical industry that strongly influence product life cycles, and it is essential that these are fully understood if one is going to be successful in designing lifecycle management (LCM) strategies.

Four of the important special features of the pharmaceutical industry that influence LCM are the following:

1. *Drugs Are Easy to Make.* Most drugs are rather cheap and easy to manufacture, so the entry barriers as far as manufacturing is concerned are low. Furthermore, the cost of goods sold (COGS) of high-priced branded drugs represents a relatively low percentage of sales. Dozens if not hundreds of companies are perfectly capable of making exactly the same drug as is contained in the vast majority of branded products. This is particularly true of small molecules and somewhat less true of large biological molecules, as we shall see later. In most cases, however, a brand company cannot rely on competitors not being able to manufacture the same molecule, to the same quality standards. Contrast this with another industry with high development costs, aircraft manufacture; Boeing does not have to worry that dozens of other companies will copy the Dreamliner!

   Not only is it easy to copy a drug, but the capital investment needed to set up labs and manufacturing facilities capable of developing the copy product and then producing it in large quantities is not very high. The innovator has to spend heavily to prove that a new molecule is safe and effective, but these investments do not have to be repeated by the

Pharmaceutical Lifecycle Management: Making the Most of Each and Every Brand, First Edition. Tony Ellery and Neal Hansen.

developers of copy products, as they are using the same molecule and can rely on referring to the data of the originator to gain regulatory approval, just as long as the copy product behaves in the same way in the body, that is, is bioequivalent. This is, of course, the basis for the generic drugs industry, and as we shall see later, it was the concept of bioequivalence in the Hatch–Waxman legislation in 1984 that allowed the generics industry to take off in the United States.

2. *Patents Prevent Copy Products.* Key to the very existence of the branded pharmaceutical industry is therefore the ability to patent a new molecule and thus obtain the exclusive rights to sell it. Only so can the brand company demand prices that are high enough to recover the high costs of developing the molecule. We will be looking at patents in considerable detail later in the book. From the point of time at which a new molecule is first discovered, the innovator company can expect about 20 years of protection during which time no other company is allowed to commercialize the same molecule, and such a patent is valid in most countries of the world.

3. *Consumers Do Not Pay for Drugs.* Branding in the consumer goods industry is very different from branding drugs. Consumer-goods advertising seeks to create an image of the brand in the eyes of the consumers which convinces them to pay a much higher price for the product than they would be willing to pay if that image was absent. This concept is called "value creation"; simply put, it convinces a consumer to accept a price higher than could be justified by the costs of raw materials plus manufacturing and distribution, and more than could be justified by an objective, nonemotional comparison of the value of the brand compared to alternative, cheaper product offerings. In some cases, the added value created is in the brand name of the company, in other cases, it is in the individual products. As an example of branding at the company level, customers will pay high prices for a Mercedes-Benz automobile, and the individual model descriptions (CLK, G550, etc.) are of secondary value; consumers would not pay premium prices for a Dodge G550. A good example of branding at the individual product level would be products like Lipton, Flora, Omo, Vaseline, and Lifebuoy. They are all made by Unilever, but how many consumers are aware of that? If Unilever changed the Lipton brand name to "Smith Teas" tomorrow, their sales would plunge as the value is in the individual brand name. Indeed, when Kellogg's decided to rebrand its kids breakfast cereal Coco Pops to Choco Krispies in the United Kingdom, to bring the brand name in line with the United States, Germany, and Spain, sales plummeted. In the end, the Coco Pops brand was restored after research suggested 92% of consumers wanted the old brand back.

There is much less value in a brand name in the prescription pharmaceutical industry for the simple reason that the consumer, the end user of the drug, is in many cases not the person making the buying decision. Until comparatively recently, the physician made the buying decision; he decided what to write on the prescription, and the pharmacist had to dispense it as written. It is reasonable to suppose that physicians, with their scientific education, made their choices based mainly upon the extensive controlled scientific data generated for the different drugs, as well as upon their own experiences with the alternative therapies. Of course their choices were influenced by advertising and detailing by pharmaceutical sales forces, and by consumers exposed to direct-to-consumer advertising requesting specific products, but the objective, data-driven component of their choices was likely to be much more than, say, a housewife choosing between Omo and Persil, or a smoker choosing between Marlboro and Camel cigarettes. But the prescribing decision was certainly not driven by price—indeed in most cases, the prescribing physician did not even know what the price was! However, in recent years, in many countries, the individual physician is no longer the decision maker. Medical insurances determine which drugs will be reimbursed and which will not, and this limits the physician's choices; once the patent on the drug has expired, the various government measures that we have already considered activate, and the patient is likely to receive a generic rather than the brand. The medical insurers are not interested in the brand name, at either the company or individual product level. They are only interested in choosing the cheapest drug available—or the cheapest available version of the same drug—unless there is solid, numerical evidence that an alternative brings enough additional benefit to justify any price premium. In the case of generics, the price premium of the original brand is huge and a bioequivalent represents a much better deal for the payer. Third-party payers are very unresponsive to advertising, and there is effectively no emotional component of their decisions.

In self-pay markets like India and South America, pharmaceutical branding is more effective, because the patient can decide whether to pay the incrementally higher price for their preferred brand, or for the brand over the generic, and then the emotional factors come into play just as they do with other categories of consumer goods. There is a moral issue here, of course, as paradoxically, the more expensive original drugs thus tend to retain a higher market share than the cheaper generics in precisely those poor countries which can least afford it. This is compensated for to some extent by the fact that the price differential of the brand to the generics tends to be smaller in such countries.

As we shall see later, one option for a brand which will soon be facing generic competition in countries where prescription drugs are paid for by insurers rather than the consumer may be to move the brand to nonprescription, self-pay status ("over-the-counter" [OTC] drugs), thus again directly addressing the emotional preferences of the consumer. Not all OTC switches are commercially successful, and of course, many categories of drug cannot be obtained without a physician's prescription. Nevertheless, there have been several examples of very profitable OTC switches, including Zantac®, Advil®, Claritin®, and Prilosec®.

4. *Governments Set Prices and Support Generics.* We have already considered this in the previous chapter, and will be looking at it in much greater depth later in the book. Suffice it to say here that in most developed markets, the prices that a branded pharmaceutical company can ask for a patented new drug are not determined solely by competition and by market forces, but by government policy. After patent expiry, governments provide many different kinds of incentives for physicians to prescribe generics, pharmacists to dispense them, and patients to use them.

3.1 LIFECYCLE CURVE OF PHARMACEUTICALS

These, then, are four features of the branded pharmaceutical industry that determine how the lifecycle curve will appear for a patent-protected drug. The curve varies considerably from case to case, the indication for which the drug is used and the geography under consideration being the main two determinants. The curve shown in Figure 3.1 is fairly typical for a mass-market drug (family practitioner-prescribed) in the United States.

Let us compare this with Figure 2.2, the curve for a typical industrial product, to see where the main differences are and what causes them.

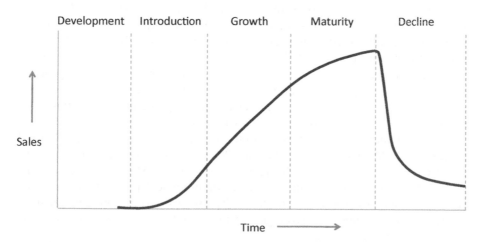

FIGURE 3.1. Lifecycle curve of a mass-market drug in the United States. *Source*: Ellery Pharma Consulting.

3.1.1   Slow Rate of Growth during the Growth Phase

Growth tends to be slower for drugs than for many other industrial products. Why should this be?

Physicians are understandably reluctant to move patients to a new drug until it has proven its worth. Buying the newest cell phone obviously involves a lower risk than moving a sick patient from a therapy that is controlling the disease to one that might or might not prove to be better, but which might have side effects. Understandably and justifiably, the growth curve will be steeper in the case of a new therapy for a hitherto untreatable or uncontrollable disease and slower for a me-too drug or for a new drug class where established drug classes are already performing well.

Added to this, drug companies are severely limited regarding how much they can promote a new drug until it has been approved, so the kind of pre-marketing that is performed with a new Hollywood film or a new model of automobile is not possible with a new drug. There are a limited number of ways that brand companies can legally premarket their new brands. For example, large clinical trials are necessary to get health authority approval for a new drug, and selecting clinical centers for the trials in the major target markets, and utilizing physicians who are opinion leaders ("early adopters") in these markets, will increase awareness of the new brand even before it can be sold and promoted. And careful selection of the patient population to be treated, the parameters chosen to demonstrate efficacy and safety, and the comparator drugs selected for use in the trial all serve to position the new drug in the minds of its future prescribers and payers. The Internet facilitates the rapid spread of information about drugs that are in development even before approval, so that patients will also have a much higher awareness of new drug introductions than was the case in the past.

Lately, and especially following the withdrawal of Vioxx®, the Food and Drug Administration (FDA) and other health authorities have become much more cautious about letting new drugs be introduced initially to broad populations. This means that the rollout of the new drug is increasingly only in patients with special need of it, which is often a rather small subgroup of the broader patient population that may ultimately use the drug. Only later, once an extensive safety database has been established, will health authorities allow the drug to be used in broader populations where the benefit may be less pronounced and the risk–benefit ratio therefore less favorable. In the United States, the FDA Amendments Act of 2007 gave the FDA the authority to require a Risk Evaluation and Mitigation Strategy (REMS) from manufacturers to ensure that the benefits of a drug or biological product outweigh its risks. These REMS programs can vary in their severity from simple medication guides and communication strategies to full monitoring and registry systems to ensure appropriate use.

An additional factor contributing to the relatively slow initial growth is that more and more biologics are being developed in place of small molecules.

Often these drugs target multiple smaller indications, which are introduced successively over the life of the drug. Novartis's Gleevec® would be a good example. Initially launched to treat chronic myeloid leukemia (CML) in 2001, by 2006 Gleevec was also approved for the treatment of a whole portfolio of other orphan indications. All were small, but added together they meant annual global Gleevec sales of over US$3 billion. Gleevec is included in this book as one of our case histories. As another example, biologics developed to treat autoimmune diseases may be tested first in psoriasis patients, where clinical trials are cheaper and faster to complete than, for example, in the bigger and potentially more profitable indication of rheumatoid arthritis.

3.1.2 Lack of a True Maturity Phase

With many drugs there is often no true Maturity Phase, no real plateauing of sales, as sales continue to grow right up to the moment when a sudden decline sets in. The reason for this is that branded drugs are frequently still in their Growth Phase when this is "artificially" cut short by patent expiry, successful challenge to the patent or "at-risk" launch by generic companies, and the subsequent appearance of multiple low-priced generics on the market. Increasingly, it is not even necessary that the patent on the brand itself expires to trigger the start of the Decline Phase. Because of the multitude of me-too drugs on the market, as soon as the basic patent expires on the first brand in a drug class, generic pressure is exerted on all the patented brands in that class too. This relatively new phenomenon of therapeutic substitution was first seen with the statins in Germany, and it is starting to reduce the attraction to companies of developing late-entry "me-too" compounds.

3.1.3 Precipitous Decline Phase

The loss of sales as the Decline Phase is entered is precipitous in many markets and has been likened to falling off a cliff. At patent expiry (or in the United States in the special situation of expiry of 180-day exclusivity, which we shall consider later), cheap generics flood the market. Because the entry barriers after patent expiry are low, because third-party payers do not have brand loyalty, and because government incentives promote the use of generics, brand sales are quickly lost. Usually, it is not a viable strategy for the brand company to attempt to match the generic prices, as margins are so low. Instead, the originator is likely to stay with the high price—or even try to increase it—and continue to sell to the small, non-price-sensitive "laggards" who are suspicious of generic drugs.

While sales decline rates are generally steep and getting steeper in the United States, Europe, and Japan, different factors do determine the rate of sales decline.

3.2   FACTORS AFFECTING RATE OF CONVERSION TO GENERICS

3.2.1   Government Policy

As we have seen earlier, some governments are more aggressive about promoting generics than others, and this fact leads to different rates of generic substitution after patent expiry. The United States remains to this day the most aggressive generic market, with generics often taking 95% of volume share within the first 12 months. One remark is necessary regarding any observed generic erosion figures for the United States, which are often an average of two very different situations. In the United States, it is possible for one generic company to get 180 days co-exclusivity with the originator following patent expiry. This generic company maintains a high price, so that sales erosion of the brand is much slower. We will be looking at the whole issue of 180-day exclusivities later in the book. Where this effect is not present, generic erosion in the United States is faster than in any other major market. For example, sales of Novartis's antifungal treatment Lamisil® in the United States were eroded by 93% within 6 months of patent expiry and the entry of generics in July 2007, following the simultaneous launch of 14 generics upon patent expiry.

Outside the United States, generic erosion rates can vary significantly between countries. In Northern European markets, such as Germany, the United Kingdom, and Scandinavia, generic erosion rates are high, with specific policies such as pharmacist substitution and generic prescribing and dispensing targets all used aggressively to drive generic uptake. In these markets, erosion rates of greater than 50% after 12–18 months can be expected, with some drugs seeing much greater erosion. By contrast, in many of the Southern European markets, generic erosion rates are much lower, with Spain and Italy often seeing generic erosion rates of less than 20% after 12–18 months. In these markets, reference pricing policies that often see the branded companies reducing their prices to stay within a reimbursement bracket lead to cost savings without extensive generic penetration. In general, individual country dynamics play a huge part in the impact of patent expiry and the speed and depth of generic erosion—the classic pharmaceutical life cycle with its precipitous patent cliff is true of the United States but hides the reality of a stronger afterlife in the rest of the world.

3.2.2   Disease

In addition to national market factors, therapeutic market dynamics also play a role in determining likely generic penetration. There are disease states where physicians have little hesitation in switching patients from the brand onto the generic, because the perceived risk of doing so is low and the results of the switch are easy to monitor. A good example would be hypertension. The physician can monitor the patient's blood pressure after the switch and return to the original brand if unhappy with the performance of the generic. The majority of patients are in no danger if their blood pressure is elevated above its previous level for a week or so. At the other end of the spectrum, a transplant surgeon will be very reluctant to switch a renal patient to a generic. If the generic were not to perform as well as the brand, then the patient might start to reject the transplanted organ and become seriously ill. This has also been the case in the past with epilepsy drugs, where concerns over narrow therapeutic indices and the risk of losing seizure control kept generic penetration rates low. However, when generic competition launched against newer new antiepileptic drugs, such as UCB's Keppra® where the low therapeutic index issues are not so apparent, penetration was still swift and deep, highlighting that even in traditionally "protected" markets, payer pressure will win through.

3.2.3 Size of Brand

All other things being equal, the larger the brand, the more generic companies are likely to enter the market at patent expiry. What is the lower brand sales limit below which no generic is likely to enter the market? As competition heats up in the generic industry, almost any brand is going to attract generic competition. According to analysis presented in Datamonitor's PharmaVitae Explorer, there is virtually no brand sales threshold below which genericization is unlikely to happen; however, there is a definite trend for brands valued at over US$100 million sales to be more severely eroded. In a separate benchmarking study, Datamonitor highlighted that in Germany, after 2 years of generic competition, brands that generated sales of between US$50 and US$100 million per quarter before patent expiry experienced competition from 26 generic manufacturers on average while brands that generated less than US$10 million faced competition from only four generic manufacturers (Datamonitor, "Generic benchmarking: Brand erosion at patent expiry," March 2009, DMHC2496).

3.2.4 Hospital versus Nonhospital Drug Usage

Whether a drug is used in a hospital or retail market can also influence the impact of generic competition, but in two contrasting ways. On the one hand, generic competition can be more intensive for a hospital brand, as the decision makers tend to be hospital pharmacists choosing what to stock rather than individual physicians. Hence, in traditionally brand-loyal markets such as France and Spain, where individual physician preference for brands will limit retail generic erosion, hospital generics can succeed, and indeed this is where many of the first generic players cut teeth. On the flip side, many brands sold into hospitals are already heavily discounted as part of bulk procurement deals, so the price differential between the generic and the brand will often be smaller, creating less of an incentive to use the generic. The net result would seem to be a slightly higher overall erosion in the hospital space, at least in terms of value.

3.2.5   Active Substance and Other Barriers to Entry

We have already stated that drugs are usually rather easy to manufacture, and that neither manufacturing know-how nor the size of the investment needed to create a copy product is likely to deter a generic competitor. Occasionally, there are exceptions to this rule, with Wyeth's Premarin®, extracted from mare's urine, a classic older example. Fundamentally, such barriers to entry will either come from an ability to source the raw material or to successfully formulate the drug without infringing on patents that remain in place. This latter topic will be discussed later in the book and forms a key tenet of the drug industry's goal of maximizing exclusivity where possible. The branded pharmaceutical industry had hoped that the greater complexity and higher levels of investment necessary to create the generic of a biological would mean fewer generics on the market and thus less sales erosion, and to a certain extent this is true; also, regulatory hurdles are higher for "biogenerics" or "follow-on biologics," and we will look at the special aspects of LCM of biologics later in the book.

One misunderstanding, however, that must be cleared up is the belief that generics companies do not like barrier-to-entry products, and that by raising the barriers to entry companies can deter generic competitors. While this may be true for some mass market generic players, the opposite is actually the case for most of the main generics companies. These companies actively seek out barrier-to-entry products for the very same reasons that brand companies try to raise barriers—to limit the generic competition they will face. For a generics company, being the only generic on the market, or at least one of only two or three players can be the ticket to much higher profits and market share, as price competition will not be as aggressive.

3.3   THE LIFE CYCLE OF A PHARMACEUTICAL BRAND

Bearing in mind all of what we have so far written, let us finish off this chapter by looking at some of the issues we will need to address when designing the lifecycle plan for a specific brand. We will be looking more closely at all of these LCM strategies and all of these questions in detail in subsequent chapters, and we will be offering advice on how to create what we will call an integrated LCM strategy, where the interdependence and timing of lifecycle strategies from cradle to grave will be considered. It goes without saying that each brand will benefit most from a specific portfolio of LCM measures tailored to optimize the life cycle of that particular brand. There is no ideal LCM plan template that can be used blindly for every brand.

THE LIFE CYCLE OF A PHARMACEUTICAL BRAND

Development Phase. Different companies define the border between research and development in different ways, often with a bridging period of "early development" or "translational medicine" linking the two. We will assume that the Development Phase starts at the point at which positive results are obtained in a proof-of-concept (PoC) trial, a small clinical study which has shown that the new molecule is active against a specific molecular target or that it is efficacious in a particular disease state. For molecules that are aimed at targets common to different diseases, the selection of the indication or indications to be included in the PoC trials should already include LCM considerations, although at this stage they should be in the background, and scientific and clinical aspects should determine the population to be studied. Based on the results of the PoC trial, the company will generally decide its lead indication, and considering LCM aspects with new drugs which have the potential to target multiple indications will help ensure that the right decisions are taken regarding indication sequencing, which is one of the most important LCM areas of them all. So what are the questions that we as LCM managers must answer at this early stage of the life cycle? Very importantly, what is the level of resources we are willing to invest in the molecule? Do we want to share the risk—and later the revenue—by taking a development partner? Will we already be investing in follow-on indications and improved formulations during development of the initial indication/formulation, or do we want to manage risk by waiting until we have got a first approval before investing more into the brand, even though this means that the subsequent indications and formulations will not generate revenue until later in the life cycle? Here we need to remember that the first indication to enter development will not necessarily be the first indication to reach market, as different indications demand clinical trials of very different lengths. Our answers to the questions will be influenced by what other drugs we have on the market and in our development pipeline, and we will be looking into that aspect in Part G of this book. Can we identify potential responder and nonresponder patients using biomarkers? Biomarkers may also help us to identify patients that might show side effects. Should we think about parallel development of a companion diagnostic? Would it be best to get to market fast in a limited indication, or invest more time and resources to be able to address a wider patient population right from the start? What clinical trials will be needed to get approval and market access at a premium price? What comparators should we use in our trials? They will have to be drugs that we think our molecule can beat, but they will also have to be drugs that are widely used in our target markets, ideally the gold standard. If we have other advantages, for example regarding convenience, it may be enough to match the safety and efficacy of the gold standard. But this is unlikely to be sufficient if the gold standard is going generic soon after our launch because the price differential will be too big to be bridged by merely claiming better convenience. And where should we conduct the clinical trials? Probably we will want to select centers in our major target markets, to ensure that awareness of the new brand is high even before launch. Choosing top opinion leaders to run the trials may be attractive, but less so if their centers are overcrowded with other trials which could delay our patient recruitment and thus our launch. It may then be better to look for early adopters who will champion our product as they strive to build their reputations. What clinical end points should we select? They need to be adequate to gain approval, but not so stringent that the probability of success is significantly reduced. What data will be needed to ensure that we get premium pricing? And that reimbursement is granted? And that the drug is listed in formularies? Are we sure that our lead indication will not make it more difficult to get subsequent indications approved, or negatively impact the price for those subsequent indications? One of the additional patient populations we should be considering now are children, as quite apart from incremental sales, there are exclusivity benefits of testing drugs in this often neglected population. Have we looked at the option of seeking an orphan indication, which could also be of advantage if our molecule has a limited patent life as we could obtain orphan drug exclusivity in the main markets? Have we adequately protected the exclusivity of our molecule otherwise? How strong is our primary patent? How broadly have we been able to patent potentially related products from the same drug classes, and especially modifications of our own molecule, to prevent competitors coming to market with me-too products? What is the situation regarding prior art? Do we need additional patents to protect the molecule more strongly, or secondary patents around the formulation, the use, the manufacturing process, and so on? Is our remaining patent life so short that our exclusivity will be dependent on regulatory or marketing exclusivities? If yes, do our indication and formulation strategies, and their sequencing, fully leverage this protection? We certainly do not want to trigger these exclusivities too early if our first indication is small and commercially unattractive and the bigger indications will only follow years later. As the results from our Phase IIb and III clinical trials start to appear, are they what we expected, and do they meet the requirements we set out in advance to enable the project to continue as planned? What is our strategy for publishing the results of the clinical trials, and do these results open any opportunities for additional patents, or point the way to new indications that we did not yet consider? Have we got the dosage and dosage regimen right, and if not, did our clinical design enable us to adapt the trials to adjust for any changes without having to go back and start all over again? How will we position our new brand? What is our pricing and reimbursement strategy? Have we initiated the customer relationship management (CRM) and disease management programs that will ensure maximum uptake of our brand as soon as it is approved?

Introduction Phase. So, we have just passed the first hurdle to success. We have got regulatory approval for the first formulation in the first indication in the first major market. If we have not started to do so already, that event might be enough to persuade us to start investing in follow-on indications and improved formulations, especially if we have got a good price, reimbursement, and formulary listing. If we are in a low-risk organization, if we have very limited resources, or if we are dubious about the chances of success of our brand, we might prefer to wait until the Growth Phase, to see how high sales climb. Only then can we be sure that the brand will generate enough revenue to pay for those additional programs. But the clock is running. How much time will we have to recover our investment in line extensions before the primary patent expires? Were we too cautious, did we wait too long to start those programs? And we may also be kicking ourselves at this point that we were not confident enough to invest earlier in the specific trials that we will need to get approvals in all the major markets. If we are a European or U.S. company, we probably covered both of those continents, but we may have held back with Japan, or China.

Growth Phase. Great! We have got a success on our hands! Sales are now climbing fast. They will be climbing faster, and they will reach a higher peak, if we were brave enough to start some of our LCM projects during the Development Phase. In that case, we will already have a wide geographic spread of sales, we will hopefully have more than one indication approved, and we may already be able to introduce a new, improved formulation which will further differentiate our product from the future competitors which are now being developed. Perhaps we have a new, once-daily form, and the competitors are stuck with twice-daily products. New indications will be most valuable to us when they enable the drug to be prescribed by a different physician specialty, or to a completely different patient population. If a different route of administration was selected for this follow-on indication, or the combination of the drug with a proprietary delivery device was developed, then we could already be building a robust sales base which may not be lost when the basic patent expires. As confidence grows in the use of the drug, it may be dosed higher, and extending the range of available dosage strengths may be a good strategy. On the other hand, if side effects have appeared in some patient groups, it may be advisable to provide a lower dosage strength. Creating a low-dose formulation may also be a good move if we want to create an OTC version of our brand. In indications where multiple drugs are prescribed with a roughly constant dosing ratio, creating fixed-dose combinations may now be an attractive LCM strategy, as it could improve patient convenience and compliance, or even move our product up the treatment hierarchy. At the very least, as we watch the brand franchise grow, consideration should be given to possible follow-up molecules in the same class which are expected to show efficacy and/or safety benefits;

if the benefits are real, and the new molecule different enough from the current one, this strategy could create a new, patented product which will replace the earlier one when its patent expires, while still leveraging the franchise that the company has built within this drug class and physician and patient population. Investigator-initiated trials may be boosting off-label sales in nonapproved indications.

Maturity Phase. Sales may be flattening off now—or at least the growth rate decreasing—as new competitors enter the market. But the far bigger risk to the continuing growth of many brands is likely to be the approaching expiry of the primary patent. As mentioned earlier, many brands never even experience a Maturity Phase, and the patent expiry hits them while sales are still growing strongly. Too often, the few years—or even the few months—before patent expiry is the time that some companies first start to think about late-stage lifecycle management (LLCM), and how they can maintain brand exclusivity for longer or retain more market share after exclusivity is lost. Very often, this is too late to put these ideas into practice before patent expiry. Some drugs may be able to rescue at least part of their sales from the impending plunge by moving to non-prescription, OTC status. It is now that brand companies, sometimes in desperation, start implementing last-minute strategies to try to delay generic entry to the market for as long as possible. The European Sector Inquiry called these strategies the "toolbox" that branded companies use shortly before exclusivity is lost in an attempt to save their doomed brand franchise. We will be looking at all of these strategies later— including raising purity and bioequivalence standards, submitting citizen petitions and white papers, trying to cut deals with the generic companies, authorized generics, spurious litigation, and much more. The purpose of the branded drug company is usually not to win against the generic threat, as this is in most cases not a realistic option, but to lose later and preferably against less generic competitors! Just before patent expiry, brand sales may be at their highest ever and profits almost certainly are, as marketing support will have largely been withdrawn in favor of newer brands in the product portfolio. For a brand selling for US$2 billion per year, with a margin of as much as 75% at this late stage, it is a simple calculation to see that every additional day of exclusivity is worth more than US$4 million profit!

Decline Phase. Despite all of our efforts, the bad thing has finally happened. Exclusivity has been lost, and generics are flooding the market. In most cases, there is little point cutting the brand price to try to chase the generics down into the basement, as the generic companies have leaner structures and lower profit margins, and can always go still lower. We will probably maintain the premium price of our brand and concentrate our efforts on the laggards. Sales may hold up rather well in countries with less sophisticated ways of forcing generic substitution, and especially in self-pay markets. Companies that are good at LCM and have thought far enough ahead may have secondary patent-protected new formulations on the market which offer enough real benefit over generics of the old formulation to get a significant share of prescriptions of the drug. But the hurdle for doing this is already high, and it is getting higher, and generic companies are becoming very efficient at designing around formulation patents. In those cases (the majority) where most of our brand sales are lost to generics after primary patent expiry, the brand will now just be managed for profit. Marketing support will be cut right back (the laggards will continue to use the brand anyway), the number of product variants will be pared to reduce manufacturing costs, and manufacturing may be moved to a low-cost country or contracted out to a third party (perhaps even to one of the generic competitors). Another possible strategy—the exact opposite of allowing a third party to manufacture the brand—is for the brand company to manufacture product for one or more of the generic companies, a so-called licensed generic. Some local LCM (e.g., new formulations) may persist in large, self-pay markets, where development costs and local regulatory hurdles are low, but generally central R&D support of the brand will be cut almost to zero. Finally, as time progresses, the brand sales drop to a level where the bother of keeping it on the market is bigger than the profits. The brand may now be withdrawn from the market, or sold or licensed to a smaller company which can make a living by selling minor brands.

In following a typical brand through its life cycle in this way, we have divided up LCM measures according to lifecycle phase. But it is evident that many of the individual measures can be applied at different stages in the life cycle. For example, a new indication may be developed concurrently with the first indication, or it may be developed during the Introduction or Growth Phases to boost sales in the middle of the life cycle, or it may be developed in the Maturity Phase when, in association with a new route of administration or some form of drug delivery device, it may be able to retain more market share from generics once the primary patent expires.

Another way of classifying LCM measures would be to look at what goals they are intended to achieve in the life cycle. Related to brand sales, there are seven possibilities:

1. Faster market introduction
2. Steeper growth curve
3. Shorter time to peak sales
4. Higher peak sales
5. Longer exclusivity
6. Slower sales decline after exclusivity loss
7. Higher brand market share after loss of exclusivity.

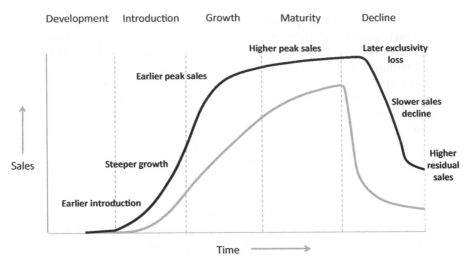

FIGURE 3.2. Effects of LCM on the lifecycle curve. *Source*: Ellery Pharma Consulting.

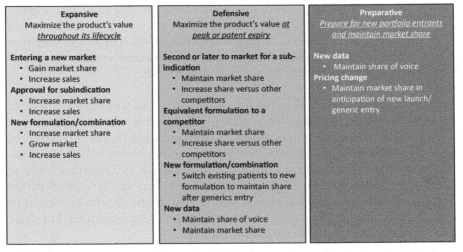

FIGURE 3.3. LCM tactic goals—expansive, defensive, and preparative. *Source*: Datamonitor.

Figure 3.2 shows these different purposes of LCM. It is important to note that Figure 3.2 only considers sales and not profit.

Again, a specific LCM measure could serve several of these different needs. For example, a sophisticated new formulation may get a higher price and this may lead to higher peak sales, and if securely patented, it may lead to a slower sales decline and a higher market share after patent expiry.

Yet another way of classifying LCM strategies is that used by Datamonitor, as shown in Figure 3.3. Datamonitor divides LCM strategies according to whether they are "expansive," "defensive," or "preparative," reflecting the primary goals of the tactic or strategy in question.

For this book, we have decided to categorize LCM measures according to the functional department in the company that is likely to have the lead responsibility for a particular measure. This has the advantage in a long book of this kind that it enables functional specialists to concentrate on "their" chapters, while at the same time seeing how their efforts can contribute to the overall LCM program for a brand.

It is important to understand that this structure of the book is not intended to support the view that LCM is a decentralized process that should take place within the individual functions. Nothing could be further from the truth! An effective LCM program requires the highly cross-functional collaboration of a whole range of functional experts, as we shall see later when we discuss organizational aspects of LCM.

We will be looking at a whole range of potential LCM measures in the following chapters. This will include

- Legal/regulatory measures:
  - Patents
  - Regulatory exclusivities
  - Litigation and settlements
- Developmental measures:
  - Indication expansion and sequencing
  - Dosage strengths and regimens
  - Reformulation and combinations
  - Delivery devices
  - New route of administration
  - Biomarkers/diagnostics
  - Raising technical hurdles for generics
  - White papers and citizen petitions
  - Next-generation products
- Commercial measures:
  - Geographical expansion and optimization
  - OTC switching
  - Brand loyalty and service programs
  - Strategic pricing
  - Generic strategies (in-house, licensed, or authorized)
  - Divestiture/product withdrawal

But before we start looking at all of these measures individually, it is essential that the reader fully understands four important environmental factors that strongly influence LCM efforts, particularly in the largest pharmaceutical markets, the United States and the European Union. The next four chapters will focus on these factors, which are:

1. The Generic Approval Process (Chapter 4)
2. Hatch–Waxman Legislation and Its Effects on LCM (Chapter 5)
3. U.S. Health-Care Reform 2010 (Chapter 6)
4. European Sector Inquiry (Chapter 7)

LIFECYCLE MANAGEMENT REGULATORY AND LEGAL ENVIRONMENT

The Generic Approval Process

This chapter will describe the processes that generic companies follow for getting marketing approval for their products in the major markets.

4.1 UNITED STATES

Section 505 of the Federal Food, Drug and Cosmetic Act recognizes three different types of New Drug Application:

1. Applications containing full reports of investigations of safety and effectiveness (Section 505(b)(1)). These applications are made using a New Drug Application (NDA).
2. Applications containing full reports of investigations of safety and effectiveness but where at least some of the information required for approval comes from studies not conducted by or for the applicant and for which the applicant has obtained a right of reference (Section 505(b)(2)).
3. Applications that contain information to show that the proposed product is identical to a previously approved product (Section 505(b)(j)). These applications are made using an Abbreviated New Drug Application (ANDA).

The basis for approval of a bioequivalent generic medicine in the United States is thus the ANDA. Such an application contains all of the data necessary to allow the review and ultimate approval of the generic drug product by the Food and Drug Administration (FDA)'s Center for Drug Evaluation and Research, Office of Generic Drugs. Once the ANDA has been approved, the applicant is permitted to manufacture and market the generic drug product.

A generic drug product is one that is comparable to an innovator drug product in dosage form, strength, route of administration, quality, performance characteristics, and intended use. All approved products, both innovator and

Pharmaceutical Lifecycle Management: Making the Most of Each and Every Brand, First Edition.
Tony Ellery and Neal Hansen.
© 2012 John Wiley & Sons, Inc. Published 2012 by John Wiley & Sons, Inc.

generic, are listed in the FDA's Approved Drug Products with Therapeutic Equivalence Evaluations (Orange Book).

Generic drug applications are termed "abbreviated" because they are generally not required to include preclinical (animal) and clinical (human) data to establish safety and effectiveness. Instead, generic applicants must scientifically demonstrate that their product is bioequivalent to the original drug (i.e., that it performs in the same manner). One way of doing this is to measure the time it takes the generic drug to reach the bloodstream in 24–36 healthy volunteers. This determines the rate of absorption, or bioavailability, of the generic drug, which can then be compared to that of the original drug. The generic version must deliver the same amount of active ingredients into a patient's bloodstream in the same amount of time as the innovator drug.

Using bioequivalence as the basis for approving generic copies of drug products was established by the original Hatch–Waxman Act of 1984, which we will look at more closely in the next chapter.

This is the complete list of the requirements that the FDA places on a generic drug:

- Generic drugs must have the same active ingredients and the same labeled strength as the brand-name product.
- Generic drugs must have the same dosage form (e.g., tablets, liquids) and must be administered in the same way.
- Generic drug manufacturers must show that a generic drug is bioequivalent to the brand-name drug, which means the generic version delivers the same amount of active ingredients into a patient's bloodstream in the same amount of time as the brand-name drug.
- Generic drug labeling must be essentially the same as the labeling of the brand-name drug.
- Generic drug manufacturers must fully document the generic drug's chemistry, manufacturing steps, and quality control measures.
- Firms must assure the FDA that the raw materials and finished product meet specifications of the U.S. Pharmacopoeia, the organization that sets standards for drug purity in the United States.
- Firms must show that a generic drug will remain potent and unchanged until the expiration date on the label.
- Firms must comply with federal regulations for good manufacturing practices and provide the FDA a full description of facilities they use to manufacture, process, test, package, and label the drug. The FDA inspects manufacturing facilities to ensure compliance.

A Section 505(b)(2) application enables companies to obtain FDA approval of a new drug by relying partially on the agency's findings for a previously approved drug, and is used to request approval for products which incorporate a limited change compared to an existing approved drug. A 505(b)(2) application thus lies between an NDA and an ANDA. The FDA only requires that the safety and efficacy of the change be demonstrated. Here are examples of some of the changes that would fall under the 505(b)(2) process (taken from the FDA's guidelines on 505(b)(2) applications):

- Changes in dosage form, strength, formulation, dosing regimen, or route of administration
- New combination products, including substitution of an active ingredient
- Modified active ingredients (e.g., salt, chelate, ester, complex)
- New indications for previously approved drugs
- Over-the-counter switch of an approved prescription drug.

The advantages of pursuing the 505(b)(2) route rather than the NDA route are those of expense and time. There are also advantages for generic companies taking the 505(b)(2) route instead of going for an ANDA. First and foremost, the 505(b)(2) route will lead to the launch of an "improved" version of the original drug. This will give the new product an advantage in the market over the "ordinary" generics, and very importantly, it will make the new product eligible for a 3-year period of exclusivity, or even 5 years if the change can be claimed to create a new chemical entity. We will be looking at these types of exclusivity later in the book. The best an ordinary generic can hope for is 180 days of exclusivity as first filer (as described in the next chapter).

However, companies sometimes cut corners in estimating how many data are necessary to adequately document the change, and the commonest reason for rejection of 505(b)(2) applications by the FDA is a lack of an appropriate data. To avoid this problem, the guidelines recommend that the sponsor should submit its plans to the Center for Drug Evaluation and Research (CDER) before embarking on the development program. The plans should make clear where the sponsor will be referring to the FDA's findings for the previously approved drug and what studies the sponsor will conduct to ensure adequate documentation of the change. An additional source of data to support the application are published studies on the previously approved drugs, and generic companies using this source wherever possible avoid disputes with the sponsor of the original NDA filing regarding the legality of the FDA using data from their filing as a reference.

4.2 EUROPE

The generic approval process in the European Union (EU) is in principle similar to that in the United States, but it is complicated by the number of different national health authorities. There are currently 27 member states, all with their own distinct regulatory histories and varying degrees of acceptance of generic drugs.

As in the United States, generic companies can submit abridged applications and are not obliged to repeat the safety and efficacy studies already performed by the brand company. As in the United States, bioequivalence studies are required to demonstrate the "essential similarity" of the product.

There are four alternative authorization procedures available in Europe. Marketing authorization for a pharmaceutical product in more than one country in the EU must be applied for through one of three procedures, the "Centralised Procedure" (CP), the "Mutual Recognition Procedure" (MRP), or the "Decentralised Procedure" (DCP). The last of these is relatively new, having come into force with the newly revised EU Pharmaceutical Directive in November 2005. Companies only wishing to market their product in one country can employ a "National Procedure."

CP. The CP is administered by the European Medicines Agency (EMA) in London. It consists of a single application which, when approved, grants marketing authorization for all markets within the EU. This procedure is obligatory for biologics, for orphan drugs, and for products used for treating AIDS, cancer, neurodegenerative disorders, diabetes, autoimmune diseases, and viral diseases. The procedure may be also used for products containing new chemical entities as their active substances, and for all other products bringing therapeutic or scientific progress and which are considered to be important for patients within the EU. The procedure may also be used for generic medicine applications once the data exclusivity periods have expired.

MRP. Most authorizations for generic medicines are obtained using the MRP process or the DCP. Under the MRP, the assessment and marketing authorization of one Member State, the "Reference Member State" (RMS), should be "mutually recognized" by other "Concerned Member States" (CMSs). There is a statutory 90-day assessment period after which each CMS has to grant a marketing authorization with an identical summary of product characteristics to that in the RMS, unless they disagree with their original assessment of the product. If a CMS raises objections and does not recognize the original marketing authorization, the matter may be referred to the EMA for discussion among the parties and resolution. Binding arbitration is imposed if these discussions fail to reach a conclusion.

DCP. The DCP can be used where an authorization does not yet exist in any EU Member State. Identical dossiers have to be submitted in each Member State where marketing authorization is sought. The applicant chooses an RMS, which drafts assessment documents and sends them to each involved CMS. These either approve the assessment, or an arbitration procedure is triggered. The DCP has the advantage of involving each targeted CMS earlier in the evaluation process than under the MRP process, thus minimizing later disagreements and arbitrations.

More information on the MRP and DCP can be found on this website: http://ec.europa.eu/health/documents/eudralex/index_en.htm

National Procedure. In this case, marketing authorization will only be valid for the one country in which the regulatory submission is made. The National Procedure can still also serve as the first phase of an MRP if the country is selected to act as the RMS for that procedure.

4.3 JAPAN

The Japanese generics market was relatively underdeveloped until recently. Then, in 2007, the Japanese Ministry of Health, Labour and Welfare (MHLW) announced an "Action Program for the Promotion of the Safe Use of Generics," setting a target of achieving a 30% market share (by volume) for generic drugs by 2012, an increase from 18.7% in September 2007. The government predicted that achieving this target would save 500 billion yen (US$5 billion) over the 5 years.

Generic products are reviewed for bioequivalence by the Pharmaceuticals and Medical Devices Agency (PMDA) which reports its findings to the MHLW. The MHLW will only approve generics once the branded product patent has expired. Any disputes are treated by the Patent Office, or taken to court if no agreement can be reached. As in Europe—and unlike the United States— there is no equivalent of 180-day exclusivity for the first company to challenge a patent. Review times are long in Japan because of resource bottlenecks, so generic products may not become available until months or years after the patent has expired. These delays cause unnecessary health costs and are being addressed by the government.

CHAPTER 5

Hatch–Waxman Legislation and Its Effects on LCM

In this chapter we will look at the initial Hatch–Waxman legislation, and at follow-on legislation which came into force subsequently.

5.1 HATCH–WAXMAN ACT OF 1984

The concern in many countries that health-care costs are spiraling out of control and that reducing drug prices is an important element of cost containment is not new. Indeed, this was the motivation for the original Hatch–Waxman Act of 1984 or, to give it its full title, the Drug Price Competition and Patent Restoration Act of 1984. The main purpose of the new Act was to expedite and encourage earlier market entry of generic drugs, although some crumbs of comfort were also offered to the branded industry to aid in their digestion of the new legislation. The main provisions of the Act were as follows:

> *Establishment of an Abbreviated New Drug Application (ANDA) Process.*
> Prior to Hatch–Waxman, a generic company wishing to market the copy of a branded drug had to repeat all of the efficacy and safety trials that had been the basis of the original regulatory approval of the branded drug. The costs and time involved were considerable, and there were not many companies willing or able to make this investment. Prior to Hatch–Waxman, there were at least 150 off-patent branded drugs which did not have any generic competition, and this was causing an unnecessary cost burden on the health-care system. Hatch–Waxman stated that it was sufficient for the generic company to show that their drug was bioequivalent to the original and to submit an ANDA as the basis for approval. The costs and time involved in conducting bioequivalence studies are minimal, and the likelihood of being successful is very high. This one

Pharmaceutical Lifecycle Management: Making the Most of Each and Every Brand, First Edition. Tony Ellery and Neal Hansen.
© 2012 John Wiley & Sons, Inc. Published 2012 by John Wiley & Sons, Inc.

provision of Hatch–Waxman changed the face of the generic industry completely, with far more companies entering the market, competing on price, and thus driving down the costs of older, off-patent drugs.

Bolar Provision. In early 1984, Roche had sued a generic manufacturer, Bolar, for infringement of Roche patents covering Roche's brand, Valium®, based on Bolar's testing of samples to assess whether their generic of the drug was bioequivalent to the original brand at a time when the Roche patent was still in force. Bolar argued that they were entitled to use Valium in their experiments, that they were not commercially exploiting the drug, and that they were therefore not infringing the Roche patent. However, the Court of Appeals for the Federal Circuit rejected Bolar's contention, holding that Bolar was conducting its experiments because it intended to sell its generic after the Valium patent expiry, and that Bolar's experiments therefore had a business purpose. This ruling had the effect of ensuring that no generic would be able to enter the market immediately after the brand patent expired, as the generic company could not start its bioequivalence testing until after patent expiry. In reaction to this situation, the Hatch–Waxman Act was amended so that the use of a patented drug solely with the intention of creating a file for the submission of an ANDA did not infringe the patent of the patented drug. This "Bolar" provision established a "safe harbor" in which generic companies could develop their generic copies, and meant that generic drugs could enter the market on the day that the patent expired instead of many months later.

180-Day Exclusivity. The first two provisions of the Hatch–Waxman legislation, the ANDA process and the Bolar provision, were designed to ensure fast generic entry after patent expiry. But the legislation went one important and controversial step further. It determined that the first filer of an ANDA under Paragraph IV would obtain 180 days of market exclusivity to compete with the original brand. We will describe this process fully in Chapter 9. Suffice it to say here that it offered a significant financial reward to generic companies which were able to successfully attack and invalidate brand patents even before they expired.

These, then, were the provisions that aided the generics industry. What was offered to the branded industry by Hatch–Waxman? There were three points, all of which we will examine in Chapters 8 and 9.

- Patent term restoration
- NCE exclusivity
- New clinical trial exclusivity

These measures provided some degree of protection for the branded companies, but the overall purpose of the legislation was to get more generic drugs to market more quickly, preferably even before patent expiry.

5.2 MEDICARE MODERNIZATION ACT OF 2003

In late 2003, some amendments to Hatch–Waxman became law as part of the Medicare Prescription Drug Improvement and Modernization Act, the so-called Medicare Modernization Act or Medicare Act.

Limit of One 30-Month Stay. As we will see in Chapter 9, any attempt by a generic company to invalidate an existing brand patent utilizing the Paragraph IV process addressed by the Hatch–Waxman legislation triggered a 30-month "stay" period during which the generic could not be sold, and during which time the brand and generic companies were expected to resolve their patent dispute. In an attempt to delay generic approval even further, brand companies reacted by entering additional, "late-listed" patents into the Orange Book long after new molecular entity (NME) approval, and even after Paragraph IV certification. Each of these additional patents entitled the brand company to a new 30-month stay, so generic approval could be delayed almost indefinitely. The Medicare Act stated that there could only be a single 30-month stay, and that even this one stay would only be granted if it was based on a patent which had already been in the Orange Book when the first generic filer submitted its ANDA. Furthermore, approval of a generic by the Food and Drug Administration (FDA) could occur even before this 30-month stay had elapsed if a district court or the appeals court decided that the patent was invalid or not infringed. It is important to note that generic companies still had to notify the innovator of any Paragraph IV filing against additional patents, and the innovator could still sue, but the FDA could no longer impose additional 30-month stays.

Definition of the First Filer. The Hatch–Waxman Act had led to the bizarre sight of generic company representatives standing in line at FDA in an attempt to be the first filer and thus gain 180 days of exclusivity. The Medicare Act put an end to this by stating that any company filing on the same day as the first filer would also be given first-filer status.

Restriction of First-Filer Status to One per Product. The Hatch–Waxman Act had allowed first-filer status to be granted to any generic company filing Paragraph IV Certification against a patent in the Orange Book. But products are often protected by more than one patent, and different companies might file against different patents. This led to confusion as to which company really should enjoy first-filer status. The Medicare Act determined that there could only be one 180-days exclusivity grant per product instead of one per patent, and that this status would be granted to the first company to file against any patent in the Orange Book.

Registration of Deals with the Federal Trade Commission (FTC). Following the Hatch–Waxman Act, there were cases of brand companies paying the holders of 180-day exclusivities not to enter the market, or to delay their entry and thus also the start of the 180 days. This practice not only eliminated the price competition between the originator and the first filer, but other generic companies were blocked from entering the market. Effectively, the profits being made on the brand while it enjoyed exclusivity remained the same, but were simply shared between the originator and the first filer. Any financial benefit to the health-care system which should have ensued as a result of the expiry or invalidation of the patent was lost. The Medicare Act required that any such "pay for delay" or "reverse payment" settlement agreements be reported to the FTC.

Declaratory Judgment Actions. The Medicare Act gave generic companies the right to file a declaratory judgment if the innovator did not sue the generic company within 45 days of their filing the Paragraph IV Certification. Without going deep into the legalese, this meant that if the innovator did not sue within the 45 days, he would lose the 30-month stay.

Orange Book De-Listing Counterclaim. Generic companies were given the right to bring a counterclaim in an infringement action to de-list—or to correct—a patent that they believe should not have been listed in the Orange Book, because they do not claim either the approved drug or an approved method of using the drug.

180-Day Exclusivity Forfeiture. Finally, the Medicare Act determined that the first filer forfeits exclusivity in certain situations, including if it fails to market its product within 75 days of FDA approval (or expiry of the 30-month stay, whichever is earlier) or within 75 days of a court decision or settlement.

5.3   FDA AMENDMENTS ACT OF 2007

Several amendments to the foregoing legislation became law in 2007:

Citizen Petition Modification. This part of the FDA Amendments Act blunted a weapon that innovators had sometimes used against generic companies. A Citizen Petition is a formal request to the FDA to take an action on an issue, and the FDA is required to consider and reply to this request publicly. This may be a valid request, as when a company truly believes that a generic copy will not reproduce the safety or efficacy of the original, but originators sometimes submitted spurious petitions merely to delay generic approval while FDA considered its response. The FDA Amendments Act determined that the FDA would not delay the approval of a pending ANDA or a pending 505(b)(2) application as a result of a Citizen Petition unless it determined that "a delay is necessary to protect the public health."

Authorized Generics Database. We will look at authorized generics later in the book. Suffice it to say here that innovators use authorized generics as a way of capturing more postpatent expiry brand value, and there is controversy as to whether or not this benefits the consumer. This part of the FDA Amendments Act committed the FDA to create an authorized generics database to assist the FTC as it moves ahead with its study of the competitive effects of authorized generics.

5.4 Q1 PROGRAM SUPPLEMENTAL FUNDING ACT OF 2008

This legislation extended Hatch–Waxman provisions regarding patent listing, patent certification, 30-month stay, and exclusivity to antibiotics, to pave the way for generic antibiotics.

5.5 DISCUSSION OF HATCH-WAXMAN LEGISLATION

What has been the result of all of the legislation described in this chapter? The original stated purpose of the Hatch–Waxman legislation back in 1984 had been to establish a balance between the competing interests of innovators and generic drug companies, with the public as the ultimate beneficiary. But even then, in signing the bill, President Reagan had indicated that generic drugs might save American consumers US$1,000,000,000 over the following 10 years. This confirmed that the government's primary interest in passing the "Drug Price Competition and Patent Restoration Act" was drug price competition, and the resulting lower prices, rather than restoring patents. Supporters of the Act claimed that it would compel branded drug companies to concentrate their R&D efforts on creating innovative new drugs. Again, it is hard to see how this could be consistent with President Reagan's statement. Predictably, the generics industry rejoiced when the Hatch–Waxman Act became law, while the brand industry looked for loopholes that would enable them to keep generics at bay and extend the exclusivity of their brands. Loopholes were found, and the subsequent amendments closed some of them.

Today, a quarter century after the Hatch–Waxman Act was passed, it is clear that the primary intention of the legislation in promoting generics has been realized. Before 1984, only about 35% of off-patent drugs had generic competition; today almost all do. Eighty percent of U.S. prescriptions are for generics, compared with 15% pre-Hatch–Waxman. There has been a dramatic increase in the number of ANDAs and Paragraph IV challenges in the years since 1984, and the success rate of generic companies in invalidating patents, especially formulation and polymorph patents, has been high. Where no generic company enjoys 180-day exclusivity, brand sales erosion is precipitous after patent expiry, in some cases over 90% within weeks.

The branded pharmaceutical industry has benefited less, as was to be expected. Brand life cycles can effectively end when the primary patent expires, and patents themselves are less secure than they used to be. Quite simply, brand companies cannot expect to evergreen their older brands and are completely dependent on their new product pipelines. Peter Drucker once wrote "Innovate, or die," and Hatch–Waxman has placed Big Pharma in the United States in precisely that position. The jury is still out for several large companies on which of Drucker's alternatives will come to pass.

In a speech honoring the 25th anniversary of the Hatch–Waxman legislation in September, 2009, Representative Henry Waxman said the following: "Madam Speaker, twenty-five years ago, President Ronald Reagan signed the landmark Waxman-Hatch law, delivering generic drug competition to the American marketplace. Since that time, generic drugs have provided millions of American consumers with access to low-cost, yet safe and effective drugs. In the last decade alone, generics have saved consumers, businesses, and state and federal governments US$734 billion. American consumers fill more than six of every ten prescriptions with safe and effective generic medicines. During these difficult economic times, generic pharmaceuticals are critical to assuring that patients continue to have access to life-saving medicines. Making sure that Americans have access to, and can afford, life-saving medicines has been one of my chief goals as a Member of Congress, and I am proud of the success of generic competition in helping achieve that goal. Since passage of the Hatch–Waxman law, we have seen a shift in the pharmaceutical marketplace to permit greater competition and innovation—a win-win for purchasers and manufacturers alike. As a result, millions of Americans have access to safe and affordable generic medicines and our health care bill is much lower than it otherwise would have been. There is still much more we can do to increase savings from generic drugs. We should not only celebrate the 25th anniversary of Hatch–Waxman, but we should use it as motivation to ensure there is real generic competition for biotech medications. Let us show Americans that we understand that they deserve access to affordable medicine and give them a pathway that provides reasonable incentives for innovation, but does not pose unnecessary barriers to competition."

At about the same time, one of the authors asked Henry Waxman during a teleconference whether he had any plans to stimulate innovation. He replied that the original Act provided sufficient incentive, and that the main priority was still to increase generic competition. He presented the diagram shown in Figure 5.1, which makes this intention eminently clear. Ensuring that generics get to market, and then dominate it, as soon as possible in the brand life cycle means one of two things, or more probably, both:

- Shorter exclusivity periods
- More rapid generic penetration

In this situation, compounded by their depleted development pipelines, it is not surprising that branded pharmaceutical companies try to find additional ways of prolonging exclusivity and slowing postpatent brand sales erosion, and these two aims are the whole purpose of late LCM (LLCM).

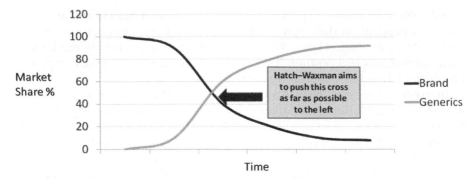

FIGURE 5.1. The main goal of Hatch–Waxman Act of 1984 is to encourage generic competition earlier. *Source:* Adapted from Markus Meier, HNC's World Generic Medicines Congress Americas in 2008.

There are still opportunities for LLCM, although the US government and especially the FTC, continue their efforts to close these "loopholes" in the legislation at the earliest possible time. As we will be discussing later, this rapid evolution of LLCM hurdles means that managers responsible for lifecycle management in brand companies must always be looking ahead when deciding what LLCM measures, initiated today, are still likely to be effective in the future. Indeed, this is much of the science and art of late-stage lifecycle management (LLCM).

CHAPTER 6

U.S. Health-Care Reform 2010

Heath-Care Reform in the United States comprises a far-reaching compendium of different legislation passed at different times which, depending on what is included in the term "Health-Care Reform," can be dated right back to the introduction of Medicare and Medicaid by the Johnson administration in 1965.

Unlike the Hatch-Waxman legislation and its modifiers described in the previous chapter, health-care reform is not concerned only with reducing costs, and particularly by promoting the use of generics. Instead, the main focus of Health-Care Reform is to provide health coverage for individuals who have hitherto been denied it by the U.S. system. We will not attempt to cover the whole field of Health-Care Reform in our book. Instead we will restrict ourselves to the two latest building blocks of Health-Care Reform: the Patient Protection and Affordable Care Act (PPACA) and the Health Care and Education Reconciliation Act, which amended the PPACA, and both of which became law under the Obama administration in March 2010. And we will only look at those aspects of the new legislation that may affect lifecycle management (LCM). We will group them according to when they come into force during the 5-year scope foreseen for the enactment of the legislation.

Immediate. Insurance companies may no longer drop patients from coverage when they get sick. Uninsured patients with preexisting disease conditions can now obtain health coverage supported by funds from high-risk pools. A reinsurance program enables companies to provide health coverage for early retirees up to their official age of retirement. Small businesses are granted tax rebates to enable them to provide health coverage for their staff. Some of these early measures are only temporary, as they will be replaced by more effective measures as enactment proceeds over the subsequent 3 years. Branded drug companies

Pharmaceutical Lifecycle Management: Making the Most of Each and Every Brand, First Edition.
Tony Ellery and Neal Hansen.
© 2012 John Wiley & Sons, Inc. Published 2012 by John Wiley & Sons, Inc.

may no longer delay approval of generic products by making label changes to the brand name or listed drug—prior to the new legislation, the labeling of a generic drug was required to match the labeling of the referenced brand name or listed drug, or would not be approved. From now on, an Abbreviated New Drug Application (ANDA) can be approved despite last-minute changes to the labeling of the listed drug, provided that the labeling change does not affect the "Warnings" section of the listed drug's labeling.

By End of 2011. An annual fee will be imposed on drug companies proportional to their market share. The annual fee is a stepwise annual increase, starting at US$2.5 billion in 2011, increasing to a maximum of US$4.1 billion in 2018, and decreasing to US$2.8 billion in 2019 and onward.

2013. The threshold for claiming medical expenses on tax returns is raised to 10% from 7.5% of income (except for the elderly, where the increase comes into effect in 2016).

2014. Patients with incomes up to 133% of the federal poverty level (FPL) will qualify for Medicaid coverage. Health-care tax credits will be introduced that help patients with incomes up to 400% of the FPL to purchase health coverage. A premium cap, on a sliding scale, will be provided for maximum "out-of-pocket" pay for patients with incomes up to 400% of FPL. Citizens failing to obtain health insurance will have to pay increased taxes. Health plans will no longer be permitted to exclude patients from coverage due to preexisting conditions. Companies failing to provide health coverage will be liable to be fined. Health insurance companies will start paying fees based on market share.

Finally, the new legislation authorizes the Food and Drug Administration (FDA) to create a new regulatory pathway for biosimilar biological products, allowing licensure of biological products as biosimilar or interchangeable to products with current licenses. Innovator manufacturers of reference biological products are granted 12 years of exclusive use before biosimilars can be approved for marketing.

What will be the impact of Health-Care Reform on the branded pharmaceutical industry, and especially on LCM? Long term, most of the measures enacted in 2011–2012 look beneficial to the pharmaceutical industry in general, including the generics industry, as they serve to increase the number of U.S. citizens with health coverage by about 30 million, including patients with preexisting disease who in the past could not afford to pay for the drugs necessary to treat their conditions. However, this increase in the number of patients receiving drugs at a time when the U.S. economy is in severe trouble is bound to exert a downward pressure on drug prices to compensate for the increased usage. In the same way, the pressure to avoid high-priced branded drugs when a generic drug will do the same or virtually the same job is sure to increase. In the midterm, the annual fee that will be imposed on drug companies starting in 2011 will be painful, especially as it hits at a time when the industry is already suffering the effects of patent expiries and a shortage of major new drugs. The legislation regarding biologics is a two-edged sword. On the one hand, the United States will now create a route to market for "generic biologics," but on the other, this will only kick into effect after a very generous 12-year exclusivity period for the original brand, which is much longer than the generics industry had hoped for and much longer than the 5 years granted to small molecules. In the short term, the branded drug industry has benefited from something that the Health-Care Reform did *not* do, namely, reducing or freezing the price of drugs. Thomson Reuters MarketScan reported in March 2011 that prices for the 15 best-selling drugs rose by much higher rates in 2010 than they did in each of the previous 5 years.

CHAPTER 7

European Sector Inquiry

Just as in the United States the Hatch–Waxman Act and subsequent related legislation targeted legal loopholes that brand companies use to maintain exclusivity and delay the entry of cheaper generic products to the market, the European Sector Report into the pharmaceutical industry, which was released in July 2009, looked at the same issues in Europe. The inquiry had concentrated on two areas of concern to the European Commission:

1. The entry of generics to the market is often delayed until well after brand exclusivity has been lost, so that the health-care systems incur unnecessary expenses. Examination of the competitive relationship between brand and generic companies was expected to show to what extent company behavior contributes to this situation.
2. How does the competitive relationship among brand companies impact innovation?

The report was based on the in-depth investigation of 219 products. These were selected on the basis of their patent protection having expired in recent years, and/or generic entry having recently occurred for the first time. For purposes of comparison, some top-selling drugs were also included which still benefited from exclusivity, but where exclusivity was due to expire in the near future. The investigation studied the situation in all 27 European Union Member States.

The main finding of the inquiry was that competition does not function as well as it should. The Commission concluded that there was both a delay in the market entry of generic drugs and a decline in innovation as evidenced by the fact that less novel medicines were reaching the market. Both company behavior and regulation were determined to play a factor in this. The Commission made a series of recommendations to correct the situation, which would lead to a reduction in health-care costs.

During its inquiry, the Commission uncovered many documents regarding brand company strategies to limit generic competition. Passages from three of these documents, which were included in the report, are quoted below:

1. One company executive stated: "We identify options to obtain or acquire patents for the sole purpose of limiting the freedom of operation of our competitors . . . Rights covering competitive alternatives are maintained in major markets until risk of competing products appearing is minimal."
2. Another admitted "I suppose we have all had conversations around 'how can we block generic manufacturers.' (. . .) Don't play games in patenting new salt forms too late, the generics are starting earlier and earlier. Get (. . .) claims on key intermediates that cover a number of routes. Process patents are not the biggest block but can put generics off if a superior chemistry job is done."
3. And a third was happy to claim that: "Interchangeability issues were used in (several countries) to limit generic erosion. (. . .) Outcome: extra (. . .) sales of USD 61 m compared to expected generic erosion."

The report highlighted several different specific delaying measures aimed at generic companies, which together constituted what the report called a "tool-box" of brand company late-stage lifecycle management (LLCM) strategies:

- Originator companies file "patent clusters," a large number of Europe-wide patents covering each single brand (up to 100 patent families and 1300 patents per brand).
- There have been nearly 700 cases of patent litigation with generic companies, with each case lasting an average of 3 years. In more than 60% of these cases, the generic company ultimately prevailed. Originator companies obtained injunctions restraining generic entry in 112 cases, but in nearly half of these cases, the final judgment was favorable to the generic company.
- Brand companies signed over 200 settlement agreements with generic companies; these set out the terms for ending ongoing litigation or disputes. In 50% of these settlements, generic entry was restricted, and in approximately half of these, there was a value transfer from the brand to the generic company. More than 10% of the settlements were so-called reverse payment settlements which provided for direct payments.
- Brand companies intervened in national procedures for the approval of generics in a significant number of cases, which on average led to 4 months of delay before the generic could enter the market.

The report concluded that there were a variety of reasons for the delayed market entry of generics. Some of these were caused by regulatory delays in marketing authorization and in pricing and reimbursement procedures, while others were caused by brand company behavior such as the use of certain patent application and enforcement strategies, certain patent settlements aimed at the restriction of generic market entry, as well as interventions in marketing authorization procedures.

The solutions proposed by the report to solve these problems included:

- Increased scrutiny under the European Community (EC) Treaty antitrust law to the sector, bringing specific cases where originator companies use certain strategies which may infringe Article 81 or 82 of the EC Treaty. Increased scrutiny of defensive patenting strategies that focus merely on excluding competitors rather than on innovative efforts. The two most relevant passages from the Final Report were as follows:
  - "Defensive patenting strategies that mainly focus on excluding competitors without pursuing innovative efforts and/or refusal to grant a license on unused patents will remain under scrutiny in particular in situations where innovation was effectively blocked."
  - "It should be noted from the outset that enforcing patent rights in court is legitimate and constitutes a fundamental right guaranteed by the European Convention of Human Rights. However, the inquiry's findings show that, like in any other industry, litigation can also be an efficient means of creating obstacles in particular for smaller companies. In certain instances, originator companies may consider litigation not so much on its merits, but rather as a signal to deter generic entrants."
- Focused monitoring of settlements that limit or delay the market entry of generic drugs, at the expense of consumers. The Final Report indicated which settlements were likely to come under the microscope in the following passage: "Settlement agreements that limit generic entry and include a value transfer from an originator company to one or more generic companies are an example of such potentially anticompetitive agreements, in particular where the motive of the agreement is the sharing of profits via payments from originator to generic companies to the detriment of patients and public health budgets."
- Reaching agreement on an EC patent and a specialized patent litigation system.
- Leveling the playing field for generic medicines through different actions, including:
  - Ensuring that third-party submissions do not lead to delays in the approval of generic medicines.
  - Encouraging Member States to provide automatic or immediate pricing and reimbursement status for generic medicines that are equivalent to the original brands.
  - Introducing legislation that encourages generic uptake, for example, prescription by generic active substance name rather than by brand. The

Final Report concluded that, all other things being equal, having a compulsory substitution policy increases the market share of generic drugs by 12–25%.

◦ If there are clear indications that a company intervention before a marketing authorization body was made primarily to delay the market entry of a competitor, then any injured parties are invited to bring the appropriate evidence to the attention of the relevant competition authorities.

The complete report can be found on http://ec.europa.eu/index_en.htm.

This completes the section of the book devoted to legal and regulatory environment in which lifecycle management decision must be made. In the following chapters, we shall be considering the different tactical measures that can be employed by project and brand teams to optimize a product life cycle, from the patents and exclusivities that can be sought to drive exclusivity to the developmental and commercial measures that can drive competitive differentiation and meet medical needs.

PATENTS AND EXCLUSIVITIES

CHAPTER 8

Patents and Other Intellectual Property Rights

We start off with three chapters on Legal/Regulatory Strategies. This chapter covers Patents, Chapter 9 examines Regulatory Exclusivities, and Chapter 10 considers Litigation and Settlements.

This chapter must start with a disclaimer. We are not patent attorneys, although we have obtained advice from them. This does have the advantage that what we write should be easy to understand for nonattorneys, which is not always the case in books and articles on patents. If we have understood it, you should be able to do so as well! But you are warned not to use just this chapter uncritically as the basis for determining your patent strategy as part of your overall LCM strategy. Please do consult an experienced patent attorney, firstly because you will want to be 100% sure that you are making the right patent interpretations and decisions, and secondly because patent law as it relates to pharmaceuticals is a fast-evolving field so that the half-life of this chapter may be shorter than the average for the whole book.

Before we consider patents, let us briefly consider other forms of intellectual property rights. They do not usually figure in discussions on LCM, but they are important and they are worth mentioning here.

8.1 NONPATENT INTELLECTUAL PROPERTY RIGHTS

Trademarks. A trademark or trade mark is a distinctive sign or indicator used by an individual, business organization, or other legal entity to identify that the products on which the trademark appears originate from a unique source, and to distinguish these products from those of other entities. Recently, the word "products" even covers certain clinical trials that companies have trademarked (e.g., the ONTARGET and PROFESS trials conducted by Boehringer with Micardis). The

---

Pharmaceutical Lifecycle Management: Making the Most of Each and Every Brand, First Edition.
Tony Ellery and Neal Hansen.
© 2012 John Wiley & Sons, Inc. Published 2012 by John Wiley & Sons, Inc.

trademark can comprise a word or group of words, or a design, or a word-plus-design combination. Prozac®, for example, is a trademark owned by Eli Lilly and Company for its brand of fluoxetine. Generic drugs carry the name of the active principle of the product—in this case, fluoxetine—but cannot use the trademark. A strong trademark is less important for pharmaceutical products than for consumer products, especially as the payer is usually not the user, but can be important after patent expiry in self-pay markets, where the consumer often wants to buy the original product, and in over-the-counter (OTC) switching. Furthermore, the company trademark can inspire a degree of confidence in physicians and patients. It is worth remembering that generics are prescribed by International Nonproprietary Names (INNs). Brand directors are good at thinking up catchy names for brands, and this helps to reduce market share loss after patent expiry. Researchers seldom consider the counterpart. Making the INN as long, unpronounceable, and difficult to spell as possible can have a similar effect, proving once again that it is never too early to start thinking about LCM. In any case, trademarks must be considered early enough during development—not later than Phase II—as it is getting increasingly difficult to find names that are internationally acceptable, and there are few things worse than discovering that the new trademark you have been promoting, and perhaps already printing on packaging, is not acceptable in a major market. An important restriction when considering a new trademark is that it is not allowed to be either descriptive or misleading. Thus, you would not be able to call an antihypertensive "Pressurdrop," as this would monopolize a descriptive term and prevent other companies from using it. Equally, you could not call an antibiotic "Bacteriogrow" (not that you would want to) as the term is misleading.

Trade Dress Rights. A trade dress right protects the commercial design of goods offered for sale, for example, the shape, configuration, pattern, or color, in two- or three-dimensional form of pills or their packaging. Like brand trademarks, the importance of trade dress to the pharmaceutical industry is less than with consumer goods, but a good trade dress design can also be part of the overall LCM strategy in clever hands. We will be referring to the Nexium® (esomeprazole) case history repeatedly in this book, and AstraZeneca were undoubtedly very clever regarding the design rights of their antacids. They wanted to establish continuity between their off-patent drug, Losec® (omeprazole), and its patented successor, Nexium. They therefore gave Nexium capsules the same color as Losec capsules—purple—and continued to talk about "the purple pill" as the best treatment of heartburn. Patients who had been using Losec identified more with Nexium than they did with the generic omeprazole, which was prevented from being purple by AstraZeneca's design rights, and this helped AstraZeneca in converting patients to their new drug. The website of Nexium is actually called http://www.purplepill.com.

Copyright. This intellectual property right protects artistic expression in textual and visual works, and can be used to protect things like patient leaflets, artwork that is used in packaging, and advertising content.

Domain Names. A domain name is a locator (or, to give it its full name, a "Uniform Resource Locator" or "URL") used to identify the home page of a website accessible on the Internet. An example of a domain name is www.purplepill.com.

Know-How or Trade Secrets. Confidential or "closely held" information in the form of unpatented inventions, formulae, designs, procedures, and methods which have not been patented, together with accumulated skills and experience.

8.2 WHAT ARE PATENTS?

A patent is a set of exclusive rights granted by a national government to an inventor or assignee thereof for a limited period of time in exchange for the public disclosure of an invention. Patents are the foundation upon which the innovative pharmaceutical industry is built. Without patents, there would be no commercial basis for companies to research and develop new pharmaceuticals. We have already looked at why this is so:

- Drugs are extremely expensive to develop, and these costs must be borne by the originator company that first markets the drug.
- Gaining marketing approval for a generic of this original drug is generally cheap and easy; the development work done by the originator does not have to be repeated, as long the generic is bioequivalent.
- Third-party payers do not care about brand names—they are only interested in getting a drug at the cheapest possible price.

Without patents, soon after a brand company put a new drug onto the market, and depending upon its commercial success, literally dozens of generic companies could introduce identical copy products and compete on price—the most important differentiator in the generic drugs industry. Within a very short time, the price of the drug would drop to only slightly above the costs of manufacture and distribution. In such a situation, the brand company could not make enough profit to recoup the development costs invested in putting the original version of the drug onto the market.

A patent is a document, issued upon application by a government, which describes an invention and ensures that it can only be exploited (manufactured, used, sold, and/or imported) by the owner of the patent or with his authorization. The term "invention" means a solution to a specific problem in the field of technology. An invention may relate to a product or a process. The protection conferred by the patent is limited in time, generally up to 20 years.

The idea of patenting inventions is very old. The first recorded example of what we today think of as a patent dates from 500 B.C. In the Southern Italian city of Sybaris (at that time part of the Greek Empire), a statute was passed in which "encouragement was held out to all who should discover any new refinement in luxury, the profits arising from which were secured to the inventor by patent for the space of a year."

The first example of "modern" patent legislation dates from 1474, when the Republic of Venice enacted a decree that new and inventive devices, once put into practice, had to be communicated to the Republic to obtain the right to prevent others from using them.

The purpose of a patent is to provide an inventor with an incentive to make public his invention without fear that somebody else might steal it from him. A patent results from a bargain between the government and the inventor. In exchange for disclosure of his invention to the public, if the government determines that the invention is indeed new and nonobvious, the government gives the inventor a patent. This is the right for a limited period of time to exclude others from making, using, or selling what he invented. This disclosure must be detailed enough so that a person of ordinary skill in the field of the invention can implement the invention. This arrangement has several benefits for society:

- There would be little motivation for inventors and thus little progress if new ideas could immediately be taken and utilized by third parties.
- The patent protects the inventor when he demonstrates his invention to potential investors, so that the invention can be developed commercially in cases where the inventor is unwilling or is unable to do this himself.
- Other inventors have the opportunity to create improvements of the initial invention which can themselves in turn also be patented, increasing the value to society of the original invention.

A patent must contain the following information:

- Cover page:
    - Title of the patent and abstract of the invention
    - Names and addresses of all inventors
    - Name and address of the patent owner or assignee (the owner/assignee is often the company which employs the inventor)
- Specification: This typically contains two parts:
    - Description of the field of the invention and what was already known in this field before the invention was made ("prior art")
    - General description of the invention
- Detailed description of how the invention works, including examples. In the case of a new drug, this description will include the chemical formula, the manufacturing process, and the physical properties of the drug.

- Claims: The claims define the scope of the protection given to the invention by the patent. Claims, therefore, define a protective boundary line around the subject of the patent. Claims may be broad or narrow. Generally, a patent attorney will try to formulate the broadest possible claims, but where there is significant prior art, the claims will have to be narrower, because claims of a patent cannot be so broad as to cover things that are old. One patent may contain several separate claims, but each must be supported by the description of the invention in the previous section. It is important to understand that the invalidation of one claim in a patent does not automatically imply invalidation of other claims and thus of the whole patent; a claim may be lost, but the rest of the patent can still remain valid.

Usually we think of a patent as granting the inventor a monopoly, or the exclusive right to exploit his invention, but actually this is incorrect. Rather, the patent merely grants the patent holder the right to prevent his invention from being exploited by third persons without his permission. Thus, the patent holder is not given the right to practice the invention, but is given the right to prevent others from practicing it. This "right to exclude" others from making, using, or selling the invention is the most important right that a patent confers. This may seem at first sight like a subtle distinction, but it is an extremely important nuance, as we shall see later.

Furthermore, although a government grants this right to exclude others, it neither monitors whether third parties infringe the patent nor does it prosecute infringers. It is up to patent holders both to ensure that their patents are not infringed and to take legal action against anyone who does so.

8.3   WHAT IS PATENTABLE?

For a patent to be granted, a number of conditions must be met:

- The subject matter must be patentable
- The invention must be new ("novel")
- It must involve a nonobvious, inventive step
- It must be industrially applicable
- The disclosure of the invention in the patent must meet defined standards

8.3.1   Patentable Subject Matter

Because so many different things *can* be patented, it is easier to define what cannot:

- Discoveries of materials or substances already existing in nature; laws of nature. Here—as in other points listed below—there are exceptions. It is possible in some cases to patent substances which are present in very small quantities in nature where the inventor has succeeded in both identifying the substance and isolating it in practically useful quantities. The key distinction is between technical innovations and mere discoveries which are not the result of an inventive process. At the present time, it is still possible to patent the unexpected result of doing something obvious, but there is some criticism of this situation.

- Scientific theories or mathematical methods.
- Plants and animals other than microorganisms, and essentially biological processes for the production of plants and animals, other than nonbiological and microbiological processes. Genetically engineered mice have been patented, however.
- Schemes, rules, or methods, such as those for doing business, performing purely mental acts, or playing games. However, in the United States—but not in Europe—it is possible to patent certain business methods, such as "one-click" ordering of merchandise on the Internet.
- Methods of treatment for humans or animals, or diagnostic methods practiced on humans or animals (but not products for use in such methods). There is an important exception. In the United States, methods of treatment can be patented, although patents in these areas cannot be enforced directly against the treating physician.
- Inventions already inherent in the prior art. This is best illustrated by an example. If a marketed drug with an unknown mechanism of action is effective against a disease, a person who discovers the mechanism of action will not be able to patent it because the mechanism of action was already "inherent" in the use of the drug.

8.3.2 Novelty

An invention is considered new if it is not anticipated by prior art. Prior art can be defined as all the knowledge that existed in the field prior to filing of the patent application, whether in writing or by oral disclosure. In the United States, however, prior art is determined as the date of invention, which is presumed to be the date of filing of the application unless the inventor can prove an earlier date. An earlier invention enters the realm of prior art in one of several ways:

1. Publication, including on the Internet
2. Public oral presentation (but not in the United States, where an oral presentation by itself is not considered prior art)
3. Use of the invention in public, or public knowledge of the invention, or offering the invention for sale (in the case of a U.S. patent, the public use or public knowledge or offer for sale must be in the United States)

Lack of novelty can be found only if the publication or presentation contains all of the characteristics of one of the claims in the patent, thus anticipating the subject matter of that claim.

Just about the biggest mistake an inventor can make is to publish his invention before patenting it. Then the publication is already in the public domain, and the invention is no longer patentable. In the United States, almost alone among patent authorities, a 1-year grace period is afforded to the inventor after the first publication of the invention or its public use or offer for sale within which period the inventor can still apply for a patent. One of the authors experienced a painful example of an inventor waiting too long to file a patent several years ago. This inventor tried to sell a clever and very simple way of administering one common substance to eliminate the troublesome side effects of a top-selling drug. Developing this combination product would have been expensive, involving multiple clinical trials, but the financial rewards and the benefit to patients would have been significant. Shortly before the deal was signed with the inventor, it was realized that he had already published his work but not patented it prior to doing so. The deal fell through, as there was no way of preventing others from immediately copying the combination therapy once it reached market and destroying the high-price strategy that would have been necessary to recover the development costs. The invention never got to market, to the detriment of both the inventor and those patients who would have benefited from his invention.

8.3.3 Inventive Step

The question of whether a nonobvious and therefore inventive step has been made by the invention is one of the trickiest areas in determining the patentability of an invention. If it can be considered that the invention "would have been obvious to a person having ordinary skill in the art," then it will be concluded by the patent examiner that no inventive step has in fact been achieved. The expression "ordinary skill" is key. Most inventions are based to some extent on prior art, and if one was to refer to "top experts" instead of "persons with ordinary skill," then many worthy inventions would be deprived of a patent.

It is important to understand that "inventive step" is not the same criterion as "novelty." The question of "inventive step" only arises if the "novelty" criterion has already been met. "Inventive step" implies that the invention is not merely new, but that it is the result of a creative idea that advances prior art in some way.

In determining novelty, it is enough to compare the invention singly with each individual publication or other item that constitutes the prior art. In determining whether an inventive step has been made, on the other hand, the entirety of the prior art must be considered. If it is concluded that an invention could be obvious to a person of ordinary skill by combining the teachings of two separate publications, for example, then the inventive step criterion will not be met even though novelty has been shown. We will see how important this distinction can be later in the chapter when we examine in detail the landmark KSR versus Teleflex case.

In evaluating whether an invention has achieved the necessary inventive step, it can be useful to look at it successively from three perspectives:

1. The problem to be solved
2. The solution to the problem
3. The advantages of the invention over prior art

If the problem is known or obvious, the examination of the patent will concentrate on how original the proposed solution is. If the solution is obvious, then a patent may still be allowed if the *result* of the invention is unexpected. If the problem is known, the solution obvious, and the results as could be expected by that "person having ordinary skill," then there has been no inventive step. Let us take a concrete example here. Combining two antihypertensives in a fixed-dose combination tablet to reduce blood pressure is an obvious solution to an obvious problem. But could a patent be obtained if the resulting blood pressure drop was much greater than the sum of the effects of the two components? That would be an unexpected result. We will look deeper into this issue later.

8.3.4 Utility

This is the term often used by patent attorneys to signify "industrial applicability." To be patentable, an invention cannot be merely theoretical. It must be capable of being utilized for practical purposes. Thus, a patentable product must be capable of being manufactured. And a patentable process must be capable of being carried out in practice. So you cannot patent Peter Pan's fairy dust or a flying carpet.

8.3.5 Disclosure

The last requirement of patentability is whether the invention is adequately disclosed in the patent application. Here, again, our old friend, the "person having ordinary skill in the art," makes a reappearance. The disclosure must be made in such a manner that he can carry out the invention. To go back to the start of the chapter, a government awards a patent in exchange for the inventor making his invention public. The public derives no benefit from the government's bargain with the inventor unless the text of the patent has enough detail so that the public really could carry out the invention after the patent expires.

For this reason, examples must be described in the patent, often including drawings or diagrams. The United States requires that the "best method" known to the inventor for carrying out the invention be included.

To allow third parties to comment on whether or not all of the above conditions have been met, some governments provide for a so-called opposition procedure which may be initiated before or after the patent is granted. This procedure allows third parties to register any objections they may have to the validity of the patent.

8.4   HOW LONG DOES A PATENT LAST?

A patent normally lasts 20 years from the date of filing until the date of expiry. Prior to harmonization in 1995, U.S. patents lasted 17 years from the date of issue, so some older U.S. patents have a slightly different term; U.S. patents that were in force on June 8, 1995, or that were issued on an application that was filed before June 8, 1995, have a term that is the greater of the 20 years from filing or 17 years from issue.

Pharmaceutical companies have to patent their new molecular entities (NMEs) very early in development. Otherwise, they risk losing the invention to competitors, or losing the ability to file a patent because of publication. And the whole drug development process from patent filing until regulatory approval and approval of the price and of reimbursement can take more than 10 years. This would leave pharmaceutical companies a relatively short time of less than 10 years to recover their investment before the patent expired and generics entered the market. To compensate for this long development process, legislation in both the United States and Europe has been passed which can extend patent protection beyond 20 years.

8.5   PATENT TERM RESTORATION IN THE UNITED STATES

As we have already seen, the Hatch–Waxman Act came into force in the United States in 1984. The main purpose of the legislation was to provide the foundation for generics to get to the U.S. market quickly after patent expiry, but it did also offer some compensation for the branded pharmaceutical industry. The most important of these was Patent Term Restoration, a mechanism to lengthen the patent to compensate for that part of the patent term lost while the drug was still in development. The formula for determining by how much the patent term should be extended is as follows:

- 50% of the time spent in initial clinical trials (investigational new drug [IND]), plus
- 100% of the time spent in the New Drug Application (NDA) approval process at the Food and Drug Administration (FDA)

There are, however, restrictions in how this rule would be applied:

- The patent extension is for a maximum of 5 years.
- The patent extension will be reduced, if necessary, to preclude protection beyond 14 years after FDA approval.
- The patent must still be valid and unexpired when the patent term restoration is requested.
- There could have been no previous extension under this provision.
- If a number of patents cover the drug, only one of them is subject to extension. Thus, in the case of a new drug with a new mechanism of action, each protected by separate patents, the drug composition of matter patent might still be in force through term extension after the patent for its mechanism of action has already expired. Patent term restoration is thus a good defense against early genericization, but might not prevent competitor drugs with the same mechanism of action entering the market after the mechanism of action patent has expired.

8.6   SUPPLEMENTARY PROTECTION CERTIFICATES IN EUROPE

There is a similar provision in Europe, called the "Supplementary Protection Certificate," abbreviated to SPC. Again, an SPC is awarded for a maximum of 5 years, providing protection for up to 15 years after regulatory approval. What this means in practice is easier to understand in a diagram (see Figure 8.1).

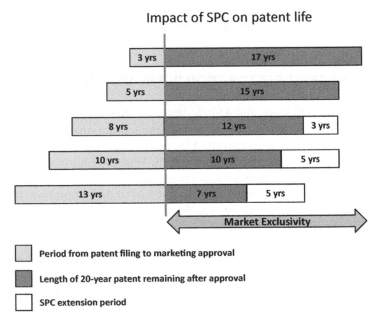

FIGURE 8.1. How European supplementary protection certificates work. *Source*: Ellery Pharma Consulting.

The diagram would look the same for the United States, except that the maximum period after FDA approval is only 14 years in the United States instead of the 15 years in Europe. The SPC is issued on a country-by-country basis and—unlike patent term extension in the United States—is administered outside of the European patent system.

8.7 PATENT TERM EXTENSION IN JAPAN

Patent term extensions can also be obtained in Japan. The maximum extension that can be granted is the time that elapses between the start of clinical testing or the date on which the patent was registered, whichever is later, and the approval date. As in the United States and Europe, the extension may not exceed 5 years. Unlike in the United States or Europe, however, patent term extensions may be granted to multiple patents on the same product, for example, to the composition of matter, the use, the formulation, and the manufacturing process.

The patent term extensions available in the United States, Europe, and Japan are very important LCM tools. Whenever product development from patent filing until regulatory approval takes longer than 5 years (Europe) or 6 years (United States)—which is usually the case in the branded pharmaceutical industry—these instruments can provide for longer market exclusivity.

8.8 HOW ARE PATENTS OBTAINED?

We will not go into the details of how to file a patent, as this varies from country to country and would lie outside the scope of this book. However, it will be helpful to mention a few points regarding the filing of patents.

Typically, patents are first filed in a company's country of domicile (a so-called priority application). Where a regional body such as the European Patent Office (EPO) is available, filing the patent there has the advantage in that it allows patents in a number of countries to be obtained without having to prosecute separate applications in each of those countries. This saves both money and complexity. The EPO has effect in 38 European countries (as of October 1, 2010), including all EU Member States. It examines and grants "European Patents" which have the same status as national patents under the national laws of the participating states.

The Patent Cooperation Treaty (PCT) operated by the World Intellectual Property Organization (WIPO) provides a centralized global application process. The PCT system enables an applicant to file a single patent application in a single language to obtain what is effectively an option to file in almost all countries in the world. The PCT application typically must be filed within a year after filing the initial patent application, and its option lasts 2.5 years after the initial filing of a patent application, or about 1.5 years after it is usually filed. The option of obtaining patents in a wide range of countries around the world is retained, while the cost of a large number of applications is deferred.

A patent application consists of the specification of the invention together with the appropriate official forms and correspondence relating to the application. If the patent specification complies with the laws of the office concerned, a patent may be granted for the invention described and claimed by the specification.

Before granting the patent, the patent office will examine the form and substance of the patent application, and conduct a search to see what prior art pertains to the patent.

The process of negotiating with the patent office for the grant of a patent, and interaction with a patent office with regard to a patent after its grant, is known as "patent prosecution." This term can cause confusion as it is often mistaken by lay persons for "patent litigation," which relates to legal proceedings for infringement after the patent has been granted.

As stated earlier, there is considerable variation in how patents are handled in different countries. In the past, the "Big Three" of the United States, Europe, and Japan have been the most important markets, and these so-called Trilateral Offices have dominated the global patent landscape. Today, however, other markets are gaining in importance, especially the BRICT countries (Brazil, Russia, India, China, and Turkey).

Although the EPO covers an area with a much greater population than either the United States or Japan, the latter two agencies handle far more patent applications. The United States Patent and Trademark Office (USPTO) handles around 400,000 patent applications per year, something like twice that in Europe, for a number of reasons including lower filing fees and a somewhat more favorable treatment of patent eligibility in the United States, where courts have stated that "anything under the sun that is made by man" can be patented. Although the United States has later retrenched somewhat from this view, the "industrial utility" criterion is interpreted much more broadly than in Europe. For example, some business methods are patent eligible in the United States but they are not in Europe.

As mentioned earlier, in the United States, the "first to invent" is entitled to the patent whereas in Europe, Japan, and most other countries, this right is given to the "first to file." Both systems have strengths and weaknesses. As the "first-to-file" system is based on an objective criterion, there is less scope for challenge as the filing date of a patent can only rarely be challenged, and therefore, there is less likelihood of expensive and time-consuming administrative cases, so-called interference proceedings. In the United States, documents like signed and countersigned laboratory journals become very important in establishing priority. Supporters of the U.S. system counter by saying that the "first-to-file" system benefits large companies at the expense of individual inventors, as the large companies can afford to file multiple patents early. In practice, the "first-to-file" party is usually in the stronger position in any such dispute in the United States as well, so both in the United States and Europe, early filing is generally recommended. But one should still bear in mind that the earlier the filing, the earlier the expiry of the patent, and therefore, the earlier the arrival of generic competition.

The Japanese Patent Office (JPO) also handles far more patent applications than the EPO, but this is due to a procedural difference; the EPO grants only one patent for any given invention, while the same invention in Japan could be divided up between as many as 10 different patents, with every technological aspect of the invention filed independently.

There is a huge backlog of patent applications in both the United States and Japan, so that first action on a patent application in the United States and Japan takes a number of years compared to a year or so in Europe.

Patents are increasingly utilized on a global scale, so it is only logical that patent laws are in a slow process of harmonization around the world. Meeting the requirements of the World Trade Organization's (WTO) Trade-Related Aspects of Intellectual Property Rights (TRIPS) Agreement, which contains an aligned set of patent laws, is a prerequisite for a country to be admitted to the WTO.

8.9 PATENT ENFORCEMENT

As we stated earlier, a patent gives the patent holder the right to exclude others from practicing the invention. While a government awards a patent, it is up to the patent holder to enforce it. Patent enforcement is thus the process of legally maintaining the granted patent by taking action against persons considered to be infringing the patent.

A third party that manufactures, imports, uses, sells, or offers for sale patented technology, during the term of the patent and within the country that issued the patent, is said to be infringing the patent unless it has obtained the prior permission of the patent holder (e.g., by taking out a license).

Outside of the United States, when an inventor has plausible (prima facie) evidence that his patent is being infringed by a third party, the burden of proof that the patent is not being infringed lies with the infringer. There is thus a presumption of validity and therefore of infringement. This might be considered to be a reasonable approach, as the very granting of the patent in the first place has shown that, in the opinion of the patent office, the invention is worthy of a patent. In the United States, on the other hand, the patent holder has the burden of producing evidence of infringement and also bears the risk of nonpersuasion if the preponderance of the evidence weighs in favor of the alleged infringer.

When an inventor accuses a third party of infringement, the infringer will try to defend his action in one or more of several different ways:

- Deny practicing the patented invention, that is, claim that his actions lie outside the scope covered by the patent

- Claim that the patent is invalid, that is, that it should not have been granted because it did not meet the criteria discussed earlier in this chapter as being prerequisites for patentability
- Claim he was only practicing the invention in countries not covered by patents
- Claim that the patent has expired
- Claim that he has obtained a license to practice the invention

The first two are the most common causes of legal conflicts.

In general, the patent holder only has the option of opening a civil lawsuit against an infringer, although in some countries (e.g., Austria and France), criminal penalties can be imposed for willful infringement.

It is important to bear in mind that patent infringement only occurs if all of the claim's elements are practiced in the technology used by the infringer. If a single element is missing, then the patent has not been infringed with respect to that claim.

To determine whether it is possible to practice a technology without infringing an existing patent, it is necessary to carry out a "clearance search," which is also known as a "freedom-to-operate search." This will ascertain whether the technology infringes any of the claims of issued patents or pending patent applications. This search is normally carried out by specialized patent attorneys.

We mentioned earlier that it is possible to get national patents granted in most European countries based on one application to the EPO. However, it is important to remember that any multinational infringement cases would have to be duplicated in all of these countries, as the EPO patent effectively becomes a separate patent in each of the participating countries. It is perfectly possible to lose a case and have the patent invalidated in one European country while it is upheld in others.

If an infringer loses a patent case, he is liable to have to pay damages to the patent holder. These may take the form of compensating for lost profits or paying a royalty. The infringer is likely to have to pay most of the patent holder's attorney fees as well, though in the United States only if there was "willful infringement" of the patent.

8.10 TYPES OF PATENTS

There are three types of patent:

Utility Patent. This is the most common type of patent, and most of the patents that are of concern in the branded pharmaceutical industry are of this type. Utility patents cover new inventions, and last for 20 years, as already discussed.

Design Patent. Design patents cover the ornamental design of useful objects and may have some value in the protection of drug delivery devices in the United States, although the most important features are best protected by utility patents. Design patents only last for 14 years.

Plant Patent. This includes cultivating different types of plants to create mutants or hybrids and also newly found seedlings. In the United States, plant patents can be awarded to newly developed or discovered plants that are reproduced asexually. Plant patents last 20 years.

Let us have a closer look at utility patents. In the branded drug industry, they can cover a wide range of inventions, including drug compounds, their intermediates and metabolites, drug combinations, manufacturing methods, treatment and dosage regimens, formulations, delivery devices, biomarkers, diagnostic kits, and so on. There is a clear hierarchy of utility patents according to how much protection they are likely to provide for a pharmaceutical product. There are three main types of utility patent of interest to us here, and they are presented below in order of preference:

8.10.1 Composition of Matter Patent

This is the strongest type of utility patent. It claims an active drug compound, and usually variations thereof (e.g., salts, hydrates, esters). As with most patents, the narrower the claims, the more likely the patent is to be granted, and the more robust the patent is likely to be if challenged. For this reason, pharmaceutical companies often apply for at least two separate patents, one covering the specific compound that they intend to develop and one covering a broad range of similar compounds in an attempt to prevent competitors developing "me-too" drugs from the same compound family. In this way, they can be sure that no generic company can copy their product until the composition of matter patent expires, while also having a good chance of blocking competitors with similar compounds entering the market before exclusivity expires on their own brand.

The composition of matter patent—often called the "basic" or "primary" patent—is the strongest defense for a brand. This is because it stops any competitor from developing the same compound, whatever the process, indication, route of administration, or formulation.

The number of primary, composition of matter patents issued to protect new molecules is relatively small and declining. The vast majority of patents are secondary patents.

8.10.2 Medical Use Patent

This kind of secondary patent claims an indication for the drug compound, and can also be a strong defense for the brand. Medical use patents may not only cover the indications for which the drug is approved and sold, but can also cover nonapproved indications. But a medical use patent is generally not as strong as a composition of matter patent. In the absence of a composition of matter patent, a generic competitor may develop and market the same compound as is in the brand but is forbidden to label it or promote it for the protected indication, as this would be interpreted as active inducement by the generic company of physicians and patients to infringe the patent. However, nothing prevents physicians from prescribing the generic copy "off-label" for the patented indication, and it is difficult for the brand company to stop this unless it can prove that the generic company was actively encouraging the off-label use.

As cost containment measures in health care become ever more drastic, a brand company expecting courts to allow its brand to be sold at a high price in a patented indication when an identical generic is already available is likely to encounter increasing resistance.

8.10.3 Formulation Patent

This form of secondary patent claims a specific formulation in which the compound is delivered to the patient. The literature is full of examples of formulation patents protecting brand sales after expiry of the composition of matter patent on the active compound. Unfortunately, the vast majority of these examples are out of date, and they therefore do not reflect the situation today, let alone the situation as it is likely to develop in the future. To be effective as protection, a formulation patent must be broad enough to prevent a generic competitor from being able to develop an alternative formulation which allows them to meet the regulatory requirements for pharmaceutical equivalence and bioequivalence. If the generic company is unable to show bioequivalence without infringing the formulation patent, then it would have to conduct its own extensive clinical trials to gain regulatory approval of its formulation. But as we shall see later, the questions of whether or not a patent will be granted, and whether it will be broad enough to prevent generics getting to market on the basis of bioequivalence studies, is only one aspect of the factors that must be considered when deciding whether it is worth developing a new formulation for a brand approaching the end part of its patent life.

These, then, are the three main types of utility patent that are of interest to branded pharmaceutical companies. But many other things can be patented, and it is up to the ingenuity of the project/brand team and their patent attorney to decide which, if any, of these patents would be helpful in growing, maintaining, or protecting the brand.

8.11   KSR VERSUS TELEFLEX—RAISING THE NONOBVIOUSNESS BAR

A landmark legal ruling in the U.S. Supreme Court in April 2007 is likely to have a lasting effect on what constitutes nonobviousness in deciding whether a patent should be granted, and subsequently whether it is likely to stand up to generic challenge. It is therefore worth looking at the case in some detail.

Teleflex held the exclusive license to a patent on an electronic device that allows car drivers of different height to adjust the position of the car's accelerator and brake pedals to make them easier to reach. KSR also manufactured an adjustable pedal assembly, which it initially supplied only for cars with cable-actuated controls. As electronic controls grew more popular, KSR introduced an electronic pedal position sensor to their assembly, and Teleflex promptly filed a patent infringement lawsuit, asserting that KSR's new design came within the scope of their claims. KSR countered that Teleflex's patent was invalid, as a "person having ordinary skill in the art" would have found it obvious to combine an adjustable pedal assembly with an electronic sensor for it to be effective in an electronically controlled car.

The District Court ruled in favor of KSR, ruling that the nonobviousness criterion had not been fulfilled by the Teleflex patent. Teleflex appealed, and the U.S. Court of Appeals reversed the decision, finding in favor of Teleflex. The case was again escalated, this time to the U.S. Supreme Court, and the decision was once again reversed, this time definitively. The Supreme Court was of the opinion that granting patent protection to advances that would occur in the ordinary course of things anyway, and which do not involve any real innovation, retards progress, and may, in the case of patents combining previously known elements, deprive prior inventions of their value or utility.

In October 2007, as a result of this case, the USPTO published "Examination Guidelines for Determining Obviousness." The guidelines list seven rationales for declaring an invention to be obvious:

1. Combining prior art elements according to known methods to yield predictable results
2. Mere substitution of one known element for another to obtain predictable results
3. Use of known technique to improve similar products in the same way
4. Applying a known technique to a known product ready for improvement to yield predictable results
5. "Obvious to try"—choosing from a finite number of identified, predictable solutions, with a reasonable expectation of success
6. Known work in one field of endeavor may prompt variations of it for use in either the same field or a different one based on design incentives or other market forces if the variations would have been predictable to one of ordinary skill in the art
7. Some teaching, suggestion, or motivation in the prior art that would have led one of ordinary skill to modify the prior art reference or to combine prior art reference teachings to arrive at the claimed invention

If these rationales are applied consistently in the future, they will negatively impact several of the LCM strategies that companies have successfully practiced in the past. As an example, combining two antihypertensives in a fixed-dose combination to treat high blood pressure is unlikely to pass scrutiny under Rationale 1. And how will sustained-release formulations to turn twice-daily drugs into once-daily fare under Rationales 2 and 3? And is it even conceivable that "me-too" drugs may in future be deemed obvious? Several strategies have been proposed as a way around the consequences of the KSR versus Teleflex ruling. Here are two of them:

- Making the forum dealing with the invalidity issue aware, if possible, of an increased universe of options that were available, from which the invention was chosen, for example, identifying and pointing out a large number of alternative drugs that could have been used in a fixed-dose combination
- Arguing, where possible, that the prior art urged as a basis for invalidation in fact "teaches away from" the invention, for example, when the invention is a formulation that an earlier publication claimed or suggested would not work

The rulings in two case histories in this book relied heavily on the precedent set by KSR versus Teleflex, namely Famvir and The Yasmin Family. Readers interested in examining the implications of the KSR versus Teleflex ruling in more depth are encouraged to look up the following United States Federal Circuit cases: Crocs, Inc. v. US ITC (2010); DePuy Spine, Inc. v. Medtronic Sofamor Danek, Inc. (2009); Ecolab v. FMC Corp. (2009); Wyers v. Master Lock (2010).

8.12   PATENT STRATEGY

It should be evident from everything that we have written in this chapter that the overall patent strategy for a brand is one of the most important but also one of the most complex aspects of LCM. Each element of the patent strategy needs to fit exactly into the jigsaw puzzle of measures taken to protect the brand as securely and for as long as possible.

The first patent applications will have been made before the compound entered development. They will cover aspects like the compound class, the specific compound being developed (composition of matter patents), and possibly the process for manufacturing the NME itself and any key intermediates. The physical/chemical properties of the NME may also have been patented. The broad patent claiming as much of the substance class as possible will refer to a chemical structure with multiple functionally equivalent chemical entities allowed in one or more parts of the compound. It may thus include thousands, even millions of potential compounds, the vast majority of which have never been synthesized or tested and whose very existence may only be theoretical. Such claims—so called Markush claims—may not result in a patent being granted and may be very vulnerable to later challenge, but they can be narrowed down in the 18 months between filing and publication of the patent application. Companies take out a much narrower, and therefore stronger, patent on the compound(s) of the class that actually have been synthesized and tested. Companies with me-too compounds will be restricted to such narrower patents, and must ensure that their patents adequately cover their differentiators. One should never be too specific in these early patents about potential line extensions which could be introduced later in the life cycle, as this can create prior art which prevents later secondary patents which would extend beyond the expiry date of the composition of matter patent.

Once the drug has entered development, the next patent that may be considered is for protection of the initial formulation. Changes to the formulation during development should also be reviewed for patentability, especially where these changes lead to unexpected results regarding the way the molecule is stabilized, absorbed, or metabolized. Other aspects that should be considered include scale-up strategies, changes in the route of synthesis, treatment protocols, changes in dose, timing and mode of administration, and potential use in combination with other drugs.

Once the drug has entered clinical trials, additional opportunities for patent applications may emerge. Perhaps the drug has a unique and unexpected plasma concentration curve, or unexpected effects on the body that were not "obvious" based on the preclinical work. New patentable methodologies may be developed in the course of the clinical trials, such as biomarkers and companion diagnostics. Unexpected results where the drug is used with other therapies may emerge. Continuing work on the molecule back in research, including efforts to identify follow-up drugs, may uncover new, patentable forms of the molecule such as new crystalline forms, polymorphs, stereoisomers, prodrugs, or active metabolites.

After the drug has been launched and attention swings to indication expansion and improved formulations, new patent opportunities are likely to emerge. These could include new indications or new uses, new routes of administration, new formulation, combinations, and drug delivery devices.

The team managing the brand should never lose sight of what is being done with the molecule back in research or in manufacturing. For example, new routes of synthesis may produce a higher purity product and this route—or the key intermediates generated in this process—may be patentable. New excipients used in the formulation may have a positive effect on bioavailability and can also be patented if these effects were unexpected.

Generally speaking, the longer the product has existed and been studied, the less likely it is to find something new and patentable. But anything that is found can be of immense value. Never forget that the later something is found which protects the brand, and the later it is patented, the longer this additional protection will extend beyond the expiry of the composition of matter patent.

Finally, on September 16, 2011, President Obama signed into law the America Invents Act (AIA). It is too early to judge what effect this will have on the international patent landscape, and the reader is encouraged to acquaint himself with this legislation. What it does do is to move the United States closer to the "first-to-file" system used elsewhere in the world.

CHAPTER 9

Nonpatent Exclusivities

We have discussed patents, and how the protection provided by them can be extended by patent term restoration (in the United States), Supplementary Protection Certificates (in Europe), and patent term extension (in Japan).

There also exists a range on nonpatent exclusivities that can have a huge positive impact on the life cycle of a pharmaceutical brand, especially in cases where there is no composition of matter patent or where the remaining patent life of the brand is short.

9.1 NCE EXCLUSIVITY (UNITED STATES)

New Chemical Entity Exclusivity (also known as New Molecular Entity Exclusivity) was a provision of the Hatch–Waxman legislation. It states that the Food and Drug Administration (FDA) cannot accept any generic drug application (Abbreviated New Drug Application [ANDA] or 505(b)(2)) for the same drug until 5 years after the first approval date of the new molecular entity (NME). In other words, no generic company can submit an application which refers to the data generated by the innovator in the original New Drug application (NDA) during this 5-year period. An exception is made for drugs where there is still a patent listed in the Orange Book, that is, where the generic company is filing under Paragraph IV and thus challenging the validity of a patent. In this case, the FDA can accept a generic submission after only 4 years. The rationale here is that the ANDA applicant thus gains an additional year to litigate the patent if the innovator sues. As the FDA typically takes around 18 months to approve an ANDA, NME exclusivity in reality provides longer protection than the nominal 4 or 5 years.

However, it is important to realize that the protection provided relates to the data generated by the company that gained the first approval, and not to the composition of matter of the NME. A competitor could still perform a full

Pharmaceutical Lifecycle Management: Making the Most of Each and Every Brand, First Edition. Tony Ellery and Neal Hansen.
© 2012 John Wiley & Sons, Inc. Published 2012 by John Wiley & Sons, Inc.

development, generating its own data for the filing, and submit an NDA. In this case, NME exclusivity would not provide any protection, as the new NDA would present its own data rather than referring to that in the original NDA.

9.2 NEW CLINICAL STUDY EXCLUSIVITY (UNITED STATES)

This is also known as "new use exclusivity," "new formulation exclusivity," "label exclusivity," or "other significant change exclusivity," but the term New Clinical Study Exclusivity is a more accurate descriptor of what the extra exclusivity actually rewards. New Clinical Study Exclusivity was also a Hatch–Waxman provision.

This form of exclusivity is granted for changes in an approved drug product, including changes in indications, dosage strength, dosage form, route of administration, patient population or conditions of use, which require new clinical investigations that are essential to gain FDA approval. Bioavailability studies do not count as new clinical studies in this context.

New Clinical Study Exclusivity prevents the FDA from approving an ANDA or 505(b)(2) submission for 3 years from the date of FDA approval of the change. Again, it does not prevent approval of a new NDA. Note that NME exclusivity prevents submission of a generic during the exclusivity period while New Clinical Study Exclusivity only prevents approval of the generic. Thus, the extra exclusivity provided is in practice only 3 years or so. Note also that the protection only covers the new indication or the new formulation. The other indications and formulations are not protected.

9.3 DATA AND MARKETING EXCLUSIVITY (EUROPE)

Prior to 2003, data exclusivity in Europe was not handled in a uniform way. Legislation existing at that time stated that an NME would be awarded a minimum of 6 years exclusivity before a generic company could refer to the data in the original submission when filing for generic approval, and this period was extended to 10 years in the case of high-technology medicinal products. In practice, different countries interpreted this in different ways. For example, Germany, France, and the United Kingdom granted a 10-year period of data exclusivity, while Austria, Greece, and Spain allowed only 6 years.

This situation was harmonized in December 2003. The new legislation is popularly known as the "8 + 2 + 1" formula. According to this legislation, NMEs are entitled to 8 years of exclusivity during which time no generic manufacturer may refer to the innovator's data in making a submission ("data exclusivity"). At the end of the period, a generic submission can be made, but there is then a period of 2 years during which the generic drug may not be marketed ("market exclusivity"). An additional 1 year of protection is awarded if a new indication is submitted during the first 8 years. This extension can only

Category	United States	EU	Japan
NCE	5 years	8 + 2 years	8 years
New indication	3 years	1 year	4–6 years
New route of administration	3 years	None	4–6 years
New formulation	3 years	None	4–6 years

FIGURE 9.1. NME and line extension protection in the United States, EU, and Japan. *Source*: Ellery Pharma Consulting.

be granted for one new indication; additional new indications do not result in additional 1-year extensions.

9.4 DATA EXCLUSIVITY (JAPAN)

Data exclusivity in Japan lasts for 8 years in the case of an NME and 4–6 years in the case of a new indication, a new formulation, or a new route of administration.

If we compare the situations in the United States, Europe, and Japan, we can see that the European and Japanese protection is longer for NMEs. In Europe, protection lasts for 10 (8 + 2) years and in Japan, for 8 years, whereas in the United States, NME exclusivity lasts for only 5 years (plus ca. 18 months for the ANDA review). The United States (3 years) and particularly Japan (4–6 years) provide longer protection for new indications than does Europe (1 year). The situation is summarized in Figure 9.1.

9.5 ORPHAN DRUG EXCLUSIVITY

An orphan drug is one that has been developed specifically to treat a rare medical condition, a so-called orphan disease. Certain governments provide companies with incentives to invest the resources necessary to develop such drugs. The rationale is that without these incentives, companies would not invest in developing treatments for rare diseases because the return on their investment would be negative, and the diseases would remain untreatable. There are different forms of incentive, of which market exclusivity is just one. Governments also look favorably upon orphan drugs regarding pricing and reimbursement. The incentives vary by country, as does the period of exclusivity available.

In the United States, an orphan drug is granted 7 years of market exclusivity following its introduction to the market. During this time, the FDA is not allowed to grant approval for the same drug in the orphan indication to any other company, even if the drug is no longer protected by a patent. Two conditions must be met to gain orphan drug exclusivity:

1. The disease must be rare, defined as affecting less than 200,000 patients in the United States, which equates to 7.5 patients per 10,000 population
2. It must be the first drug to be approved for this indication

Apart from the market exclusivity, orphan drugs in the United States benefit from research grants, help with the design of development programs, FDA fee waivers, and tax incentives. Critics point out that some drugs have been developed for a whole series of orphan indications, which has made them extremely profitable for their innovators, thus defeating the declared purpose of orphan drug designation. Gleevec® is perhaps the best example of a company building a blockbuster based solely on orphan indications, and is the subject of a case history in this book.

Legislation in Europe is similar to that in the United States, the main difference being that in Europe, market exclusivity is provided for 10 years instead of 7. In Europe, too, there are additional incentives including protocol assistance in preparing the regulatory dossier, easier access to the Centralized Procedure for the application for marketing approval, reduced regulatory fees, and participation in European Union (EU) research funding grants. Europe defines an orphan disease as one occurring in less than 5 patients per 10,000 population.

Japan has also introduced orphan drug legislation; the period of exclusivity is 10 years and the required disease prevalence less than 4 patients per 10,000 population.

The brand industry is taking an increased interest in orphan drugs. Around one-third of the NMEs approved by the FDA between 2004 and 2008 were orphan drugs.

Novartis drugs Zometa®, Gleevec, Sandostatin®, and Exjade® were all launched initially with orphan status. Their combined estimated sales in 2011 were likely to exceed US$8 billion. In early 2010, GlaxoSmithKline (GSK) announced the launch of a unit specializing in orphan drug research and development. In December 2009, Pfizer signed a deal with the Israeli biopharmaceutical company Protalix BioTherapeutics to develop and commercialize a treatment for Gaucher's disease, a genetic metabolic disorder, and then in June 2010, Pfizer announced the creation of a new rare disease unit to "significantly expand" their portfolio of medicines for uncommon but lucrative-to-treat diseases; the division is intended to serve as an umbrella for rare disease programs that the company is already pursuing, including the treatment for Gaucher's disease, and also drugs for hemophilia and Ewing's sarcoma.

Deciding whether to market a drug initially for an orphan drug indication, which may not even be profitable on its own, and determining which follow-on indications should be considered and in which order, is one of the earliest strategies to be considered in the life cycle of a brand, immediately after the completion of proof-of-concept studies. Based on these decisions, the subsequent clinical development plan can be designed in such a way as to optimize the launch sequence of indications and maximize the commercial potential of the molecule. The more general question for any drug as to which indications should be targeted, and in which order, is discussed elsewhere in this book.

9.6 PEDIATRIC EXCLUSIVITY

Another extension that can be obtained in both the United States and Europe is called pediatric exclusivity. Let us look first at the situation in the United States, which was the first country to introduce the concept, back in 1997.

The FDA was very conscious of the fact that many drugs were not tested in children. Because pediatric studies can be difficult to conduct and the pediatric market is in any case usually small, most pharmaceutical companies decided it was easier not to study their drugs in children and simply to note on the package insert that there were no data to support pediatric use. This meant that pediatricians had a considerably reduced armory of drugs at their disposal compared to physicians who were treating adults. Furthermore, there were no data on the side effects of drugs on children were they to swallow their parents' medicines.

The FDA therefore decided to introduce an incentive to motivate pharmaceutical companies to conduct clinical trials in children for those active substances that the FDA considered could fill a public health need. Today, the Pediatric Research Equity Act (PREA) stipulates that all new drug or biologics licensing applications (BLAs) for a new active ingredient, indication, dosage form, dosing regimen, or route of administration must contain a pediatric assessment, unless the applicant has obtained either a waiver or a deferral of the assessment until after approval has been granted in adults. How many clinical data are required for an acceptable pediatric assessment will depend on the type of application, the available knowledge on the use of similar products in adult and pediatric populations, and the disease being treated. In some cases, the FDA may decide that the pediatric effectiveness can be extrapolated from clinical studies in adults, and may then only request pharmacokinetic studies. Under certain conditions, a company may be granted a deferral and agree to conducting pediatric trials later, particularly if the drug would be ready for use in adults before the pediatric trials could be completed, and in cases where additional efficacy or safety data need to be generated before the use in children can be considered. If no waiver is granted, the pediatric trials must be conducted according to a Pediatric Written Request (PWR) issued by the FDA. The pediatric development plan must be submitted prior to or at the time of the NDA submission. The scheme was and remains voluntary, and a company may decline the FDA request. If the request is accepted and the pediatric studies are conducted according to the PWR and submitted to the FDA, then the Pediatric Exclusivity provision allows companies to qualify for an additional 6 months of exclusivity which is added to all existing patents and exclusivity on all applications held by the company for that active substance.

The scheme also works the other way around. Companies can themselves ask the FDA to issue a PWR for their product, and this is indeed what frequently happens because the FDA incentive is considerable. After all, the Pediatric Exclusivity applies to all of the company's formulations, dosage forms, and indications for which the active substance is approved. Understandably, companies have become very inventive in discovering indications where they can justify to the FDA the conduct of pediatric trials.

Timing of these pediatric studies is everything, as they must be completed and submitted to the FDA at least 6 months before the expiration date of exclusivity or patent expiry, to allow time for the FDA review.

Generally speaking, products with no remaining patent life or exclusivity do not qualify, unless the supplemental application itself qualifies for a new exclusivity period according to the corresponding amendments to the Hatch–Waxman legislation. Thus, an application to extend an approved adult indication to children for a product with no patent life or exclusivity remaining could be awarded pediatric exclusivity if new clinical studies of safety and efficacy are required for approval.

The pediatric exclusivity legislation in Europe was introduced 10 years after the United States, in 2007. It is broadly similar to that in the United States, with 6 months additional exclusivity being added to the patent or the Supplementary Protection Certificate (SPC). However, there are important differences. Some of these differences make it difficult to design a clinical program which will satisfy both authorities.

The main differences are as follows:

- It is mandatory that a Pediatric Investigation Plan (PIP)—the EU equivalent of a PWR—be approved by the Pediatric Committee of the European Medicines Agency (EMA), or no marketing authorization in the EU will be granted. This rule applies to all NMEs or new indications for patent-protected drug products. It is much more difficult to obtain a waiver in Europe.

- The PIP must be created earlier in the development process, as it must have received a positive opinion prior to submission of the Marketing Authorization Application (MAA). The legislation requires that the PIP—or the application for waiver or deferral—be submitted not later than after completion of pharmacokinetic studies in man. Waivers may be granted for medicines intended to treat conditions that occur only in adults, and for medicines that may be unsafe or ineffective, or do not offer significant therapeutic benefit, and/or fulfill a therapeutic need in children.

- A PIP is required even if a company has no intention of applying for an indication for the use of the product in children.

- The European legislation requires that specific age-appropriate pediatric formulations or routes of administration be included in the PIP if necessary. This means that companies must not only invest in pediatric trials

prior to obtaining their first approval, but may also have to develop special pediatric dosage forms.
- The 6-month additional exclusivity can be extended to 1 year if the product demonstrates a pediatric benefit for an approved indication. Where pediatric trials for orphan drugs are conducted according to a PIP, 2 years of additional marketing exclusivity are granted.

In neither the United States nor Europe is it necessary for the pediatric trials to lead to a positive outcome to obtain 6-month exclusivity, whether this be a demonstration of efficacy in the pediatric population or the recognition of safety issues. Exclusivity is awarded for conducting the trials according to the requirements of the PWR or the approved PIP, and not for any particular result of those studies.

Pediatric exclusivity is thus often a business "no-brainer" both in the United States and in Europe because the additional 6 months of exclusivity will usually more than pay for the costs of the pediatric trials. And in both jurisdictions, funding grants may be possible to support the costs of the pediatric trials. In Europe, there is generally no choice in the matter anyway.

9.7   180-DAY GENERIC PRODUCT EXCLUSIVITY

There is one more form of nonpatent exclusivity, which is unique to the United States and which is also a component of the Hatch–Waxman legislation. In this case, the benefit of the exclusivity goes to the first filer of a generic product rather than to the innovator.

The rationale behind the 180-day exclusivity is, at first sight, a strange one. As we have already discussed, patents are designed by governments to reward innovation. The 180-day exclusivity is awarded by the FDA to generic companies who succeed in invalidating patents! Consistent with the declaration of the Hatch–Waxman legislation, the motivation for the creation of this type of exclusivity was to reduce drug costs and to stimulate innovation.

- Sometimes patents are granted incorrectly for innovations that did not really meet the required criteria, particularly where no innovative step was made. Generic companies are encouraged to uncover such mistakes.
- As a result, the more incentive there will be for innovators to create truly new products with robust composition-of-matter patents.
- The earlier a patent can be broken and generics enter the market, the earlier the brand sales erode and the greater the public savings.

It is still rather an odd way of encouraging innovation. Imagine a government encouraging you to put a better lock on your front door, and at the same time incentivizing third parties to try to break into your house despite the new lock. The argument would be, of course, that this would over time improve the quality of door locks, but it would be a bit hard on today's house owners.

So how does 180-day exclusivity work in practice? When an ANDA is filed, for a drug with patents listed in the Orange Book, an ANDA applicant is required to file one of the following Paragraph II, III, or IV Certifications. (Paragraph I Certification signifies that there is no patent listed in the Orange Book.)

- *Paragraph II*: That the patent has already expired.
- *Paragraph III*: That the generic will not be marketed until the patent has expired.
- *Paragraph IV*: That the patent is invalid or unenforceable, or will not be infringed by the manufacture, use, or sale of the drug described in the ANDA.

Filings with Paragraph II or III certification are straightforward and uncontroversial. It is in the case of Paragraph IV certification that the battle lines between the innovator and the generic company are going to be drawn. The innovator has a listed patent, and therefore has exclusivity and is not going to give up this and the resulting premium pricing of his brand without a fight. Following a filing with Paragraph IV Certification, the patent holder has 45 days to file a patent infringement lawsuit. If he does so, the FDA approval of the ANDA is automatically delayed for a period of 30 months. During these 30 months, the FDA is also prohibited from approving any other ANDA for the same drug. The purpose of the stay is to allow the parties to litigate the patent infringement claims while the ANDA filer pursues FDA approval of its generic drug. The stay may be lifted either at the end of 30 months, or when a court issues a nonappealable decision on the merits of the case, whichever comes first. The Hatch–Waxman legislation then provides a 180-day market exclusivity period for the first generic company to have filed the Paragraph IV Certification directed to that particular drug.

This 180-day period is of immense value to that first generic company because for 6 months, it will share a duopoly with the original brand. The price remains high in such a situation, and the generic company reaps enormous benefits for a relatively small investment. Once the 180 days have expired, generics flood the market—just as they would have done at patent expiry were there to have been no Paragraph IV Certification—and prices plunge.

The original legislation has been amended during the years since the Hatch–Waxman Act became law in 1984, especially to close certain loopholes that the brand companies were using to delay market entry of the generics.

■■■■■■ **CHAPTER 10**

Patent Settlements

One of the most controversial areas in the whole field of lifecycle management (LCM) is that of patent settlements, especially in the United States. To understand why, it is worth looking at the cost dynamics of a new molecular entity (NME) around basic patent expiry.

Before the patent expires, the branded drug company has a monopoly on the sales of the NME and can charge very high prices. Let us put a notional figure to what one unit of the NME costs the payer at this time—US$100. This is our baseline. Once the patent expires, in the absence of 180-day exclusivity, a number of generic companies will enter the market with exact copies of the NME. Although some of these companies will try to leverage additional advantages over their competitors (generic branding, deals involving other products, etc.), the primary basis for competition at this stage will be price. As generic companies have lower costs and accept lower profit margins than branded drug companies, they are capable of reducing the price of the NME considerably before the business becomes uninteresting for them. The higher the number of generic companies that are competing, the faster the price of the NME will drop and the lower it will plateau. In a matter of months or even weeks, one unit of the NME may now cost the payer only US$20, a saving to the payer of 80% compared to the prepatent expiry situation. The figure is in reality often even lower than this.

In the United States, where 180-day exclusivity has been granted to a generic company, the difference to the situation described above is one of degree rather than principle. In a duopoly situation, the generic company only has to reduce the price of the NME marginally compared to the original brand to get a share of the business. The cost of one unit of the NME may only drop, say, 30% to US$70, and again the payer benefits from the patent expiry.

Pharmaceutical Lifecycle Management: Making the Most of Each and Every Brand, First Edition.
Tony Ellery and Neal Hansen.
© 2012 John Wiley & Sons, Inc. Published 2012 by John Wiley & Sons, Inc.

From the perspective of the branded drug company, the biggest win that it can achieve is to prevent exclusivity of the NME being lost. The second-best result would be to move prescriptions to a line extension of the brand which is protected by patent or nonpatent exclusivity and maintain the high price. In theory—and increasingly in practice—this will only work as a business strategy if the additional value offered to the payer by the line extension is at least as big as the price differential to the generics of the original drug product. The added value can be quite small during the 180-day exclusivity period, but it has to be huge once this period has expired and generics flood the market. In practice, it is very difficult to achieve.

Let us now look at the situation of the different stakeholders—the branded drug company, the generic companies, and the payer—in one specific constellation, that of NME patent expiry in the United States with one generic company holding first-filer status and thus entitled to 180 days of exclusivity. (Often the presence of a so-called authorized generic will complicate the picture further, but we will ignore that for now and address it later in the book.)

The branded drug company has lost its monopoly. For 6 months it will share a duopoly with the first-filer generic company, and then generics from multiple companies will flood the market. The branded drug company cannot compete effectively on price, so it will maintain its high price and accept a loss of sales which may not be catastrophic in the first 6 months but certainly will be subsequently. The first-filer generic company will have six very profitable months— after all, this is why they took the risk and accepted the expense of challenging the Orange Book patent—and then they will be just one of a crowd of generic competitors, though all other things being equal, they will retain a higher market share because they entered the generic market first. The other generic companies will enter what is more or less a price-driven commodity market for the NME after the 180-day exclusivity has expired. And what about the third stakeholder, the payer? Costs for the NME will reduce somewhat during the first 6 months, and precipitously afterward. The bottom line is that the branded drug company has lost heavily, the generic companies won to a greater or lesser extent, and the payer has benefited. Let us complicate the situation a little further by pointing out that both the branded drug company and the generic company will have spent a lot of time and money on the patent litigation associated with the Paragraph IV filing.

Clearly, the branded drug industry would prefer to lose less, and the generic companies would like to win more! Realizing these goals is the whole basis for so-called pay-for-delay settlements. The underlying concept is very simple— keeping the unit price of the NME as high as possible—US$100 in our example—for as long as possible and redistributing postpatent the same level of profits that were made by the branded drug company alone prepatent expiry, ensuring that as little as possible of the benefit goes to the payer (see Figure 10.1).

A "pay-for-delay" settlement in the United States is thus an agreement between a branded drug company and a generic competitor, in which the

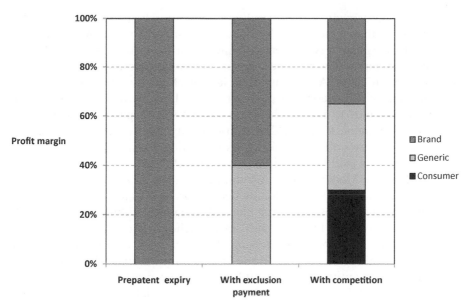

FIGURE 10.1. The loser when patent settlements are made is the payer/consumer as the drug price remains high. *Source*: Federal Trade Commission 2008.

brand company makes a payment to the generic competitor in return for the generic delaying its market entry, either by dropping its challenge of patent validity and not filing an Abbreviated New Drug Application (ANDA) in the first place, or by agreeing to delay its launch for a specific period of time. Following generic filing with Paragraph IV certification, this agreement enables the companies to avoid the costs and uncertain outcome of patent litigation, and to share in the profits of the high-price brand during the delay period. Such settlements are also known as "reverse payment" agreements. The reverse payment may take the form of a straight cash payment by the brand company to the first filer, or other noncash incentives such as the right to manufacture the brand product for the brand company, the right to launch a generic just before patent expiry, or the agreement of the brand company not to launch an authorized generic. Generally, the trend is away from direct cash payments, which attract the greatest criticism, toward other noncash incentives.

The legality of reverse payments is a current topic of heated debate, with no certainty as to what the final outcome will be. Interestingly, in the case of reverse payments, we see one of the rare situations where the interests of the branded drug industry and that of the generics industry coincide, at least for those generic companies that have made multiple first filings with Paragraph IV certification and therefore expect to profit from lucrative settlements with the brand companies. Industry argues that the practice is not anticompetitive, because the agreements usually result in competition being introduced to the market earlier than if the generic company were simply to wait until the patent expired. This argument is not very convincing for the critics, and one CEO of a brand company was very honest about the real motivation for such settlements back in 2006. According to a lawsuit filed by the Federal Trade Commission (FTC), Cephalon paid a total of US$200 million to different generic companies to induce them get them to drop patent challenges to Provigil®. Cephalon CEO Baldino subsequently boasted that these settlements kept generics off the market for six additional years and generated an additional unexpected US$4 billion in sales for Provigil.

The Medicare Modernization Act should limit the viability of the strategy in cases where an ANDA has already been approved, as it stipulates that the 180-day exclusivity is lost if the first filer fails to launch within 75 days of FDA approval (or expiry of the 30-month stay, whichever is earlier) or within 75 days of a court decision or settlement. But forfeiture has frequently been avoided by legal arguments even if the 75-day limit was exceeded. One might also expect that antitrust laws would prohibit the practice, but that is not always so as the following landmark case from 2005 demonstrates.

Schering-Plough held a patent on a microencapsulated extended-release potassium chloride supplement which it marketed in the United States as K-Dur 20®. It was protected by a patent listed in the Orange Book until 2006. In late 1995, Upsher Smith sought to introduce a generic of the product. Schering sued for patent infringement, resulting in litigation which was resolved in 1997 when the two companies signed a settlement agreement. Under the terms of this settlement, Schering agreed to let Upsher Smith market their generic from September 2001, while at the same time in-licensing several Upsher Smith development projects for US$60 million. The FTC complained that the in-licensing deal was just a front for paying Upsher Smith US$60 million to delay entry of their generic. The FTC's complaint went to court, and was alternately dismissed and approved until finally, in 2005, the Court of Appeals definitively dismissed FTC's complaint.

The latest developments regarding reverse payment settlements can be found on the FTC website. The ongoing battle between the FTC and Cephalon regarding Teva's generic of Provigil took a significant turn in May, 2011, when Teva announced it was acquiring Cephalon for US$6.6 billion. Several lawsuits also remain pending regarding a case where users of ciprofloxacin allege that a 1997 settlement between Bayer and Barr to end patent litigation concerning Bayer's Cipro® violated antitrust laws.

In May 2011, the FTC announced that it had found an "unprecedented" 60% jump in pay-for-delay deals during 2010. The deals covered 22 brand-name drug products with total annual U.S. sales of roughly $9.3 billion.

One can expect that this FTC report will be the starting point for more antitrust, antimonopoly actions, especially after President Obama had recently announced that his administration will seek to "cut spending on prescription drugs by using Medicare's purchasing power to drive greater efficiency and speed generic brands of medicine onto the market."

In the meantime, settlements continue to be made.

The reader is warned that much of this section of our book will likely have been overtaken by events before it is published. Here, more than anywhere else, the reader is advised not only to keep abreast of the current situation, but to base LCM strategies—which always take some time to implement—on how the environment is likely to develop during the time horizon of each LCM measure rather than on the situation today.

DEVELOPMENTAL LCM

CHAPTER 11

Strategic Principles of Developmental LCM

We now move into that part of the book that is concerned with developmental lifecycle management (LCM) measures, that is, those LCM activities which are led by development functions and which in most cases will require development resources and projects to realize.

It must be emphasized right at the outset that it is imperative to fully understand the fundamental drivers and resistors to successful implementation of each approach. All developmental LCM strategies seek to enhance a brand at its most basic level—its clinical profile. Critically, however, there are four fundamental principles that drive the likely success of any developmental strategy.

- The ability to provide a meaningful improvement in clinical profile
- The ability to increase the potential real-world patient base for the brand
- The ability to generate a return on investment (ROI) (as the costs of developmental LCM can be high)
- The ability to enhance the market exclusivity of the brand franchise through additional patent protection or regulatory exclusivities

The choice of developmental tactics, and the approach to implementation, is without a doubt the most influential driver of successful LCM. This is primarily due to these tactics tending to have the most significant impact, both positive and negative, on the lifetime profitability of the molecule. Additionally, this is where the greatest degree of risk is found—decisions and investments often need to be made many years ahead of tactic rollout, and they must therefore anticipate the changing therapeutic, regulatory, and competitive landscapes.

Let us now consider each of these fundamental principles in more detail and explore the factors that must be considered when planning for success.

Pharmaceutical Lifecycle Management: Making the Most of Each and Every Brand, First Edition.
Tony Ellery and Neal Hansen.
© 2012 John Wiley & Sons, Inc. Published 2012 by John Wiley & Sons, Inc.

11.1 DEVELOPMENTAL LCM GOAL 1: PROVIDE A MEANINGFUL IMPROVEMENT IN CLINICAL PROFILE

All developmental LCM measures are aimed at achieving some improvement in the clinical profile. When you invest significant funds into clinical trials, reformulations, and chemical modifications, you are expecting that the results will boost your overall offering to the market. The critical question, however, is whether the improvements provided really are meaningful to the relevant decision makers in these times of tight cost containment.

Take for example a scenario where you identify the opportunity for a new formulation of your brand (say a fast-melt tablet that ensures the patient does not need to take the tablet with water). How do you know if this will provide a meaningful improvement? As a first step, you need to consider the baseline dynamics of the indication. Such a formulation would likely be viable in two scenarios: first, where there may be a significant patient population where there is a difficulty in swallowing tablets (e.g., elderly patients, pediatrics), and second, where patients may need to take their medication at short notice, and thus may not be in a position to have a glass of water with which to take a standard tablet. Given these factors, pain indications would make viable options for such a formulation, with areas such as migraine and acute pain particularly attractive. However, if you were considering such a formulation for a daily antibiotic or an oncology drug, the value of the improvement might be negligible.

Beyond the base dynamics of the indication, the competitive landscape, both within the brand's own portfolio of indications and formulations and those of competitors, is also a critical shaping factor in determining the meaningfulness of any LCM improvement. For example, continuing with the hypothetical scenario described before, if the company developing the fast-melt tablet already has an oral solution formulation, the need for the new formulation might be significantly reduced. In this scenario, patients who simply struggle to swallow would already have a viable option, so the new fast-melt would have to target a different population. Again this could still be viable if the "on-the-move" population is big enough, or if patients were willing to pay out of pocket for the new convenient formulation, but the overall ROI for this smaller patient population is likely to be lower.

The third factor to consider in this situation is the role of different stakeholders in the decision-making process. If the new fast-melt formulation is a branded prescription drug operating in a generic world, the developing company would likely have to convince payers that the improvement provided by the new formulation is cost-effective compared with alternatives. In the world of the payer, the provision of an option for patients who cannot swallow is likely to be more viable than the "on-the-go" population, as meeting the needs of the former population could significantly improve compliance, while the latter could be seen as more of a convenience solution. If, by contrast, the new formulation would be sold as an over-the-counter (OTC) product in western markets, or indeed as a branded prescription drug in self-pay markets, the patient would have a much greater role in the decision-making process and thus, such an improvement could be seen as worthwhile and meaningful.

This played out with the success and failure of once weekly formulations in the United States within the depression and osteoporosis markets. On the successful side, Merck & Co. launched Fosamax® once-weekly for the treatment of postmenopausal osteoporosis in 2000/2001 in the United States and Europe, successfully taking more than 80% of the franchise within 2 years, and increasing the franchise growth rate in both the United States and Europe. At around the same time, Eli Lilly launched Prozac® once-weekly in the depression market, hoping to build on the success of the blockbuster Prozac franchise. However, this once-weekly failed to drive any significant market share and pretty much flopped on all accounts. So what accounted for the differential success between two very similar formulations launching at the same time in the same geographic markets to similar blockbuster brand franchises?

The reasoning behind the success and failure builds from several of the key points identified above. The first is the dynamics of the indication and patient profiles—for patients taking Fosamax once-daily, the inconvenience of having to take the drug first thing in the morning, standing up for between 30 min and 1 hour before food, was significant, particularly in moderate to severe osteoporotic patients where standing for this length of time alone can be challenging. By limiting the need to go through this process to once a week, the value of the new formulation was significant, enhancing patient compliance and therefore outcomes, in this case, fracture prevention. By contrast, there was no real issue with once-daily dosing for Prozac, and potentially a greater risk of poor compliance with the once-weekly formulation as patients could more easily forget to take their weekly tablet compared with a daily routine. The second factor influencing success will have been stakeholder behavior, in particular that of the payers. Fosamax once-weekly launched in the middle of the product life cycle, with at least 7 years of patent life remaining in the United States. As such, payers were not looking at generic alternatives at this stage, and by pricing the once-weekly at the same overall price per day as the once-daily version, the new formulation was rapidly adopted. By contrast, Prozac once-weekly launched less than a year before generic competition hit the market, and with no incentive versus the once-daily branded price, raising significant concerns with payers as to whether the additional expense of the branded once-weekly versus generic once-dailies would deliver any real value.

At the payer level, stakeholder influence on the real-world "value" of an LCM measure can be a significant barrier. However, playing to the needs of other nonclassic stakeholders can be hugely influential in driving the clinical meaningfulness of different LCM approaches. By recognizing the needs of the pharmacist, it is possible to devise a number of formulation and packaging strategies that can drive true differentiation. The introduction of split-resistant and "unbreakable" vials for difficult-to-handle compounds can drive significant value, as preventing the possibility of a toxic spillage in a hospital pharmacy has meaningful value. Similarly, the introduction of prefilled syringes that prevent both the need for reconstitution and the possibility of dosing errors can translate to real-world efficiencies and organizational cost savings.

The critical lesson to learn here is that without a deep understanding of the indication dynamics, competitive environment, and the interplay between stakeholders, evaluating the real-world meaning and value of LCM strategies will be fraught with uncertainty, and the risk profile of any investment will likely be raised.

11.2   DEVELOPMENTAL LCM GOAL 2: INCREASE THE POTENTIAL REAL-WORLD PATIENT POTENTIAL FOR THE BRAND

When assessing how much a potential tactic could increase the patient and sales potential of a brand, two critical questions need to be answered related to where these "new" sources of business will come from. For indication expansions, the key question is what proportion of the potential target patients will already be using the drug "off-label" and what the value of the label change to include the indication will really be. For formulation changes and combinations, the question is what proportion of the "newly" addressed patients are already being treated with another part of the brand franchise.

Let us look at the first of these questions—how much of the brand usage is off-label. Here it is critical to understand the fundamental driver of pre-scriber (and payer) behavior. What is needed to enable the brand to be used in a particular patient population? Does this use require an approved label, some clinical data, or just a consideration of class effect from competitor data? Regulator and payer behavior is increasingly pushing in both directions on this point. In some cases, for example, the antihypertensives, regulators are driving toward class labeling. This means that new entrants do not need to undertake clinical studies to gain the benefits of large-scale clinical trial results. Daiichi Sankyo's Benicar® is one drug that has significantly benefited from this approach, both from regulators and prescribers, driving widespread use across many different hypertension populations despite a limited overall clinical program when compared to its class predecessors. By contrast, in other indications where the general body of class-level data is lower, regulators and payers are looking to restrict off-label usage as much as possible, using programs such as Risk Evaluation and Mitigation Strategies (REMS) and prior authorization systems to ensure only patients that are deemed suitable gain access to the brand. To fully assess the potential expanded patient population that can really be accessed in practice with an indication expansion approach, it is critical to fully assess the factors that will shape uptake of a brand, both passively (off-label) and actively (on-label), and to base ROI calculations on appropriate data points.

When considering new formulations, combinations, and even generic strategies, it is critical to understand the extent to which expansion will be driven by intrafranchise cannibalization. As we touched on earlier, launching a fast-melt formulation of an oral tablet may provide an option for patients who struggle to swallow, but if you already have an oral solution available, it is likely that much of the growth of the new formulation would be cannibalistic to the existing brand franchise. For fixed-dose combination (FDC) therapies, the ability to expand the patient population will be driven by the current brand penetration of the target population. For this, let us consider three hypothetical scenarios:

In scenario 1, the brand in question, Brand A, targets the treatment of an underlying disease. Molecule B is used to treat side effects associated with treatment with Brand A. An FDC combination of A + B would be almost entirely cannibalistic to Brand A, with the only hope for expansion being if the convenience of the FDC (single pill, with side effects managed) were to be more attractive versus other potential competitors to Brand A.

In scenario 2, Brand A targets the treatment of side effects associated with a number of different agents, including Brand B (or, more probably, the generic of Brand B, Molecule B), which itself is a market leader. In this case, an FDC of A + B will almost certainly be additive for Brand A, as the focus of the FDC will be to cannibalize the market for Molecule B, in which Brand A is likely to only be partly represented.

In scenario 3, Brand A targets the treatment of an underlying disease, but the addition of Molecule B enables the drug to target a patient population not currently addressed by Brand A (e.g., a low-dose combination of the two drugs targeted to a prevention indication). Here the combination will again be additive, especially if it is not possible for the FDC to be easily replicated by a free combination.

In the case of a generic strategy, the key question of value is whether a company launching its own generic (either directly, authorized, or licensed) will increase the degree of brand erosion felt by the parent drug, or whether it will cannibalize rival generics. The balance required to successfully put a generic strategy into action is to minimize additional erosion (beyond what would happen with competitor generics anyway) while maximizing the market share of one's own generic. In some countries, for example, launching one's own generic first (even by a matter of weeks) is sufficient to drive a first-to-market generic leadership position that is maintained in terms of market share even after the launch of rivals. In this environment, the trade-off between a few weeks of additional erosion and the long-standing generic market share benefit can have a net positive effect. By contrast in the United States, decision making that relates almost entirely to price means that such generic first-to-market advantages rarely extend beyond the competitor launch (i.e., there is no loyalty to the first generic), so launching one's own generic ahead of rivals will likely only result in greater brand erosion with no upside. This latter point explains why most authorized generics in the United States only ever launch once a rival has been approved and not before.

Accurately judging the balance between expansion and cannibalization is critical to assessing ROI. Far too often, companies are blind to the source of business for their new LCM launches, getting a nasty surprise after the event when the numbers are examined in detail. Indeed this problem can become multiplied when planning an integrated LCM strategy if tactics are reviewed in isolation. If multiple tactics, approved in isolation, end up targeting the same population (e.g., multiple FDCs or formulations), then the net result will almost certainly be a drop in the effective value of the combined portfolio compared with calculated forecasts.

11.3 DEVELOPMENTAL LCM GOAL 3: THE ABILITY TO GENERATE AN ROI

The third goal of developmental LCM might seem a little trite—of course the company is looking to make an ROI. But in many cases, decision-making behaviors do not seem to follow a logical flow. Critically, there are three factors to consider here. These are when to invest, when to stop, and how to seek alternatives that might give a better ROI.

The decision to invest in potentially large-scale clinical programs to support an LCM measure can be a difficult one. How can one justify additional spending for a brand that might not even have launched yet? The key question, however, is how does the timing of that decision impact the outcome. Take for example the decision to invest in a new indication. If the clinical program will take 5 years to deliver, and the overall brand has 10 years of basic patent life, the timing of that investment is critical. If the company chooses to initiate the new program at risk, 2 years before initial approval, the new indication would deliver in year 3, giving 7 years to gain a full return. By contrast, if the company puts the plan on hold until they know the brand is successful, say 2 years after launch, the new indication will only deliver in year 7, giving only 3 years of patent life in which to gain the full benefit of the new indication. While the latter approach is not necessarily wrong, and in many cases might be absolutely correct, the ROI implications of that delay must be fully assessed.

The second decision—when to stop—is a much harder one to accept. At what point should one decide to stop an LCM development project because the market or competitive—or legal—environment has changed to such an extent that the LCM measure will no longer drive value? When must one accept that the ROI is actually better if the program is canceled, and that it is preferable to accept the losses to date rather than investing even more resources into a lost cause? In too many cases, brand companies blunder on with out-of-date LCM programs that they hope will deliver what they forecast in the original business plan 5 years previously. Keeping track of the market and competitive environment, and relating any changes to assumptions made when an original "Go" decision was made, is critical to ensure the ROI can still be realized (or even enhanced). Good LCM is a cyclical process of ideation and rechallenge, and this is essential to ensure investments are always targeted to their best opportunity for ROI.

The final decision is how to seek alternative tactics that could generate a greater ROI. Let us go back to our example of the fast-melt formulation providing an option for the "on-the-move" patient population that requires acute treatment, but does not always have a glass of water handy to take a normal tablet. If we play out the scenario where an oral solution already exists for the patients who struggle to swallow, a lower cost, higher ROI option might be to develop a single-dose packaging option for the oral solution that can be easily transported and used "on-the-go." This option would likely be quicker to market, cheaper to develop, and lower risk than the new fast-melt.

The final factor to consider when assessing the ability to generate ROI is what the company itself does outside of the pure development of the new formulation or new indication to drive success. Even today, far too many brand companies isolate their LCM projects from the normal brand development activities, only integrating the LCM project when it "delivers," as little as six months before approval. What the branded drug industry struggles with is the market shaping that in many cases is essential to prime the market for the success of the LCM measure. If a new formulation requires the market to accept a new patient stratification approach to be successful, it may take time to develop this in the mind of stakeholders, and it is not always viable for this process to only begin when the new formulation is launched. Understanding the overall story flow required for the full LCM plan to succeed is important in guiding the overall market-shaping platform for the brand franchise, and without this, ROI is likely to never be optimized.

11.4 DEVELOPMENTAL LCM GOAL 4: THE ABILITY TO ENHANCE MARKET EXCLUSIVITY OF THE BRAND FRANCHISE

The fourth goal of developmental LCM is to enhance the market exclusivity of the brand franchise either through patent protection or extended market exclusivities. As these were dealt with extensively in Chapters 8 and 9, we will not labor on these points here, only to highlight the importance of timing regarding potential implications for protectability of different LCM measures. As the regulatory environment evolves, so do the requirements that must be fulfilled to gain the market exclusivities so cherished by brand companies. For example, while pediatric exclusivity in the United States used to be a key target for mid-stage LCM, in most cases, new drugs must already have a pediatric plan in place for Europe even before launch, pushing activities focused on gaining these exclusivities much earlier in the product life cycle.

Similarly, timing can play a key role in potential market exclusivities for new formulation and FDCs in the United States. With 3 years of market exclusivity for a new formulation or combination possible, timing the approval can be critical if launch is likely to be late in the product life cycle. It can be challenging to get the timing right. On the one hand, there must be enough time before patent expiry to drive uptake. And on the other hand, one is looking to extend for as long as possible the additional period of market exclusivity that the new formulation will enjoy after basic patent expiry. This is obviously more important if the goal of the new formulation is to target patients currently on the main brand (i.e., a switch strategy). In this situation, the more patients that can be switched to the newer protected formulation, the more protection from direct generic competition there will be. However, pushing the launch too late will likely ensure the new form falls foul of the payers, as any attempt to significantly switch patients in the final 6 months before patent expiry will likely see strong resistance from payers!

CHAPTER 12

Indication Expansion and Sequencing

Indication expansion is one of the most effective lifecycle management (LCM) measures of them all when implemented in the early or mid-life cycle. If multiple indications are an option for a new molecular entity (NME), then how to sequence those indications is a crucial aspect of the LCM strategy for the molecule.

Some molecules are very specific in their actions and are only suitable for treating one disease state. As an example, methimazole inhibits the synthesis of thyroid hormones and is thus effective only in the treatment of hyperthyroidism.

Where different diseases share the same mechanism of action, however, some molecules may hold potential for approval in several different indications. Particularly, biologics have proven efficacious in multiple disease states because their targets are associated with different diseases. As an example, Centocor's TNF-blocker Remicade® is currently indicated in the United States for the treatment of psoriasis, rheumatoid arthritis, ankylosing spondylitis, Crohn's disease, and ulcerative colitis. Expanding the number of indications for which a drug is approved is one of the most effective ways of increasing brand sales and profits. The degree to which the new indication differs from the previous one will often determine how much upside the extension will provide. From this perspective, one can consider several different categories of indication extension.

12.1 CATEGORIES OF INDICATION EXPANSION

Same Physician, Same Disease. An example would be when a drug is shown to be safe and effective in combination with another drug used to treat the same disease, resulting in a broadening of the indication to cover combination usage. Combining a new molecule with a current gold

Pharmaceutical Lifecycle Management: Making the Most of Each and Every Brand, First Edition.
Tony Ellery and Neal Hansen.
© 2012 John Wiley & Sons, Inc. Published 2012 by John Wiley & Sons, Inc.

standard therapy in a fixed-dose combination may enable the new molecule to move up the treatment hierarchy and thus gain wider usage in the same target population.

Same Physician, Different Disease. This category of indication expansion is often seen with cancer drugs. A good example is Roche's Avastin® which is approved, singly or in combination, for the treatment of colorectal and lung cancer, as well as for glioblastoma and for breast cancer in Europe.

Different Physician, Same Disease. Gaining a pediatric indication puts the drug into the hands of pediatricians treating a disease for which the drug was previously only indicated in adults. As an example, Nexium® gained the pediatric indication of short-term treatment of gastroesophageal reflux disease (GERD) in mid-2009.

Different Physician, Different Disease. This was the case for Lipitor® in 2004. Up until then it was indicated only for reducing serum cholesterol and triglyceride levels, but in 2004 it gained the indication of reducing the risk of stroke and myocardial infarction in patients with Type-2 diabetes. This increased usage of the drug by diabetologists.

Novartis's bisphosphonate, zoledronate, was approved for hypercalcemia of malignancy in 2001 under the brand name of Zometa®, and a year later the indication was extended to multiple myeloma and metastases of solid tumors. This was a "Same physician, different disease" scenario as the drug remained in the hands of oncologists. But in 2007, zoledronate was approved under a new brand name, Reclast®/Aclasta®, for the treatment of Paget's disease and then for osteoporosis in postmenopausal women. This put it into the hands of gynecologists (this story is covered in more detail in Case History 32).

All other things being equal (price, size of indication, competitive position, etc.), expanding into a different medical specialty and a different patient pool is obviously going to increase the potential of a brand more than when a new indication is given to the same medical specialty or when two different medical specialties could prescribe the same drug for one individual patient.

The benefit of obtaining a new indication will generally be highest if it is achieved early in the life cycle. As clinical development for a new indication can take several years, the highest peak sales are likely to be obtained if the clinical trials for the second indication are started even before the lead indication has been approved. There are, of course, considerable risks associated with such an aggressive approach:

- Failure to demonstrate efficacy in the lead indication, which may or may not mean that development of the molecule is stopped for other indications too
- Failure to demonstrate safety in the lead indication, which is more likely to cause development of the molecule to be stopped for other indications too

- Failure to demonstrate cost-effectiveness in the first indication, which may or may not be a problem for other indications
- Failure to select the right dosage for the lead indication, which will often mean going back to dose-finding studies for other indications too
- Failure to achieve commercial targets with the lead indication, which may or may not throw into doubt the business cases for other indications

As we can see, any of these failure modes are likely to impact the chances of scientific and/or commercial success with the follow-on indication, although none of them necessarily has to be fatal. The decision as to whether to parallel develop more than one indication right from the start will be determined by a variety of factors, including:

- Estimated chance of scientific success (strength of rationale and/or track record of mechanism of action; availability of proof-of-concept results in indication or related indication; robustness of dose selection; safety signals during preclinical testing; rationale for dose selected, etc.)
- Estimated chance of commercial success (size of unmet need; patent expiry date of current gold standard; competitor pipelines; feasibility of target pricing; likely reimbursement status, depth of knowledge regarding targeted market, etc.)
- Availability of adequate funds (other pipeline requirements; company priority of targeted indication; willingness and ability to codevelop with a partner, etc.)

Large companies are more likely to parallel develop multiple indications from the start, while smaller players may have to limit themselves to one indication until this has been approved and launched, firstly because they cannot afford to take the risk of parallel development and secondly because they need the profits generated by the lead indication to finance the clinical trials for the follow-on indication. Parallel development may still be feasible for such companies if they cooperate with another company as development partner. Where resources are limited, it may be good practice to at least ensure all the proof-of-concept studies have been completed in the indications that could be targeted by the drug. This does not cost a lot of money, but it does mean that the drug will get to market faster in the follow-on indications if the development programs are approved at a later date. For a small company, a series of positive proof-of-concept trials will also increase the level of interest in the molecule among potential development partners and buyers.

In the future, the decision as to whether a follow-on indication is parallel developed or not will be influenced more and more by regulatory authorities and payers. Regulatory authorities will increasingly want to see efficacy proven and safety databases built up in high unmet need patient populations with a potentially very favorable risk–benefit ratio before allowing the drug to be used in broader populations with less need of the drug, either because their disease is milder or because other therapeutic options are already available on the market.

Although it is generally preferable to gain as many indications as possible as early as possible in the patented life of the molecule, there can be benefits of waiting until later in the life cycle, in terms of giving additional messages and materials for a sales force to promote, or providing differentiation from other class competitors. Either way, it must be remembered that developing a new indication takes a long time, and that trials must therefore be started early on in the brand life cycle even if the new indication is intended as a late-stage lifecycle management (LLCM) strategy.

Taken on its own, a new indication will do little to defend brand sales after patent expiry. Even if the new indication is patented or—in the United States—protected by 3 years of label exclusivity—there is no mechanism to stop physicians prescribing the generic or pharmacies dispensing it off-label to patients with the protected indication. The fact that the generic is not permitted to include the new indication on its label does not constitute an effective defense. Obviously, the risks to the patient are nonexistent, as the generic has already proven itself to be bioequivalent to the original brand. However, the generic company is not allowed to promote the new indication.

To be effective as part of an LLCM program, a new indication strategy must be combined with other strategies. For example, if the patented new indication is treated by a different formulation given by a different route of administration, then this can prove effective as brand defense. In these circumstances, the generic company will not be permitted to market a bioequivalent formulation suitable for the new route of administration, as this would be tantamount to infringing the indication patent. The protection is stronger if additional patents protect the new formulation and the route of administration.

A new formulation for a new indication will only be an effective LLCM measure if the formulation is patented and bioequivalence cannot be attained without infringing the patent. In other words, the fact that the indication is patented would not materially strengthen the defense because, once again, the generic would merely be prescribed off-label.

If the brand company goes to the trouble of repeating dose finding for the new indication, and can show that a different dosage is necessary for the patented new indication, this could constitute an effective defense because only the originator would be permitted to market the drug at this new dosage. A generic company offering the new dosage strengths would effectively be infringing the patent. Obviously, this strategy only really works if the new dosage cannot be replicated by using more than one tablet of the generic, or by easily dividing a generic tablet. For example if a generic is available for a 50-mg dosage, and the new indication requires a new 20-mg dosage of the brand, this would be effectively protected, as it would not be possible to replicate the dosing with the generic. By contrast, if the new indication required 150-mg dosing, then a physician could simply use three of the original generic tablets instead off-label in the new indication.

Primary patents | Secondary patents

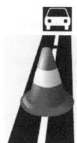 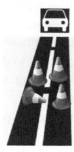

"You can block the whole road with a primary patent, but if you are relying on secondary patents, you may need several."

FIGURE 12.1. Patents as roadblocks. *Source*: Ellery Pharma Consulting.

The greater the number of individual elements that can be combined, the stronger the defense will be. A patented new indication treated by a patented new formulation delivered by a patented route of administration at a different dosage and in a different dosage regimen would be very hard for generics to attack.

In practice, it is sometimes useful to think of patents as roadblocks, blocking a generic company's path to your brand. As shown in Figure 12.1, a strong and accurately placed composition of matter patent is virtually impossible to get past. If you have to rely on secondary patents, such as indications, formulations, and dosage strengths, it is most effective to combine several different ones in your strategy as no single one can be relied upon to completely block the road.

We have looked at the relationship between lead- and follow-on indications, but what factors are involved in deciding which indications to pursue, and in which order? First, here are some of the factors that must be considered in determining which indications should be pursued:

- Likelihood that molecule will prove to be safe and effective in candidate indication (mechanism of action; preclinical safety; proof-of-concept trial results in same or related target population; efficacy/safety of marketed competitors in the same class)
- Size and cost of clinical trial program necessary to obtain regulatory approval, target price, and reimbursement
- Size of target patient population
- Growth rate of target population
- Demographics of indication (age incidence/prevalence; situation in mature and emerging markets)

- Degree of unmet need in target population; strengths and weaknesses of competitor offerings (current and expected future)
- Availability of biomarkers to identify to-treat and not-to-treat subindications/subpopulations
- Need for and capability to develop companion diagnostics
- Pros and cons of selecting an orphan indication as lead
- Competitive intensity
- Price and reimbursement policies, practices, and benchmarks in target population
- Patent expiry dates of competing products

A comprehensive indication expansion strategy will not only look at which indications it is possible and attractive to develop, but also at the best constellation of indications and the optimal sequence and timing for feeding them into the market. Here are some of the factors that need consideration.

Timelines. How long will it take to complete the clinical trials necessary to obtain regulatory approval, pricing, and reimbursement? How long will it take to reach peak sales after market introduction? The order in which clinical trials are started for different indications will not necessarily determine the launch sequence.

Regulatory Hurdles. If there is a high level of unmet need in the lead indication, then the motivation for regulatory authorities to approve the drug quickly is likely to be higher. However, the regulatory pathway (studies required, clinical end points, etc.) will be better defined in an indication where there are already similar drugs on the market. These two considerations are obviously contradictory, and it is essential that the company seek early discussions with health authorities to understand the path to market and the attendant risks and potential derailers, especially in the case of novel regulatory pathways. Regulatory approval for follow-on indications will generally be facilitated if the drug is already on the market.

Pricing and Reimbursement. It will be considerably easier to obtain premium pricing and reimbursement if the lead-indication target population is small and has a high level of unmet need. It may prove possible later to maintain at least part of the price premium when the drug is approved for use in indications with a larger target population, but this is getting more difficult to achieve unless a new dosage form or formulation can be used to clearly distinguish the new indication from the existing market. Conversely, it will be almost impossible to obtain premium pricing for a high-unmet need niche follow-on indication if the drug is already marketed in a mass indication at an (inevitably) lower price.

Potential for Side Effects in Target Population. Although a high-unmet need patient population can be attractive as the lead indication, and a higher level of side effects is likely to be acceptable, this strategy could prove unfavorable if it means treating patients who are more likely to develop side effects, for example, very sick patients. It will be necessary to include all of the information on side effects in the label, and this could discourage the later use of the drug in follow-on indications where the patients are less sick and are less willing to accept such side effects.

Safety Database for Health Authorities. As health authorities become ever more conservative and demand ever larger safety databases for new products, it may make sense to introduce the drug first in a high-unmet need population that the health authorities are more willing to accept, and generate sufficient safety data in these patients to support later submissions for indications in broader populations. This may make more commercial sense than building the safety database in the broader population before the first submission and missing out on sales while doing so.

Patent and Market Exclusivity. Gaining first approval in a niche indication and adding on mass-market indications later may make sense from the pricing, regulatory, and safety perspectives, but never forget that the patent clock is ticking and that data and market exclusivities are triggered by the first approval for the lead indication. You will not want to leave your new brand in a niche for longer than you have to if there is potential to address larger patient populations (as long as prices hold up).

Brand Name(s). Brand companies may decide to launch the drug approved for a follow-on indication as a separate brand. However, the market positioning needs to be clear, especially in a large portfolio where multiple brands exist (brand, generic, OTC). Strong differentiation is critical for establishing clear brand value in the eyes of all stakeholders.

Off-Label Use. After the drug has been approved, it is essential to monitor its use off-label, for example, where investigator-initiated trials (IITs) have proposed its use in additional indications. If use in an off-label indication is extensive, and payers are reimbursing that usage, there may be no financial rationale for conducting the controlled clinical trials necessary to get the indication onto the label.

There are thus many factors involved in determining the best sequence for developing the lead and follow-on indications. Mistakes can be very costly!

Figure 12.2 provides a helpful overview of the various questions a company should be asking when it is planning its indication expansion strategy and selecting its lead and follow-on indications, and their sequencing.

In many cases, the indication expansion strategy must be adapted during the life cycle of the drug, as new indications may emerge from use in the

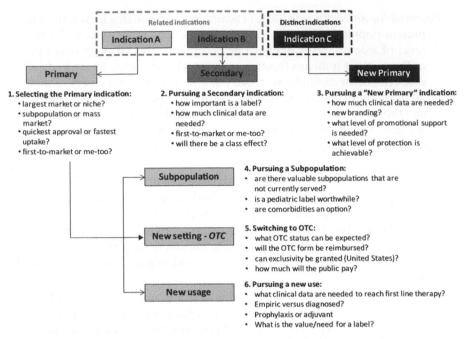

FIGURE 12.2. Multiple options exist for indication expansion.

labeled or off-label indications. Thus, although the first draft of the indication expansion strategy must be defined very early in the brand life cycle—ideally already at the time when proof-of-concept studies have been completed and the lead indication decided—it will have to be adapted as new efficacy and safety data are generated regarding the drug, and as the competitive and regulatory/reimbursement environment evolves.

CHAPTER 13

Patient Subpopulations and Personalized Medicine

In some ways the previous chapter described a happy position for a brand to find itself in. It is established in one indication, and the question is how best to expand into additional diseases. Life is not always that kind to brands. While expansion is the goal of many indication management exercises, what happens when a brand is struggling to compete even within its own indication? What happens if the clinical results coming from your traditional indication selection approaches are giving results that are far from desirable, and that will not support your desired market access strategy? Under these circumstances, there are a number of potential reasons for the "failures." It could simply be that your drug is not as good as the competition across all patients, and that you need to adopt a strategy that challenges the competition on factors outside of the pure clinical profile (presentation, price, services, etc.). Alternatively, it may be the case that your drug is better than the competition in specific patient populations, and that it is the poor performance in other patient populations that bring the results of the pooled population down to a less attractive net result.

The concept of personalized medicine comes from the perspective that if a drug can be used as a first- or second-line therapy in a fraction of the total target population, this will still be better in the long run than free access to all patients, but only ever being used in fifth-, sixth-, or seventh-line therapy (see Figure 13.1). As well as potentially increasing the number of patients that really do use the brand, the patients that are treated are likely to be more responsive to therapy, have fewer complications, slower disease progression, and therefore, potentially longer sustainability of therapy.

The role of personalized medicine in lifecycle management (LCM) stems from the observation that the vast majority of past development projects have not from the start targeted those patients most likely to benefit from the new therapy. Instead, these responders have been identified along the way and

Pharmaceutical Lifecycle Management: Making the Most of Each and Every Brand, First Edition. Tony Ellery and Neal Hansen.
© 2012 John Wiley & Sons, Inc. Published 2012 by John Wiley & Sons, Inc.

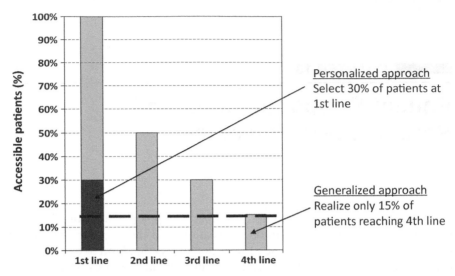

FIGURE 13.1. Increasing the accessible population through personalized medicine. *Source*: Datamonitor.

exploited late on to drive brand value. It is helpful to differentiate between two fundamentally different approaches to patient selection, depending upon whether the strategic intent of the company owning the brand or the patient selection approach is in the foreground (see Figure 13.2). In today's world, we are only just seeing the first truly designed personalized approaches, where the selection process (e.g., a biomarker) is built into the original drug-design process. An example would be a drug designed specifically for cancer patients with a particular genotype. This approach will increase in the future, but for now patient selection is typically either by default (i.e., the company has not done anything to influence the selection, and the selection has been guided by the actions of others) or learned (i.e., the company has discovered positive links between certain selection criteria and either positive or negative characteristics of therapy and has acted accordingly). It is becoming increasingly important for companies to incorporate processes designed to "learn" appropriate patient selection either into their clinical programs, or into market monitoring, to ensure that they do not end up in a default position based on the actions of others (competitors or payers).

In terms of patient selection approaches, five selection processes can be identified:

1. *Generalized.* Physicians can, and do, use the drug in any patient they deem appropriate within the scope of the indication. In today's world, a true generalized patient selection status is likely to be reserved for generic drugs and branded agents in areas with very high unmet needs

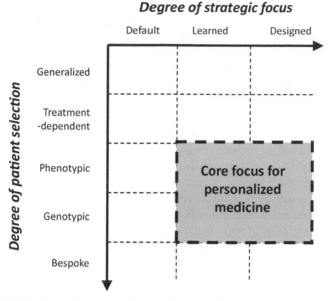

FIGURE 13.2. Patient selection and strategic focus in personalized medicine. *Source*: Datamonitor.

2. *Treatment Dependent.* This is the most common form of patient selection, driven by line of therapy, that is, a physician will only use the drug after a patient has "failed" on other lines of therapy. This is still a viable option in many indications where relatively few therapeutic options exist and so a new patient might gain access to a drug after only a few other lines of therapy have been tried, but for many other indications, the restrictive nature of the treatment-dependent patient selection has driven companies to opt for a more active patient selection process.

3. *Phenotypic Selection.* This is a mainstay of today's active patient selection process, where a specific marker for success with a target drug is used to aid patient selection. Many different marker systems can be used to drive patient selection, from demographics (age, sex, etc.) to diagnostic questionnaires (e.g., FRAX® for osteoporosis) to symptomatic selection (e.g., exacerbates for asthma/chronic obstructive pulmonary disease [COPD] therapy) and specific biomarkers. The critical goal here is for the generalized patient population to undergo the selection procedure before therapy is initiated and the selection of the most appropriate therapy to follow the results.

4. *Genotypic Selection.* Genotypic selection follows two potential approaches, one already a reality, and the other a consideration for the future. At present, genotypic selection is focused on the identification of genetic markers present in tumor cells to aid the selection of appropriate cancer

therapy. By understanding the interplay between tumor genetics and therapeutic response, appropriate therapies (both in terms of efficacy and lack of side effects) can be identified early in the treatment paradigm. While this form of genotypic selection is increasingly common today, in the future, the potential for therapy selection based on the patient's genotype is something that is raising interest (both positive and negative) from a number of parties. The concept that a patient's genotype, alongside the disease history, will determine the response to a medicine is a concept that is relatively simple to visualize, but increasingly difficult to realize. As the forthcoming section on selectivity and specificity of selection criteria will highlight, unless the link between genotype and response is very strong, the concept of limiting access to a patient based on a genetic test will be difficult for many to swallow (except the insurance companies)!

5. *Bespoke Selection.* The final selection category is the truly bespoke therapy, where each patient receives a truly customized drug, tailored to his own specific disease. This concept became a reality with Provenge® from Denreon, a patient-specific therapeutic vaccine for the treatment of advanced prostate cancer. This vaccine uses the patient's own immune cells as a critical active agent in treating the disease, so each treatment regimen is truly bespoke to the patient from which the cells were harvested.

From a patient selection perspective, the real interest for LCM comes from the phenotypic and genotypic approaches, as these can be applied during the product life cycle to drive improved brand value.

The drive for patient-selective approaches to indication management is coming as much from the regulatory and payer environments as it is from advances in understanding the molecular mechanisms of drug action.

- *Regulators*: Their focus is on safety and concerns over adverse events. This has led to a requirement for massive studies if broad patient populations are being targeted, and this drives companies to more selective indication strategies, using risk evaluation and mitigation strategy (REMS) programs to limit initial access as needed.
- *Payers*: The increasing availability of generics makes it more difficult to find convincing arguments for generalized use of branded therapies. Convincing arguments have to be based on identifying two groups of patients, those least likely to succeed with existing standards of care—and thus by default who are more likely to benefit from a new approach—and those most likely to respond well to new therapies. This creates a divergence in strategic goals for drug companies and for payers in patient selection. The payers want to identify which patients they should not use generic drugs in (negative selection for new brands), while drug companies want to identify which patients their brands should be used in (positive selection for new brands).

• *Advances in Science*: Today's greater understanding of the molecular mechanisms underlying diseases enables selection of therapy on the basis of specific responsiveness to a target that may not be fully represented in a heterogeneous patient population.

13.1 WHAT DOES A GOOD PATIENT SELECTION STRATEGY LOOK LIKE?

Executing a successful patient selection strategy can work wonders for a brand as part of its LCM strategy. Ultimately, the goals of such a strategy are twofold:

1. To build a unique competitive position for the brand, one where the drug can be seen as superior and differentiated from rivals in a target population
2. To secure appropriate market access (price and formulary position) for the brand that enables physician and patient access.

For such a strategy to be successful, companies must consider a number of factors that should be built into the design:

• *Fit with Market and Competitive Landscape*: For a patient health care (PHC) approach to be successful, it must fit in with the market and the competitive dynamics of the disease. The severity of disease, the speed of disease progression, the level of competition, and the level of unmet medical need will all shape the demand for and likely uptake of a personalized approach. The more severe the condition, the more likely that physicians will be receptive to a selection process that helps them choose the right therapy rather than accepting a cheaper alternative. A fast-progressing disease is also likely to be a better candidate for a more aggressive selection process, as there is less time to experiment before a patient deteriorates. For example, if we compare management of aggressive lung cancer with that of rheumatoid arthritis, the former takes weeks and the latter months or even years for the disease to progress. In terms of competition, it goes without saying that the more competitors there are, the more likely a patient selection strategy will be required, as differentiating from the competition is more likely to be necessary. Finally, the level of unmet need will be likely to shape the focus for any patient selection arguments. In areas with high unmet need in terms of efficacy, patient selection may focus more on identifying nonresponders to current therapy earlier and using these to target new therapies. By contrast, in an area of low unmet need for efficacy, focusing the selection criteria toward patients who are more or less likely to experience side effects may be a more effective approach.

- *Convincing Pharmacoeconomics*: Possibly the most important factor in driving a patient selection process is the development of strong pharmacoeconomic arguments to help persuade payers to support a brand. Payers are the most critical stakeholders in the acceptance and uptake of a selection strategy, and they must be convinced that the additional costs associated with selection will be associated with a greater return somewhere down the line. This is obviously easiest in the case where selection will lead to reduced drug costs (e.g., where implementing a test will lead to patients likely to experience costly side effects being excluded from the treated pool), but more challenging when the cost savings may come further down the line in terms of improved outcomes. This balance between near-term expenditure and long-term savings is a critical factor influencing the uptake of personalized medicine strategies between different markets, with some payers happy to focus on the long game, while other seek only to use personalized medicine to save money in this year's budget. In some cases, however, it is not necessary for a personalized strategy to actually demonstrate long- or short-term cost savings. A cost-neutral (or even slightly incremental) strategy can still be viable if it improves the predictability of a result. For example, if a test can highlight which 30 patients from a pool of 100 will respond to therapy, but the net cost of the test for all 100 equals the savings made by not treating the other 70, the test will likely still be accepted based on the greater predictability of outcome.

- *Viability of Selection Procedure*: One key factor influencing the real-world viability of a selection process is the dynamics of the selection procedure itself. Selection processes based on demographic criteria, a patient questionnaire, or symptomatic presentation are unlikely to bring any form of cost or time barriers to the patient process, so will likely see easy adoption if the outputs are meaningful in terms of patient outcomes. By contrast, biomarker testing can throw up multiple challenges to real-world adoption, including cost of testing, logistics of test implementation, and the delay between testing and results. In terms of cost, the critical factor is how many patients will need to be tested to gain a positive result. At a most basic level, the cost of the test relative to the cost of the treatment must be balanced—a US$1000 test for a drug that only costs US$50 for a course of therapy is unlikely to fly. Even if the costs of testing are reasonable, if you have to test 10 patients to get one positive result, the cost of nine negative tests needs to be added to the system costs of the one patient who succeeds, because the other nine will now have had an additional procedure that has not improved their chances of a good therapeutic outcome. Even when a test can identify six out of ten patients that are viable for therapy, if the cost of the test is very high, adoption might also be low as payers may see trial and error as a more "cost-effective" option. On top of cost, the logistics of testing can be a major barrier. A simple in-office diagnostic test can be easily integrated into a treatment paradigm, while a test that requires specialized out-patient clinics may face much greater barriers. Indeed, the great success of one of the earliest patient selection strategies, Bone Mineral Density (BMD) testing for postmenopausal osteoporosis, was enabled by Merck's investment in getting BMD testing machines into as many physician practices as possible. Finally, the link between the timing of test results and disease progression must be considered. Using a test for an infectious disease condition that takes 2 weeks to get back a result is not likely to be viable as the physician will want to act quickly. Indeed, this was one of the major real-life barriers to H1N1 testing in influenza patients at the height of pandemic scares of recent years. In this situation, physicians would reach for a therapeutic approach immediately rather than wait for the results of a test, which were then used merely to confirm a diagnosis rather than select appropriate therapy.

- *Sensitivity and Specificity of Selection Criteria*: While cost, timing, and logistics of a selection process are indeed critical, perhaps the most important factors associated with the test itself are the sensitivity and specificity of the result. Sensitivity relates to how well the test picks up patients that will respond to the therapy, or will experience the side effect being tested to avoid. The more sensitive a test, the lower the number of false negatives (patients screened out that should have been screened in) that will be found. Specificity relates to how specifically the test identifies only patients that will respond to therapy. In this case, the more specific the test, the lower the number of false positives (patients screened in that should have been screened out) that will occur. In the real world, payers hate false positives, as they are paying for patients who will not respond, while physicians hate false negatives, as they are withholding drugs from patients who would respond well to them. In contrast to the selection focused on cost, logistics, and time, it is generally the rule that biomarker testing will have a much greater sensitivity and selectively than demographic- or questionnaire-based selections. The latter group may be cheaper and easier, but their true diagnostic value may be much more limited than their more advanced rivals.

- *Uniqueness of Test*: The final factor to consider here is the uniqueness of the testing procedure and the applicability of the result. The decision to invest in diagnostic testing to support a brand can be a costly one, and the drive to push a test out into the market to secure better market share for a brand will only be effective if the test results cannot be applied to a competitor brand. Take for example a scenario where four brands could be used to treat an indication, with three biomarkers identified to help patient selection (see Figure 13.3). In this situation, if the company promoting Brand A were to design a specific test for Biomarker X, it would indeed help to select patients that would not only respond to Brand A, but would also identify responders to Brands C and D as well. By contrast, the owners of Brand C would be able to tie the results of a test for

	Marker X	Marker Y	Marker Z
Drug A	✓✓		
Drug B		✓✓	
Drug C	✓		✓✓
Drug D	✓✓	✓✓	

Diagnostic for X – Drug A, C, or D
Diagnostic for Y – Drug B or D
Diagnostic for Z – Drug C
Diagnostic for both X and Y – Drug D

FIGURE 13.3. The value of uniqueness in biomarker testing. *Source*: Datamonitor.

Biomarker Z to the specific need for Brand C, while the owners of Brand D would need to develop a test for both biomarkers X and Y to ensure their brand is used ahead of all competitors.

13.2 PATIENT SELECTION WITHOUT PREDICTIVE CRITERIA: POST HOC APPROACHES

What can a company do to get good market access for its drug, when it knows that only some patients respond to the therapy, but there is no way of identifying which ones will fail until they fail? In this situation, we are moving more into the territory of commercial strategies rather than developmental strategies, but it is appropriate to consider these within this context. Many companies have found themselves in just this situation when trying to launch new oncology drugs. The only way to gain generalized usage is to agree to a price that is too low for the company to accept, because the payers will not accept the desired price without some form of reassurance that accurate patient selection can be made. In such situations, companies may need to turn to "pay for nonperformance" agreements. In these agreements, the payer only has to pay for patients who respond to therapy, and will be reimbursed by the drug company for patients who fail. This form of retrospective patient selection can be very painful for the drug company as it must carry the cost of treating the nonresponders, but it can be an effective short-term measure to enable usage while the proactive patient selection strategies are being developed. Indeed, these agreements will often mean the difference between some usage and none at all, so the companies involved often have no choice in the matter if they want any form of reimbursement. As payers focus more and more on aggressive cost containment, such agreements are on the increase, further pushing the need for proactive patient selection strategies to be brought earlier in the product life cycle.

13.3 WHAT ABOUT THE PATIENTS WHO ARE NOT SELECTED?

One ethical dilemma posed by excessive patient selection is what happens to patients who do not meet the criteria for active selection, as companies will aim to select only the patients that give the best response with the lowest risk of side effects. Moving forward, this may leave populations of patients who are not eligible either by label restriction or reimbursement criteria for any therapy based on their risk of nonresponse. How can the drug industry ethically address these patients without compromising its overall strategy?

This challenge is likely to increase the demand and need for expanded access programs, enabling patient access outside of approved labels on a specific named-patient basis and driven by medical need. Building such programs into the LCM plans for a drug ensures that drug companies can meet their ethical obligations to provide access to their medicines in a responsible manner without impacting their optimal patient selection strategy.

CHAPTER 14

New Dosage Strengths, New Dosage Regimens

We will be devoting a lengthy chapter to new formulations, which constitute one of the most important areas of lifecycle management (LCM), but it is also worth first looking briefly at the twin strategies of making more dosages available (in essentially the same formulation) and of changing dosage regimens using existing formulations.

14.1 NEW DOSAGE STRENGTHS

Adding dosage strengths can be a useful strategy in the growth phases of the brand's life cycle. These new dosages will help physicians to customize dosage according to the needs of individual patients, and this may help to gain market share from alternative brands that do not offer the same flexibility. In the absence of significant side effects, physicians will become more comfortable over time in increasing the dosages that they prescribe, and compliance and adherence may well be improved if patients are then not forced to swallow multiple tablets to reach the prescribed dose. This effect is demonstrated nicely in Case History 9 in the Appendix, which covers Diovan®. The opposite may also occur. Physicians may wish to reduce the dosage in particularly susceptible patients, such as children, elderly patients, or patients taking multiple drugs. In other cases, they will wish to start a patient on a lower dosage, increasing this gradually over time if the patient is responding to the therapy and not showing side effects. Such dose titration is going to be more accurate if there is an adequate range of dosages available.

Providing a range of dosages sufficient to allow physicians to titrate the optimal dosage for individual patients can be an effective late-stage lifecycle management (LLCM) strategy as well, enabling the brand to maintain a higher market share after exclusivity expires. Generic companies may only develop

Pharmaceutical Lifecycle Management: Making the Most of Each and Every Brand, First Edition. Tony Ellery and Neal Hansen.
© 2012 John Wiley & Sons, Inc. Published 2012 by John Wiley & Sons, Inc.

the best-selling dosage strengths, and it may well be that the optimal dosage for an individual patient lies between two dosages offered as generics. Furthermore, if the physician is obliged to use the wider range of dosages offered by the original brand to titrate the right dosage for a new patient, then he is more likely to remain with the brand and not switch the patient to the generic even in cases where the selected dosage is available as a generic. This will not help, of course, in markets where the brand is removed from the formulary once a generic becomes available or where the pharmacy can switch the prescription from the brand to the generic.

The benefits of providing a wide range of dosage strengths in the mature phase of the brand life cycle must be weighed against the extra cost of multiple stock keeping units (SKUs) at a time when the brand is being milked for profit. It is important to quantify the commercial upside provided by each dosage strength and not just to assume that more is better. When a new dosage is introduced, this does give sales representatives the opportunity to talk about it with physicians and get some attention for an older brand.

As mentioned in the previous chapter, combining the strategies of new indication and new dosage strength can be effective as part of an LLCM program. Generic companies will only be able to get approval for the dosages used in the indications on their label. If the brand company has patented a new indication which requires a different dosage, neither can be included on the label of the generic, as this would be tantamount to encouraging infringement of the patent.

14.2 NEW DOSAGE REGIMENS

New dosage regimens are usually the result of reformulations, as when a twice-daily oral form is replaced by a once-daily oral form in a controlled release formulation. However, there are cases when existing or new dosage strengths in established formulations can be utilized in new dosage regimens as part of an LCM program. And the new dosage regimen may be patentable.

Here is an example from the European Patent Office (EPO) in 2003. Genentech had applied for a patent on a new dosage regimen for Insulin-like Growth Factor-1 (IGF-1). Under this new regimen, IGF-1 was injected discontinuously in a cyclic "on/off" fashion. Genentech's patent application was initially rejected during prosecution, but the Technical Board of Appeal then ruled in Genentech's favor.

The value of a new dosage regimen can be threefold—differentiation, protection, and cost-effectiveness. From a differentiation standpoint, a new dosing regimen can distinguish one class competitor from a rival or aim to close a gap. The approval of the bisphosphonate Actonel® in its 2CD dosing regimen allowed once-monthly dosing by giving two high doses on consecutive days. This enabled competition with the once-monthly rival Boniva® from Roche/GlaxoSmithKline.

By demonstrating effectiveness in reduced-frequency dosing regimens, companies can also improve their cost-effectiveness arguments with payers. Genentech and Novartis's Lucentis® was approved for the treatment of wet age-related macular edema as a one monthly fixed dosing regimen. However, in the real world, the drug is more commonly dosed PRN (*pro re nata*, or as needed) and many subsequent studies have observed effectiveness with this approach, reducing the number of annual doses significantly, and thus improving overall cost-effectiveness.

CHAPTER 15

Reformulation, New Routes of Administration, and Drug Delivery

15.1 REFORMULATION AND NEW ROUTES OF ADMINISTRATION

Reformulating drugs has been one of the most widely used lifecycle management (LCM) strategies of the last two decades. Reformulations have been effectively used in the growth, maturity, and decline phases of the life cycle, and many of the examples of successful LCM cited in the literature and described at LCM conferences are based on reformulation.

The same active substance can be presented in a variety of different dosage forms. Many secondary patents claim formulations, often including specifications of dose or concentration, and these patents invariably expire later than the basic patent on the new molecular entity (NME) that they contain.

The majority of reformulations are aimed either at reducing the dosage frequency of the drug or at changing the route of administration.

While reformulation will continue to be a cornerstone of brand LCM, the environment for successful reformulation strategies has changed considerably in recent years and many of the success stories of the past will not be reproducible in the future. This is particularly true where reformulation is used as a defense strategy against generics.

The motivation for a company to reformulate its brand varies according to when in the life cycle the reformulation is implemented. Figure 15.1 summarizes the different strategies that may underlie the decision to create a new formulation.

15.1.1 Switch and Grow Strategy

The "Switch and grow" strategy is utilized during the growth or early maturity phase of the life cycle, when the brand is still securely protected by a patent.

Pharmaceutical Lifecycle Management: Making the Most of Each and Every Brand, First Edition.
Tony Ellery and Neal Hansen.
© 2012 John Wiley & Sons, Inc. Published 2012 by John Wiley & Sons, Inc.

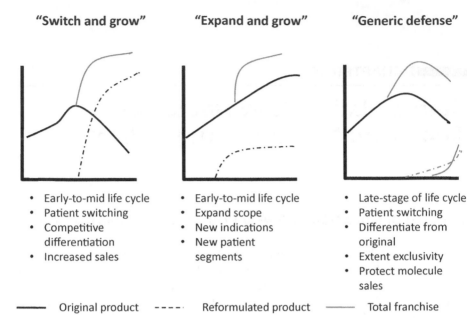

"Switch and grow"	"Expand and grow"	"Generic defense"

- Early-to-mid life cycle
- Patient switching
- Competitive differentiation
- Increased sales

- Early-to-mid life cycle
- Expand scope
- New indications
- New patient segments

- Late-stage of life cycle
- Patient switching
- Differentiate from original
- Extent exclusivity
- Protect molecule sales

——— Original product   - - - - Reformulated product   ——— Total franchise

FIGURE 15.1. Reformulations are developed with different aims depending on the phase of the life cycle. *Source:* Datamonitor.

There can be different motivations for pursuing this strategy. The challenges and timelines of bringing a new drug to market for the first time are such that companies will often elect to follow a low-risk, fast-to-market strategy by first introducing a simple formulation. A typical example would be when a company decides to go to market with a thrice- or twice-daily oral preparation and to tackle the issue of controlled release later to develop a once-daily tablet. This decision will be influenced by the technical difficulties associated with the better formulation, and by the competitive situation. In other cases, the technology required for a better formulation may not even become available until after the drug has already been introduced in its first formulation.

The purpose of creating the improved formulation is to switch patients away from the old, competitively less attractive formulation and thus gain more market share from other companies with competing molecules. In past years, higher prices could often be obtained for the improved formulation so that profits increased even in cases where unit sales of the new formulation merely replaced those of the old formulation. Thus, it was possible to recoup the development costs of the new formulation even if no significant additional market share could be gained. Today, it is unlikely that the reformulation will command a higher price than the formulation it is replacing, so that the development costs will only be recovered if the market share can be increased at the expense of competitors, or the market expanded.

15.1.2   Expand and Grow Strategy

In the "Expand and grow" strategy, the earlier formulation is left on the market, and the new formulation is used to expand the patient population that the drug is used to treat. Fixed-dose combinations, considered in the next chapter, are one specific example of such a reformulation strategy.

Just to take one of countless examples of the use of such a strategy to expand to new indications with a new route of administration, antibiotics, antivirals, antihistamines, steroids, beta-blockers, alpha-2 agonists, immuno-suppressants, and nonsteroidal anti-inflammatory drugs (NSAIDs) have all been developed as eye drops to treat a wide variety of ophthalmic diseases.

As an example of the benefits that a new route of administration can some-times bring to an existing indication, Novartis's Exelon® was available as a tablet for treating Alzheimer patients but sales only really took off when it was introduced as a dermal patch, as this enabled nursing staff and family members to visually confirm that the patient really was getting the medicine (Exelon is described in Case History 1 in the Appendix). As an example of using reformulation to address the needs of a specific patient subpopulation, presenting oral drugs as syrups as well as capsules or tablets enables them to be dosed to small children, which might not be feasible in solid form. Such pediatric reformulations are sometimes necessary to obtain pediatric exclusivity, especially in Europe.

15.1.3   Generic Defense

Reformulation has a key role to play in the controversial area of generic defense, although the opportunities to extend exclusivity or retain more post-patent expiry market share are now less than they used to be.

Composition of matter patents can be applied to formulations rather than only to the active substance when they claim carriers or excipients, such as fillers, binders, disintegrants, and lubricants. Generic companies are still free to market the same active substance in a different formulation once the basic patent has expired, just so long as this formulation does not infringe the patents on other aspects of the new formulation. But even where it is possible to create a bioequivalent generic using formulation technologies and sub-stances that lie outside of the patent, brand companies may still be able to delay generic entry to the market by alleging infringement and requesting provisional injunctions that block commercialization until a final court ruling is made. Sometimes a claimed formulation may lead to a specific effect, such as delayed release of the active substance, but such effects tend to be obvious to an ordinary person skilled in the art and are generally unlikely to warrant a patent. An exception would be when a new excipient produces a completely unexpected effect. But even where a new formulation does result in an unexpected result, for example, a synergy between the active substance and one of the excipients, this may not be enough in the future to warrant a patent if it could have been expected that an ordinary person skilled in the art would have tried mixing that active substance with that excipient. Patent claims relating to parameters like pharmacokinetic profiles, particle distribution or micronization may not be admissible for the same reason. Only where a non-obvious element of the formulation leads to a surprising and significant result—such as a dramatically better efficacy or safety profile—is a robust patent likely to be granted.

Reformulation as "Generic defense" has probably been the most commonly used late-stage lifecycle management (LLCM) strategy of them all during the last 30 years. Obviously, this reformulation strategy is utilized late in the life cycle, during the latter part of the maturity phase. The concept was originally a very effective one. As patent expiry on the drug approached, the company introduced a new, improved, and patented formulation, switched patients from the old to the new and withdrew the old formulation from the market so that no generic manufacturer could refer to it as the Reference Listed Drug (RLD) in its Abbreviated New Drug Application (ANDA). This resulted in an extension of the drug's exclusivity beyond patent expiry.

This generic defense strategy has become much more difficult in recent years for a number of reasons:

- As already stated, an "obvious" reformulation may be denied a patent, or its patent may be vulnerable to generic challenge. Generic companies increasingly adopt an aggressive legal stance against secondary patent barriers raised by innovators.
- Generic companies have become more adept at designing around patents, that is, at creating formulations that enable bioequivalence to be demonstrated without infringing the patent on the branded reformulation. The number of companies offering drug delivery platforms has increased in recent years, so that generic companies lacking in-house expertise can easily access a wide range of me-too formulation platforms.
- Generic companies in the United States can now use a withdrawn RLD unless it had to be withdrawn for reasons of safety or effectiveness. In Europe, too, generics can be approved even if market authorization has been withdrawn in a European Union (EU) country, provided that the marketing authorization was still valid when the generic was filed.
- Third-party payers are unlikely to reimburse an expensive reformulation when a generic is available in the original brand formulation, unless the reformulation offers benefits that can be proven to result in improved disease outcomes. This issue is very important and cannot be overemphasized. It is no longer sufficient to come to market with, for example, a once-daily formulation and expect to retain significant market share from generic offerings of the twice-daily formulation. Payers just won't accept this. Taking specifically this case of once daily versus twice daily, the real-world evidence is far from overwhelming that the improved convenience to the patient of once-daily dosing will result in improved compliance,

and it is in any case extremely difficult to prove that occasionally missing a dose will negatively affect most disease outcomes. The argument has even been advanced that twice-daily dosing offers better security than once daily, as a patient missing a dose will only be without adequate blood levels of the drug for up to 12 h compared to up to 24 h.

However, if all of these caveats are borne in mind, a well-planned reformulation strategy can protect at least some market share by providing a new patent and market exclusivity. It will be more effective when combined with a change in dose form, dosing regimen, or route of administration, where a combination of several patents and exclusivity provide a barrier which may prove difficult for generic companies to cross. To increase the chances of success, generic defense reformulation strategies are shifting away from controlled release-style products toward more radical approaches for improving bioavailability and compliance, in the hope that this will be more effective in combating generic competition.

Some companies flood the market with different formulations and dosage strengths in the hope that generic companies will not copy all of them. They may not, but it is still essential that a careful business case be developed to compare the costs of each of these multiple developments and the negative impact of cross-cannibalization between the different presentations with the profits to be made from the additional postpatent market share.

Even after patent expiry, there may still be situations where it is worth going to the expense of developing a new formulation. After all, a genericized brand often retains a low proportion of its sales for a long period of time after patent expiry, and for a multibillion dollar brand this can be a lot of money. As an example, Novartis's Voltaren® still had worldwide prescription sales of US$800 million in 2010, decades after the basic patent expiry. Under these circumstances, there may be a business case for developing new formulations, if not globally, at least locally. This can be especially attractive in self-pay markets where sales are still respectable, thanks to consumer preference for the original brand. Moreover, these countries usually have lower regulatory requirements than the United States, Europe, and Japan and this, together with a lower local cost base, can make the development of a line extension, alone or in partnership with a local company, quite attractive. To continue with the Voltaren example, Novartis developed Voveran Thermagel® in India (Voveran® is the local brand name of Voltaren) long after the basic patent expired on diclofenac. Alongside diclofenac, this product contains capsaicin and is used to treat strains and sprains.

When considering reformulation strategies, it is important to remember that a new formulation can be granted 3 years of exclusivity in the United States. The maximum of 1 year in Europe if it is associated with a new indication is less of an incentive.

We will be considering the importance of starting LCM early in the brand life cycle later in the book, but nowhere is it more important than in reformulation strategies. Especially in the case of generic defense, the switch to the new formulation must be made early enough for the sales force to convince physicians to move patients onto the new formulation before exclusivity expires and cheap generics in the old formulation flood the market. Sales forces will need 2 years or even longer to accomplish this, and adding the time it takes to create the new formulation and test it clinically demonstrates how early the development project must be initiated.

Another important reason for completing the development early is that physicians are growing increasingly suspicious of the motivation of companies that introduce reformulations shortly before patent expiry, and may be reluctant to prescribe them. This is vividly illustrated by the comments of a U.S. key opinion leader on Pfizer's Zmax® reformulation of its antibiotic Zithromax® (azithromycin): "It's a marketing ploy. Don't get me wrong, I live in a capitalist country and I understand the way the market works, but if it was an improvement that truly made the drug of great benefit they wouldn't wait until after the patent is off on the first. These are ways of prolonging their market." ("Commercial Insight: Antibacterials," Datamonitor, 2006, DMHC2253)

This reaction is typical for the United States, where LLCM has received a lot of exposure and a bad press. Countries with less mature generic markets are more likely to tolerate reformulation strategies late in the life cycle.

In recent years, the central nervous system (CNS) and alimentary and metabolic therapies have been those most frequently targeted for reformulation. Respiratory, anti-infective, and genitourinary and sex hormone therapies have also experienced frequent reformulation. This reflects the large patient populations within the major indications of these therapeutic areas, the high commercial value of many of the products, and the highly competitive nature of the markets. All of which drive companies to be more active in seeking to expand their franchises, gaining a competitive advantage within the respective markets.

There is a wide range of different dosage forms that might be considered when deciding the reformulation strategy for a brand. There follows a list of the most important ones.

Oral Dosage Forms. Pill; Tablet for swallowing (fast release, extended release, or delayed release); Effervescent tablet; Oral disintegrating tablet; Capsule (soft or hard; fast release, extended release, or delayed release); Granules; Liquid (syrup, solution, or suspension); Thin film

Topicals. Cream; Gel; Lotion; Ointment; Paste; Salve; Eye drops; Ear drops; Patches (fast release, extended release, or delayed release)

Injections. Intradermal; Intramuscular; Intravenous; Subcutaneous

Respiratory Inhalants. Powder; Aerosol; Nebulizer; Vapor

Suppositories. Rectal; Vaginal

A more comprehensive list of alternative formulations and routes of administration may be found on the Food and Drug Administration (FDA) website.

Success drivers	Success resistors
• Improving efficacy or compliance, or meeting an unmet need through reformulation can achieve high uptake among physicians and payers • Launch early enough prior to patent expiry to switch patients before generic entry • Lower investment than new product development and launch • Maintains sales of brand franchise when patients switched to reformulation ahead of patent expiry • Capitalizes on brand equity established for original product	• Generic companies with the capabilities to develop own noninfringing reformulations • Increasing use of tiered and/or restrictive drug plan formularies may limit uptake • Effectiveness of withdraw and switch strategy blocked by EU regulations • Reformulated products risk being included in jumbo reference pricing in Germany • Physicians are increasingly skeptical of reformulated products as they are seen as ways to extend the market life of a drug • No additional data exclusivity periods under new EU regulations (although new formulations may be patented)

FIGURE 15.2. Success drivers and resistors of reformulation as an LCM strategy. *Source:* Datamonitor.

Any of these different formulations can be valuable additions to the brand range as long as the limitations that we have already discussed are respected:

- Premium pricing for a line extension over and above the price already granted for products in the brand range is becoming increasingly difficult to obtain.
- The new formulation must offer real, quantifiable benefits in safety or efficacy over competitive brand offerings if it is to recoup its investment.
- After composition of matter patent expiry, the hurdle for the level of benefit required becomes much higher as the generics will be available very cheaply.
- Secondary patents protecting the new formulation must be strong enough to withstand challenge by generic companies.
- There should be no alternative route for obtaining a bioequivalent generic product using other technologies that lie outside the scope of the protecting patent(s).

Summarizing and expanding this section, Figure 15.2 shows the main factors that drive and resist reformulation as an LCM strategy.

15.2 DRUG DELIVERY DEVICES

In a broader sense, reformulations are just part of the field of "drug delivery," which can involve sophisticated mechanical and electronic devices. The FDA defines drug delivery devices as "modern technology, distributed with or as a part of a drug product, which allows for the uniform release or targeting of drugs to the body." Here is a list of some of the devices that can be used to deliver drugs to the body, and which can therefore form part of the LCM program for a drug:

- Drug-eluting stents
- Drug-eluting beads (DEB)
- Implants
- Inhalers (vaporizer, dry powder, or nebulizer)
- Infusion pumps
- Injectors, prefilled syringes, needle-free injection
- Implants
- Electronically controlled skin patches
- Antimicrobial catheters
- Antibiotic-loaded bone cements
- Photodynamic therapy

The use of drug delivery devices can differentiate drugs from competitive offerings. It can also provide additional patent protection, both regarding the device itself and in many cases the route of administration too. Differences in device design which generic companies would have to make to circumvent the device patent often change drug bioavailability so that the bioequivalence route to market is no longer an option for the generic drug.

Competitive differentiation in drug/delivery device combinations has shaped many different therapeutic markets over the last decade. In the respiratory markets, competition is fierce for the best inhaler, with GlaxoSmithKline (GSK), AstraZeneca, Boehringer Ingelheim, Pfizer, and Novartis all competing in many cases with agents that by themselves have limited differentiation. Indeed, one of the key players in the respiratory segment moving forward will be the Israeli generics giant Teva, combining its expertise in generics with a focused development program of next-generation inhalers. The failure of inhaler/drug combinations was one of the key contributing factors to the failed race to the first viable inhaled insulin, where some of the proposed solutions looked closer to a scuba diving apparatus than a traditional inhaler!

Injectable drugs have for many years been the target for strong device differentiation. In diabetes, the evolution from vial and syringe, to prefilled syringe to pen formulations has enabled leaders such as Sanofi-Aventis and Novo Nordisk to drive further competitive differentiation and meet patient needs. It remains to be seen whether such developments will effectively protect these franchises once generic, or biosimilar, insulins become available, but the platform for differentiation has at least been established. We will look more closely at injection devices when we consider the LCM of biologics in Chapter 26.

More advanced technological innovations are difficult to find to date, although the continued development of smart patches and implantable devices, many with built-in diagnostics could open up new opportunities for the future. The development of the artificial pancreas, combining blood glucose monitoring with suitable drug delivery, is the goal of many in the diabetes space that will likely be realized within the next decade. A variety of recent publications have suggested that the drug–device combination is likely to grow much faster than the prescription drug market in the coming years. This will offer opportunities for LCM, although the cost of the drug is generally only a small part of the overall cost of the combination, and in many cases this will be restrictive in realizing sufficient return on investment. This and the modest size of the drug–device combination market mean that this area is likely to remain a minor factor in brand LCM in most therapeutic areas for the foreseeable future.

CHAPTER 16

Fixed-Dose Combinations (FDCs) and Co-Packaging

Combination strategies have traditionally been used in the growth and maturity phases of the brand life cycle, although increasing competition is driving use much earlier to gain optimum returns. There is a trend in many indications to use free combination therapy—that is, two different drug products—to treat disease. There are several rationales for combination therapy as opposed to just increasing the dose of a monotherapy. First, if two or more drugs with different mechanisms of action but the same therapeutic end point are given to treat a disease, then the overall therapeutic effect is likely to be additive, while side effects are likely not to be. This is very much the case in conditions such as hypertension and Type 2 diabetes, where patients are rarely able to reach their goal with one therapy alone, so they need efficacy that can only be gained through combination approaches. In the case of infectious diseases, the rationale is frequently that it is less likely for resistant forms of the pathogen to develop.

The disadvantage of free combination therapy is that patients are prescribed two or more different drugs, and this may confuse them and cause them to make mistakes in dosing so that the treatment compliance is compromised. A typical elderly patient with metabolic syndrome may well be taking a statin, a beta-blocker, a diuretic, a calcium antagonist, an ACE inhibitor, and metformin—six different drugs—every day.

For this reason, physicians often prefer to prescribe a single tablet or a single pack that contains two or more of drugs to make dosing more convenient for the patient and thus to improve compliance. And patients may derive further benefits from lower co-pays as they are filling fewer prescriptions. Drug supply issues may also be easier to master when different drugs are combined into one fixed-dose combination (FDC) product.

Another possible rationale for developing an FDC is where one component is included to prevent side effects that could be caused by the other component. A recent example of this strategy is AstraZeneca's Vimovo®, which

Pharmaceutical Lifecycle Management: Making the Most of Each and Every Brand, First Edition. Tony Ellery and Neal Hansen.
© 2012 John Wiley & Sons, Inc. Published 2012 by John Wiley & Sons, Inc.

combines esomeprazole and naproxen, and which was approved by the Food and Drug Administration (FDA) in early 2010 and Europe in 2011. It is indicated for the relief of signs and symptoms of osteoarthritis, rheumatoid arthritis, and ankylosing spondylitis, and to decrease the risk of developing gastric ulcers in such patients. In June 2010, the FDA declined to approve a second AstraZeneca FDC, Axanum®, a combination of esomeprazole and aspirin intended for use in cardiac patients on low-dose aspirin who are at risk of developing ulcers, although it was subsequently approved in Europe in 2011.

The best examples of FDCs that really do provide undisputed benefit for patients are to be found in the developing countries, in the treatment of AIDS, malaria, and tuberculosis, where FDCs slow drug resistance, improve clinical outcomes, and facilitate logistics. In the case of antiretroviral (ARV) triple therapy, FDCs usually also offer the most affordable option.

In the developed world, FDCs usually consist of two drugs that treat the same disease. Thus, Merck's Hyzaar®, an FDC of the angiotensin receptor blocker (ARB) losartan and the diuretic hydrochlorothiazide, is used to treat hypertension. Three-way combinations are also possible. Novartis's antihypertensive Exforge HCT®, for example, contains valsartan, amlodipine, and hydrochlorothiazide.

Usually, FDC development projects involve combining the patented brand with an established active substance used to treat the same disease. Often, this second active substance will already be genericized.

An FDC development will only provide a return on the considerable investment of time and resources necessary to bring it to market successfully if a number of conditions are met.

The therapeutic effect of the FDC must at least be additive. In other words, each component drug must exert its full effect in the combination. If the effect is less than the sum of the parts, regulatory approval is unlikely to be granted. Of course, a synergistic effect is much preferable to a merely additive effect as this is an additional argument for using the particular drug combination. Furthermore, an unexpected synergistic effect can pave the way for a robust patent of the combination. In the post-KSR versus Teleflex world, simply combining two therapies approved for the same disease into an FDC and obtaining an additive effect is increasingly likely to be deemed "obvious," so that either a patent is not granted in the first place or that patent will be vulnerable to challenge.

Looking further into the future, it could become more difficult to obtain patent protection even for FDCs where a synergy has been found. After all, combining two drugs where it is obvious to do so and then observing that they have a synergistic effect could be deemed to be a "discovery" rather than an "invention," since the synergy takes place in the body and is found through clinical trials. And discoveries are not patentable. Moreover, was there really an "innovative step" or did the researcher just get lucky? Patent attorneys are not in agreement upon how this situation might develop, and the reader is advised to check up on the latest case history.

For an FDC to be commercially successful, there must be a large enough population of patients who are receiving both drugs simultaneously and at the dosages selected for the combination to make the development worthwhile. This might seem obvious, but FDCs have become such a popular lifecycle management (LCM) strategy that some companies create multiple FDCs around the same brand without clearly considering relative positioning and the impact of cross-cannibalization. In situations where physicians titrate the optimal dosage of each drug for each individual patient, FDCs are unlikely to command a significant market share as the physicians will be looking for more dose combinations than are available as FDCs. If there is little or no co-usage of the components foreseen for the FDC, or at the dosage combination foreseen, companies should not underestimate the volume of clinical data they will need to generate. It is hard work to modify the existing medical practice in such cases. This was one of the problems that confronted Caduet®, as can be seen in Case History 5 in the Appendix.

Quite simply, the FDC must be capable of taking sufficient market share from competing brands (and their FDCs) to pay for the development. In the current pricing environment, it is highly unlikely that an FDC will receive premium pricing over and above the price of the patented brand monotherapy, and in most cases, the FDC is expected to be priced significantly lower than the two individual components. The only exception might be if it can be proven that the compliance is so much higher using the FDC than the individual components in free combination that better disease outcomes can be obtained with the FDC. The likelihood that this could be proven is in most cases extremely small, and payers are unlikely to accept the argument that better compliance leads inevitably to better outcomes, let alone the argument that an FDC will automatically mean improved compliance.

After patent expiry, when both components of the FDC are available individually as generics, retaining significant market share at a premium price—that is, at a price significantly above the sum of the price of the two generic monotherapies—will be virtually impossible unless—again—improved disease outcomes compared to the free combination of generics can be demonstrated. If this extremely high hurdle can be negotiated, there will have to be a very strong patent on the FDC (formulation or FDC per se) to prevent generic companies copying the FDC. However, there are some special circumstances in which FDCs will definitely lead to significantly improved patient convenience and therefore improved compliance. We have already mentioned infectious diseases in the developing countries, but take also the example of eye drop FDCs used to treat ophthalmic diseases.

The conjunctival sac has only enough volume to accommodate one eye drop. If patients require more than one monotherapy delivered by eye drop, then they have to wait for some minutes after dropping the first drug before they can drop the second. This is inconvenient, but if the drops are given in too rapid succession, the result is that some of the fluid spills out of the eye before it can be taken up by the conjunctiva and the correct dose will not be absorbed. The inconvenience to the patient of dropping one drug, waiting several minutes, and then dropping the second is such that administering two drops instead of one is quite certain to impact compliance, especially in a disease like glaucoma where in the early stages the patient has no subjective symptoms of the disease. An example of an FDC delivered as eye drops is Merck's Cosopt® (timolol + dorzolamide). However, there are generics of Cosopt available as the formulation is not difficult to copy, and the patents on both drugs have expired.

In the case of inhaled drugs used for treating chronic obstructive pulmonary disease (COPD) and asthma, even FDCs of patent-expired molecules (steroids, long-acting beta agonists, and/or antimuscarinics) can be effectively protected. Where they are contained in a device which is itself patent protected, it may be very difficult for a generic company to demonstrate bioequivalence in another device without infringing elements of the device patent or patents. Thus, in the case of inhaled drugs, developing FDCs of two or more off-patent components may provide a positive return on investment. Furthermore, such FDCs do fill a genuine patient need. It would be very inconvenient for patients to have to carry around and use correctly two inhalers, and if they had to, compliance would undoubtedly be negatively impacted. Let us look at an example of such an inhaled FDC. Symbicort® is AstraZeneca's FDC containing budesonide and formoterol. Although the patents have expired on both active substances, no generic has so far appeared, and the product still sells at a premium price.

So far we have only considered FDCs where the component drugs all target the same disease. FDCs also exist where the component drugs target different diseases in the same patient. An example is Pfizer's Caduet, which contains the calcium antagonist amlodipine for treating hypertension and the statin atorvastatin for reducing blood cholesterol. Caduet is described in Case History 5 in the Appendix. When deciding whether or not to develop an FDC for multiple diseases, many of the points that we have already considered apply.

The first decision is, of course, whether the comorbid population really is large enough to justify the development. Again, the question of compatible dosages must be considered, as must pricing and compliance issues. Another consideration is whether the same physicians treat all of the diseases that are addressed by the combination.

Figure 16.1 summarizes some of the different factors that a company must consider before taking the decision to create an FDC as part of an LCM program.

The ultimate multi-indication FDC would be the so-called polypill, which received considerable attention following publication of the results of the Indian Polycap Study in March 2009. This randomized, controlled, double-blind study documented the outcome of 2000 patients with at least one risk factor for heart disease (diabetes, hypercholesterolemia, hypertension, obesity, or smoking). During a 12-week treatment period, 400 study participants were

Single indication FDCs—what to look for?	Multiple indication FDCs—will they be accepted?

• **Is the combination logical?**
  – Does it fit with current treatment practice?
  – Does the dosing schedule/titration of the component agents fit with an FDC?
  – If not, will it be supported by sufficient data to change treatment practice?
• **Would a brand/generic FDC improve role in treatment?**
  – Can a first-line generic be displaced by combining the same generic with a current second-line brand?
• **Which therapies would the FDC cannibalize?**
  – Will the current monotherapy brand be the primary target or is it a generic population target?
  – Will the FDC take share from the other brands in the same class?
	• **How significant is the comorbidity profile?**
	  – Is there a large enough market for this to be attractive?
	  – Is prevention a possible positioning strategy (e.g., low-dose FDCs)?
	• **What are the existing coprescribing levels?**
	  – Of the comorbid patient pool, what proportion are already on the free combination?
	• **Are the two indications treated by the same physician type?**
	  – Will the same physician initiate the therapy or at the very least, maintain it?
	• **Are the dosing schedules with each agent simple?**
	  – If physicians tend to titrate therapy, FDCs are likely to be the last line.

FDC, Fixed-dose combination.

FIGURE 16.1. Advantages and disadvantages of single and multiple indication FDCs. *Source:* Datamonitor.

given the so-called Polycap, which contained low doses of aspirin and simvastatin, and three different antihypertensives (atenolol, ramipril, and thiazide). The rest of the participants were divided into eight groups which were given either individual components or groups of them. The participants who received Polycap showed both systolic and diastolic blood pressure reductions of six to seven points. Such reductions would be expected to reduce the risk of heart disease by 62% and of stroke by 48%. The Polycap was almost as effective as the individual pills with no increase in side effects.

Other drug candidates for inclusion in a polypill to address the risk factors of metabolic syndrome could include folic acid, which has been shown to reduce the level of homocysteine in the blood and thus counter another risk factor for heart disease, and metformin, which treats diabetes and also contributes to weight loss.

The polypill concept has caused considerable controversy. Were such a pill to be taken by everybody over 55 years of age in Western Europe and the United States, it is reasonable to suppose that the overall effect on preventing heart disease would be positive. However, it would also be true that many people who did not require medication would be taking the polypill, thus being unnecessarily exposed to potential side effects and also wasting health-care resources. Furthermore, there would be a risk that some patients would be underdosing on the components that they really did need. The argument has also been raised that it would be seen to provide a *carte blanche* for people to continue and even worsen their already unhealthy lifestyles, which could in time even have a negative overall impact on public health.

Dr. Robert Bonow, past president of the American Heart Association and codirector of the Bluhm Cardiovascular Institute at Northwestern University in Chicago, said that while the treatment might be better than taking nothing, the number of medications in the pill would make tailored treatment impossible, and the treatment would fall short in the United States. He said, "This study was done in India, and we believe that this is where this kind of approach on a population basis could pay off."

Currently, the regulatory hurdle for the approval of a polypill would in any case be too high for such a development to be practicable in Europe or the United States. When Novartis obtained FDA approval for their triple FDC treatment of hypertension, Exforge HCT®, they were required to show the superiority of the product over patients receiving valsartan + HCT, valsartan + amlodipine, and amlodipine + HCT. The size of the clinical trial necessary to gain approval for a combination containing six or more active substances would be prohibitively large, and it is in any case highly unlikely that one could demonstrate the added value of the complete polypill over each of its minus variants lacking just one component.

Now FDCs are not the only route to combination therapy, and co-packaging can be a viable, lower cost option for consideration in certain circumstances. Co-packaging simply looks at providing two complementary therapies in the same box, but not in the same pill. One instance where this was successfully employed was with the bisphosphonate Actonel®, which was developed into a co-package with calcium. The rationale behind the approach focused on high levels of co-prescribing of Actonel with calcium, but a challenge of dose timing. If the calcium was taken at the same time as the Actonel, the Actonel efficacy would be lost. As such, the co-pack had blister packs with named days; on day one the blister contained Actonel, while on the next 6 days it contained calcium. In theory, the strategy worked well, but in practice, the co-prescribed calcium was so cheap that moving people to the more expensive co-pack was not seen to be enough of an advantage in many markets.

Finally in this chapter on FDCs, let us look at the situation regarding patent extensions and exclusivities for FDCs.

In the United States, at least one of the active ingredients (including any salt or ester of that active ingredient) of the product must have not been previously approved by the FDA to be eligible for patent term restoration, based on the approval of the combination product, and then only the patent covering the newly approved component or the combination of components may be extended. Thus, a 5-year period of exclusivity is granted to New Drug Applications (NDAs) for products containing chemical entities which have never been previously approved by the FDA, either alone or in combination. However, FDCs are eligible for new clinical trial exclusivity in the United States.

In Europe, Supplementary Protection Certificates (SPCs) can be granted for FDCs and may provide exclusivity which extends well beyond the 15-year exclusivity limit which applies to the patented component of the FDC.

However, an SPC will not be granted unless the combination was claimed in the original patent of the patented FDC component. Takeda's lansoprazole fell foul of this condition in the United Kingdom, where the combination with antibiotics was not granted an SPC because it was not claimed in the original lansoprazole patent. In Europe, only the specific set of new data submitted to register the combination itself is protected by data and market exclusivity (8 + 2 + 1). It is permissible for a competitor to rely on data previously submitted to register the individual active substances whose various types of protection have already expired.

CHAPTER 17

Second-Generation Products and Modified Chemistry

Modifying the chemistry of the active substance of a branded drug product has historically been one of the most successful lifecycle management (LCM) strategies of them all. The title we have chosen for this chapter, "Second-Generation Products and Modified Chemistry," covers a wide range of different strategies.

To leverage existing therapeutic area strengths, companies try to create follow-up molecules of their successful brands which they will introduce shortly before the patent on the successful brand expires, or once it becomes uncompetitive due to the appearance on the market of superior drugs from other companies. Three different strategic intents can be identified:

New Class, Same Disease. In this case the company develops or acquires a completely new molecular entity (NME) in an attempt to leverage its success in a particular disease area or with a particular medical subspecialty. As the company is recognized as a leader by its stakeholders in this arena, and as much of the company's expertise and many of its staff are tied to that disease area, it is far easier and less risky to build on existing strengths rather than to try to open up and gain critical mass and credibility in a new disease area. An example of this strategy would be Novartis's 2002 purchase of the renin inhibitor Rasilez®/Tekturna® (aliskiren) from Speedel (and subsequent acquisition of the company in 2008) in an attempt to maintain their strong position in the hypertension arena which had been built upon the success of their angiotensin receptor blocker, Diovan® (valsartan). The new drug may either be a replacement for or an addition to the existing drug. In the case of Rasilez/Tekturna® it was an addition, and a fixed-dose combination (FDC) of the two drugs (Valturna®) is already on the market. This is described in more detail in Case History 9 in the Appendix.

Pharmaceutical Lifecycle Management: Making the Most of Each and Every Brand, First Edition. Tony Ellery and Neal Hansen.
© 2012 John Wiley & Sons, Inc. Published 2012 by John Wiley & Sons, Inc.

This strategy represents LCM of a disease franchise rather than LCM of a brand, so we will not be going into it in more detail in this book.

Same Class, New Disease. In this case the company leverages its experience within a particular class of drugs to develop a new molecule of that class to address a new disease. Again, this lies outside the scope of this book. An example would be Genentech's modification of its anticancer Mab Avastin® (bevacizumab) to create the age-related macular degeneration Fab Lucentis® (ranibizumab).

Same Class, Same Disease. Here the company develops a new molecule to replace the existing product. This may be a mid-lifecycle strategy if the existing molecule is performing badly, or a late-stage lifecycle management (LLCM) strategy to shift physicians and patients to the new, patented molecule before the patent of the old one expires. The new drug may be clearly superior to the old. At the time of writing, for example, it does seem to be the case that Novartis's Tasigna® (nilotinib) may be more effective than the same company's Gleevec® (imatinib) in the treatment of chronic myeloid leukemia. Both drugs are tyrosine kinase inhibitors. The challenge for Novartis will be that Tasigna can expect generic competition when the Gleevec patent expires in 2015, and it will have to justify a very large price premium over generic imatinib.

Under the heading of "Same Class, Same Disease" there are many opportunities to slightly change a molecule in order to provide additional patient benefits or, all too often, in order merely to provide new patent protection. That is the area we will focus on for the rest of this chapter, as our book is concerned primarily with brand LCM and not with franchise LCM.

Here, again, we are in a controversial area of LCM. The brand company will always claim that the modified molecule offers incremental benefit to the patient while industry critics retort that the real reason is to gain exclusivity and higher pricing for a follow-up drug that is essentially no better than the original.

Let us now look at the different categories of chemical modification.

17.1 ISOMERISM

Isomers are compounds which have the same molecular formula but different structural formulas. Many different classes of isomers exist, such as stereoisomers, enantiomers, and geometrical isomers. Isomers do not necessarily share similar properties. The two main forms of isomerism are structural isomerism and stereoisomerism. In structural isomerism, the atoms and functional groups of the molecule are joined together in different ways. In stereoisomers, the structure of the bonds is the same, but the geometrical positioning of atoms and functional groups in space differs. This class includes enantiomers, where different isomers are mirror images of each other, and diastereomers when they are not.

Biological systems are sensitive to very small changes in structure and can respond very differently to isomers of the same compound.

Many drugs are racemic mixtures, or racemates. This means that they contain equal amounts of left- and right-handed enantiomers of a chiral molecule. Ibuprofen, thalidomide, and salbutamol are such racemic mixtures, and Teva's Adderall® is a mixture of several different amphetamine enantiomers. Different enantiomers may exert very different biological effects. One may be beneficial and the other harmful or less beneficial, for example.

This fact has been used as a way of extending the exclusivity of a racemic drug, by replacing the original drug with its patented and more efficacious isomer.

As with any patent, the applicant must prove that the invention is novel, innovative, and not obvious. Generally speaking, patent examiners are likely to assume that simply separating two isomers does not in itself constitute a nonobvious step, as there are many publications regarding the separation of isomers and the fact that isomers often show differences in biological activity. Only if the difference between the two isomers is greater than would be expected by our old friend "the ordinary person skilled in the art" is a patent likely to be granted or, if already granted, defensible. A patent might also be granted if it is very difficult to separate the two isomers and the innovation lies in the process for doing so. In one well-known old case, Lilly failed to patent the R-isomer of its own antidepressant, Prozac® (fluoxetine), and had to pay Sepracor for the rights to develop the improved version. Ultimately, the new drug did not make it to market because of an unacceptable side-effect profile. This was bad news for Lilly regarding the LCM of its Prozac franchise, but at least it saved the company the embarrassment of having to pay license fees on what should have been its own product!

A second example is probably the most famous—and infamous—examples of LLCM of recent years, when AstraZeneca succeeded in successfully transferring its proton-pump inhibitor franchise from Prilosec® (omeprazole) to the S-enantiomer of omeprazole, Nexium® (esomeprazole). This fascinating and multi-dimensional story is described in Case History 22 in the Appendix.

Today, both the Food and Drug Administration (FDA) and the European Medicines Agency (EMA) require that companies detail any isomeric properties of their drugs as an integral part of the approval process, so it has become increasingly difficult for a company to obtain regulatory approval of a racemic mixture. This LCM measure is therefore bound to lose in importance in the coming years.

17.2 POLYMORPHISM

Polymorphism is the ability of a solid material to exist in two or more different forms or crystal structures. A wide range of different factors involved in the crystallization process of a substance can be responsible for it appearing in different polymorphic forms. These include:

- Solvent effects
- Level of supersaturation
- Presence of impurities
- Temperature
- Stirring conditions

Many drugs receive regulatory approval for only a single crystal form or polymorph.

Importantly, the different polymorphs may show different solubilities or stabilities, and even different potencies, laying the way open for the granting of new patents—either for the originator or for generic companies—if these changes can be shown to be unexpected.

Worryingly for brand companies, there is a vast range of potential polymorphs for many drugs, and the increasingly sophisticated companies of the generics industry are just as likely to discover them as is the brand company itself.

Abbott's cephalosporin antibiotic Omnicef® (cefdinir) provides a wonderfully complicated example of a battle between a brand company and a whole bunch of generic companies centered on the polymorphism issue; between 1997 and 2004 Biochemie, ACS Dobfar, Ranbaxy, Aurobindo, Orchid, Lupin, and Novartis all patented different hydrated forms of cefdinir. Orchid patented the amorphous form, and the original inventors extended their patents to cover both the amorphous form and the suspension of an anhydrous formulation. Some of the patented hydrates with varying water content were characterized using basic techniques like X-ray powder diffraction (XRPD) and infrared spectroscopy which can only suggest that a different crystal structure is formed but not identify what this structure might be, or even to elucidate whether the different structure is in reality caused by impurities.

The case of Plavix® (clopidogrel), in both the United States and in Germany, is another interesting example, included as Case History 25 in the Appendix.

Several specialized companies offer high-throughput searches to identify the best polymorph of a drug early in development. More and more brand companies are utilizing these services or building their own in-house capabilities, so selection of the best polymorph is increasingly something which is done during the initial development of the drug rather than used later as an LCM strategy. As is the case with isomerism, regulatory authorities are increasingly asking for information on polymorphs when the drug is first filed with the agencies.

17.3   SALTS, ETHERS, AND ESTERS

Companies often attempt to obtain patents for new salts of known active ingredients. New salts may exhibit different stability or solubility profiles, and the latter may result in a different bioavailability profile. But it is common knowledge that this occurs, so merely deriving a salt from an acid or base will not warrant a patent claim. Not only are the salts themselves likely to be considered obvious, but the processes for creating such salts are also generally well known and are therefore difficult if not impossible to patent. Similarly, both ethers and esters of known alcohols are unlikely to support composition of matter or process claims. In rare cases, where the biological activity of the new salt is both unexpected and significant, a patent may be obtainable in some countries, or if the process for making it is extremely innovative. However, in the vast majority of cases, new salts, ethers, or esters will merely be considered as nonpatentable variants of the original molecule.

17.4 PRODRUGS AND METABOLITES

It makes sense to consider these two LCM strategies together.

A prodrug can be defined as a pharmacological substance that is administered in an inactive form, but which after administration is converted in the body to form an active metabolite. The rationale behind the use of a prodrug is usually to optimize absorption, distribution, metabolism, or excretion (ADME) of the drug.

The most common usage of prodrugs is in orally administered drugs, where the active substance is poorly absorbed from the gastrointestinal tract. Another benefit of prodrugs is that they may be less unpleasant for the patient to take than the active metabolite (e.g., unpleasant taste or painful injection). And prodrugs can be invaluable in targeted cancer therapy.

Let us look at a few examples. The ACE inhibitor enalaprilat is a potent ACE inhibitor, but it is poorly absorbed from the gut; its ethyl ester is absorbed much better, but is only a weak ACE inhibitor. This ester, enalapril maleate, is marketed by Merck as Vasotec®. It is hydrolyzed in the blood to form enalaprilat, which is thus its active metabolite. Chloramphenicol has a bitter taste because it is absorbed by the tongue, but its palmitate ester does not get absorbed and is therefore more palatable. And the succinate ester is very soluble, and therefore ideal for intravenous formulations. In the body, both esters are hydrolyzed to the active metabolite, chloramphenicol.

Another important example of prodrug usage is chemotherapy of cancer, where the active metabolites are very toxic. Where the prodrug reaches hypoxic cancer cells, it is converted by the large quantities of reductase enzyme present to the cytotoxic active metabolite. Toxic effects will be less in normal, noncancerous cells which are not hypoxic and which contain less reductase.

In today's rational drug design paradigm, it is most likely that the active metabolite will be identified first and then experiments conducted to find the best prodrug form in which it can be administered to the body. In the past, when drugs were more often discovered empirically, the opposite often occurred, the prodrug being discovered serendipitously sometimes years before the active metabolite was identified in drug metabolism studies. Once the active metabolite was identified, this opened the door to a rational search for improved prodrugs. Let us take a really old example to illustrate this, one in which the prodrug was marketed more than half a century before its active metabolite was finally identified. In 1886, acetanilide was serendipitously found to possess both analgesic and antipyretic properties, and found widespread usage in medical practice. However, it soon became clear that the drug had serious side effects, the most prominent of these being cyanosis due to methemoglobinemia. In 1947, it was finally demonstrated that paracetamol, which does not cause methemoglobinemia but which does express the same analgesic and antipyretic properties as acetanilide, was a major active metabolite of acetanilide. Later it was shown that phenacetin, which was also marketed as an antipyretic and analgesic—but which could cause nephropathy and cancer—was also metabolized *in vivo* to paracetamol. Today, paracetamol is one of the most widely used drugs in the world. It is the active substance in a wide range of headache, common cold, and flu remedies including Tylenol®, Panadol®, and Anacin®.

The significance of all of this in LCM is, of course, that prodrugs or active metabolites of known active substances may be patented, and these patents may either extend brand exclusivity or open the door to the development of a new, follow-on brand.

Novartis's Famvir® (famciclovir) is another example of a prodrug, and is included as Case History 13 in the Appendix. Famciclovir is a prodrug of penciclovir. Another good example of an active metabolite is provided by Schering-Plough's desloratadine (Clarinex®) which is the active metabolite of loratadine (Claritin®) and which is the subject of Case History 7 in the Appendix.

CHAPTER 18

Other Developmental LCM Strategies

There are several other potential lifecycle management (LCM) strategies that can be included under development measures of LCM but which do not warrant a chapter all to themselves.

18.1 MANUFACTURING STRATEGIES

Most of the focus on LCM is on what can be done to add value to the brand franchise from a development and marketing perspective, yet some significant benefits can be drawn from manufacturing-led LCM.

Enhanced Protection. Developing new, patent-protected manufacturing processes that supersede previous methods and eliminate impurities can provide valuable secondary patent protection that will raise the technical hurdles to competition.

Improved Differentiation. Brand companies sometimes try to delay generic entry by tightening the specifications on their products late in the life cycle. This is done in the hope that generic companies will not be able to meet the more stringent quality or bioequivalence standards, as they were creating their generics in comparison with the earlier, looser specifications.

Enhanced Profitability. By improving lean manufacturing processes, companies seek to minimize cost of goods and maximize profitability, giving greater flexibility in pricing later in the product life cycle. Additionally, as discussed before, companies may also look to relocate manufacturing to lower cost markets, or even outsource it completely to reduce overheads and drive a better bottom line.

Pharmaceutical Lifecycle Management: Making the Most of Each and Every Brand, First Edition.
Tony Ellery and Neal Hansen.
© 2012 John Wiley & Sons, Inc. Published 2012 by John Wiley & Sons, Inc.

18.2   WHITE PAPERS AND CITIZEN PETITIONS

White Papers are confidential communications from a company to the Food and Drug Administration (FDA) (or other health authority) regarding medical, technical, or scientific issues which may relate to safety and/or efficacy of their products or products of other manufacturers affecting the health and/or safety of patients. They are based on the uniqueness or peculiarities of the company's products, active ingredients, or labeling. They may also relate to samples of various commercially available products which the company has tested. The relevance to LCM, and particularly late-stage lifecycle management (LLCM), is that the brand company can make the health authority aware of short-comings in the quality of the upcoming generic offerings and, if the challenge is successful, delay or even prevent their market entry. This strategy can be very effective if there are real issues with the generic, and is most effective when several—or even all of—the potential generic competitors are obtaining supplies of a suspect active substance from the same active pharmaceutical ingredient (API) source. As such white papers are confidential documents, the authors are unable to give real-world examples, but white papers might be written if a brand company were to discover that the bioequivalent generic was using an excipient which could pose a health risk, or that a generic was only bioequivalent if given with meals but not if patients took it between meals.

Citizen Petitions are very similar, but are public documents filed with the FDA. Interested parties can comment to an open docket maintained by the FDA on the petition, and the FDA's response to the petition will be public. The FDA is required by law to respond within 180 days. In some cases where generic companies failed in their attempts to invalidate a patent on a new indication of a patent-expired brand, they have then pursued "carve-out" strategies where their Abbreviated New Drug Applications (ANDAs) are written in such a way that they only request approval for the earlier, nonpat-ented indications. The brand companies have reacted to this challenge by filing citizen petitions which argue that removal of safety information related to the new indication from the labeling would compromise the safety or efficacy of the drug in the new indication. Recently, brand companies have only been successful with this strategy in one case, when the FDA rejected a "carve-out" for Wyeth's Rapamune® (sirolimus). Brands which have failed with this defense strategy include Sanofi-Aventis/King's Tritace®/Altace® (ramipril) and Pfizer's Lyrica® (pregabalin). The decisions regarding some other labeling carve-outs are still pending. In one interesting case, Teva filed citizen petitions against four generic companies asking the FDA not to approve generic ANDAs of Copaxone®, their multiple sclerosis drug, based on difficulties in reliably proving bioequivalence. It is ironic that Teva, the biggest generic company in the world, uses the same LLCM weapon in its attempts to defend its biggest brand that brand companies use against companies like Teva. The case is as yet unresolved.

COMMERCIAL LCM

PART E

COMMERCIAL LCM

CHAPTER 19

Strategic Principles of Commercial LCM

As we have seen in earlier sections of this book, developmental strategies and tactics form the mainstay of most lifecycle management (LCM) activities early in the product life cycle. Commercial LCM tactics have traditionally been reserved for the later stages, close to patent expiry and beyond. However, commercial tactics are increasingly utilized throughout the product life cycle in today's world as the challenge of differentiation becomes more acute. Unlike developmental approaches, commercial LCM strategies do not focus on improving the clinical profile of the brand. Instead they focus on improving the commercial proposition of the brand family. In an idyllic world where the clinical profile of a brand is so well differentiated from the competition that usage is driven by this fact alone, such tactics can be reserved for competition with generics once they hit the market. Sadly, in practice very few brands have such an ideal and unique clinical profile, so a combination of developmental and commercial tactics is required much earlier.

Commercial tactics in general tend to be quicker, cheaper, and more responsive to market change than their developmental counterparts. There are three fundamental principles that drive the likely success of any commercial LCM strategy:

1. The ability to drive widespread and preferential patient access to the brand
2. The ability to defend market access and formulary position
3. The ability to optimize profitability of the brand franchise

The choice of commercial tactics and the approach to implementation, particularly within and across geographies, is without doubt one of the greatest challenges for LCM within the drug industry today. With significant diversity of regulatory, payer, market, and competitor dynamics across geographies, it

Pharmaceutical Lifecycle Management: Making the Most of Each and Every Brand, First Edition.
Tony Ellery and Neal Hansen.
© 2012 John Wiley & Sons, Inc. Published 2012 by John Wiley & Sons, Inc.

is essential to adopt flexible strategies that can be tailored locally to optimize success. As such, the success of commercial LCM lies significantly within the interplay between global and local teams, an area where the drug industry has not typically demonstrated its strengths.

Let us now consider each of these fundamental principles of commercial LCM in more detail and explore the factors that must be considered when planning for success.

19.1   COMMERCIAL LCM GOAL 1: THE ABILITY TO DRIVE WIDESPREAD AND PREFERENTIAL PATIENT ACCESS TO THE BRAND

It seems to be a fairly obvious statement that if a medically eligible patient (i.e., a patient suffering from a condition that the product is licensed for somewhere in the world) cannot get access to a pharmaceutical brand, then the growth of that brand will be limited. As such, it is also logical to highlight that the first goal of commercial LCM strategies is to drive widespread global access to as many patients as possible, seeking to overcome regulatory and payer (market access) hurdles to usage.

The first barrier that commercial strategies need to overcome is enabling a patient to access the drug in a regulator-approved manner. Expanding the approval base geographically is a key strategy at this stage which we will touch on later in the book, but does not represent the only way to increase patient access to the drug. For some drugs, tight regulatory restrictions at launch may lead to the need for expanded access programs to support other patients that need the drug, but cannot gain access through the open market—such programs can also be used before launch to ensure access to the drug for those patients that could truly benefit from the drug while the regulatory process is ongoing.

While the regulatory barrier is key to overcome, market access barriers are more commonly the target of commercial tactics, with the goal of driving preferential access to patients in a competitive environment. Tactics can range from pricing and discounting deals to ensure favorable formulary access, patient access programs to get the drug into the hands of needy patients who cannot afford the drug, and over-the-counter switching strategies to enable patients to purchase their preferred brands without the need to consult with a physician.

19.2   COMMERCIAL LCM GOAL 2: THE ABILITY TO DEFEND MARKET ACCESS AND FORMULARY POSITION

While commercial tactics can be used proactively to establish the optimum access, frequently, they are used reactively to defend a brand's access to patients in the light of competitive challenges that cannot be overcome with the core clinical story. Such challenges can include the launch of new competitive agents with superior clinical profiles, the release of challenging clinical data from a competitor (e.g., head-to-head trial results) or patent expiry and subsequent generic competition for a rival agent within the same class. In these situations, it is critical to develop strategic responses to overcome/circumvent subsequent stakeholder behaviors, such as the implementation of restrictive formularies, changes to tier status, and potential therapeutic substitution.

The launch of generic competition to Merck's osteoporosis agent Fosamax® (alendronate) in the United States led to just such a challenge to key competitor Actonel® (risedronate) from Procter and Gamble (P&G). With limited differentiation from the now very low-cost generic alendronate, P&G were forced to look to more radical cost-sharing deals with payers to ensure that formulary position could be maintained. Such deals are likely to become much more commonplace, alongside a broader range of commercial tactics that will be discussed later in the book, as the drug industry deals with an increasingly competitive and cost-pressured world.

19.3   COMMERCIAL LCM GOAL 3: THE ABILITY TO OPTIMIZE PROFITABILITY OF THE BRAND FRANCHISE

A critical goal of commercial LCM tactics throughout the brand life cycle is to optimize lifetime profitability; in other words, to make as much money as possible and the greatest return on investment from each and every asset. Commercial tactics play a key role in this process, particularly at the later stages of the product life cycle when the tactical choices (where to invest, where to cut investment, where to drop/raise prices) become much more heavily focused on profitability. This is also a key area where commercial LCM at the brand level overlaps with portfolio management, as companies determine which assets to support in different markets, and which assets to either sell or withdraw to maximize portfolio profitability.

The importance of maximizing profitability of late-stage assets, and the potential impact this can have on driving greater cash flow to the R&D efforts of the branded drug industry, has led to many players reorganizing and refocusing their efforts in this area. Companies including AstraZeneca, GlaxoSmithKline (GSK), Pfizer, and Abbott have all reinforced their drive through the launch of new Established Brands teams, partnering the goals of managing patent-expired portfolio in Western markets with the growth ambitions for "Emerging" markets such as China, India, and Latin America. We will discuss how such organizations are dealing with the challenge of portfolio management of late-stage assets later in this book, but at an individual brand level, the successful teams in the drug industry today are wrestling with the challenge of how to balance the right set of commercial tactics for each brand in each market to drive the elusive profitability goal.

CHAPTER 20

Geographical Expansion and Optimization

The most commonly applied commercial lifecycle management (LCM) strategy is geographic expansion. After all, it is common sense that the easiest way in which to expand your available treatable population is to ensure your product is available for use in as many countries as possible. However, drug companies are still in many cases behind the game in geographic optimization, and have some way to go in ensuring they are in the right countries, at the right time, with the right clinical and commercial proposition for their brands. Successfully executing a geographic optimization strategy for a brand is more than just expansion. It is about harmonization and rationalization of portfolios and determining when to exit a market, as well as when to enter. This concept of geographic optimization is gaining much greater traction with the need to realize growth from "emerging" markets while maximizing profits from established western markets.

The traditional brand management mentality focuses the team on the United States as the most valuable launch market. Fundamentally all prelaunch efforts should be targeted to getting the proposition right for the United States, and maybe the big five European markets (Germany, France, the United Kingdom, Spain, and Italy). As a result, the go-to-market strategy will almost certainly be heavily U.S.-centric, with other markets frequently left to do their best to adapt this approach to their local markets. Traditional lore would then see a Japan market entry strategy following some years down the line, with the need for bridging studies into the local population likely to drive delays in Japanese approval of anything between 2 and 10 years from initial Western launch. The rest of the world will follow later, but in most cases will be considered as tier-two or tier-three markets, with much less significant focus during the launch and growth phases of the life cycle. Only when the brand enters maturity will the global organization wake up to the fact that their future sales are now going to be reliant on markets where the impact of any

Pharmaceutical Lifecycle Management: Making the Most of Each and Every Brand, First Edition. Tony Ellery and Neal Hansen.
© 2012 John Wiley & Sons, Inc. Published 2012 by John Wiley & Sons, Inc.

patent expiries will be limited, and where sales can be maintained, or even grown, in a postpatent expired world.

However, this outdated view of the world is being challenged by changing country dynamics that are raising significant questions as to future priorities in global strategy. For some new brands, the United States is being deprioritized as the launch market owing to the challenge of approval by the Food and Drug Administration (FDA) and the requirement for supportive clinical data. For many of these agents, approval first in Europe is seen as a way forward, with the European Medicines Agency (EMA) seen as a more "reasonable" regulatory body to impress. Indeed, several key drugs have been successfully approved and launched in Europe ahead of the United States, including the antidiabetic agent Galvus® from Novartis, Johnson & Johnson's psoriasis drug Stelara®, and Eli Lilly/Daiichi Sankyo's antithrombotic Prasugrel®. Arguing against this trend, or suggesting a potential difference by therapeutic areas, was a report from researchers at the nonprofit advocacy group Friends of Cancer Research in early 2011. Their analysis of 35 cancer drug launches between 2003 and 2010 highlighted that of the 23 approved in both the United States and the European Union (EU), the U.S. approval was always faster, benefiting from the priority review process (allowing review within 6 months) compared with the much longer (350-day on average) EU process. Indeed, their analysis also highlighted that nine drugs had only been approved in the United States while there were only three that had EU approval but not U.S. approval.

While regulatory approval is one driver of market prioritization, a critical second is the behavior of pricing and reimbursement authorities when it comes to enabling drug access. Along this dimension, many European markets are increasingly being deprioritized, as the ability to gain reimbursement and desirable market access is becoming so challenging that launch resources could be better deployed elsewhere. Indeed, in recent years, each of the United Kingdom, France, and Germany have come under attack by the branded drug industry based on factors that decrease the potential for companies to drive growth of their new launch brands.

As early as 2004, Pfizer's then CEO Hank McKinnel attacked the European pricing policies on the back of its decision not to launch its pain agent Bextra® in France, where after a year of price negotiations, Pfizer would still have been forced to launch at a price 50% lower than elsewhere in Europe. McKinnel stated at the time that the European market accounted for only 22% of new drug launch sales, down from 50% in the 1970s, and that Pfizer was estimating Europe to drop to only 12% of launch sales in the near future.

While Europe is dropping in importance for many companies in terms of potential brand value, new markets are appearing as higher priorities for early exploitation. Southeast Asian markets such as Korea are becoming increasingly attractive, offering well-regulated competitive environments and strong growth dynamics. Meanwhile, the attractive growth dynamics of the BRICT (Brazil, Russia, India, China, and Turkey) markets are driving the drug industry to develop approaches to successful commercialization that overcome the challenges of operating within less actively regulated patent and exclusivity environments. As such, these markets are increasingly now becoming important throughout the product life cycle, not just at the end.

To explore how geographic optimization strategies can be tailored to the specific lifecycle needs of a brand and company, we will now consider the different options available and what is needed to execute a successful strategy.

20.1 GEOGRAPHIC EXPANSION

The primary geographic optimization strategy is expansion, as this enables the brand to reach more patients. Several factors need to be considered in designing this part of the brand LCM strategy:

Timing. Where is the best protection available for the brand, in terms of both regulatory and patent exclusivity? Where has the patent clock started ticking?

Growth Potential. Where are target patients located—are they more prevalent in specific geographies (e.g., hepatitis in Asian markets) or globally spread? In which markets is there greater access to medicines and reimbursement support for the drug class? Outside of reimbursed markets, where will patients be able to pay for the drug?

Competition. Where can a first-to-market advantage be gained? Where is the competition focused and can opportunities be found elsewhere? Where will generic, or copies/clones be available from launch?

Geographic Synergies. Where can synergies in regional rollout be found, for example, linking rollout in France with French-speaking North Africa taking advantage of strong intercountry links

One important element associated with geographic expansion is capability—that is, where is the company strong, and where is it weak, and thus where will it need to look to external support to drive geographic expansion. Partnerships are a common tool in driving geographic expansion, both in terms of extending reach (getting to new territories that the parent company cannot reach) and increasing share of voice in markets where the parent company is suboptimally present. The Roche organization is a clear example of a business that recognized the need to exploit different regional strengths to the benefit of the whole business. By linking Genentech, Roche, and Chugai together, the group could take advantage of therapeutic and geographic marketing experience and expertise across the globe. As such, a new drug developed by Roche in Europe could benefit from the specialist marketing expertise of Genentech in the United States and the Japanese prowess of Chugai to complement the European focus of Roche.

The Japanese pharmaceutical industry has through necessity led the way in many respects in trying to optimize partnership structures to globalize its assets. Takeda's global expansion was led through a series of different product partnerships to optimize the U.S. exposure to partner brands. The establishment of the joint venture TAP with Abbott gave the first opportunity to launch key brands such as Lupron® and Prevacid® in the United States, while out-licensing the antihypertensive candesartan to AstraZeneca in the United States provided the best route for a mass market agent. Following the setup of Takeda's North American subsidiary in the late 1990s, progression to a copromotion deal with Lilly for Actos® paved the way for future solo launches, including the gout drug Uloric® and the antiulcerant Kapidex®. Another Japanese player with a focus on geographic expansion has been Daiichi-Sankyo. The acquisition of Indian generic player Ranbaxy not only brought its fair share of challenges to the Japanese management team, but it also brought access to Ranbaxy's global distribution network through which it could launch its full range of products alongside an enviable generic portfolio.

20.2 HARMONIZATION AND RATIONALIZATION

Once a brand has been launched across the majority of markets, can one claim that the brand has now been truly geographically optimized? No, not yet. As the brand moves through the product life cycle, the challenge becomes to identify what the optimal clinical and commercial proposition is for each market, and how to realize a global strategy that provides the optimal profit balance.

For many established brands (those later in the product life cycle), significant diversity in brand-franchise composition can arise between markets, the result of different local markets taking responsibility for their own local line extension tactics (new dosage forms, routes of administration, etc.). Novartis's Voltaren® is a classic example of such a brand, now available in over 70 different formulations, combinations, and dosage forms, and rumored to have no two markets with the same set of commercially available forms! Voltaren is discussed in more detail in Case History 30 in the Appendix.

In such situations, commercial LCM strategies should focus on programs of harmonization and rationalization. Harmonization programs seek to identify where a formulation that is launched in one market or set of markets could be launched across a broader range of countries, thus driving a greater return on the original development investment. In an ideal world, such programs would be in place whenever the decision to invest in a local brand-extension strategy is made, but this is often not the case within many drug companies. By harmonizing later in the process, the target markets can assess the success of the strategy in the existing launch market, and thus be more confident of the potential value in their own markets.

By contrast with harmonization, rationalization seeks to identify where elements of the brand franchise should be withdrawn from the market once they are no longer commercially or strategically viable. This concept is much more challenging for companies to accept and adopt, and usually there is significant push back from the local markets. For the local brand manager, the thought of withdrawing part of their portfolio for any reason other than safety would be strongly resisted—after all, it is their portfolio to sell! In addition, if the brand is late in the life cycle and thus is receiving limited (or no) promotional support, any money generated is essentially free to the local affiliate. They will not see the cost of goods sold (COGS), distribution, and logistical costs which at a global level might make particular formulations unprofitable.

From a global perspective, the benefits of rationalization can be several-fold. First, by removing formulations that are no longer profitable from the market (once all costs of manufacturing and distribution have been considered), the net return from the franchise can be improved. Second, by reducing the number of individual dosage forms or stock keeping units (SKUs) within the portfolio, manufacturing and packaging efficiencies can be gained which will reduce the overall COGS of the portfolio.

One of the most significant resistors to rationalization activity, however, is the fear that withdrawing a drug for strategic, rather than safety, reasons will lead to a backlash from physicians and patients who will no longer be able to access the medicine. There are indeed a number of cases where this has proven to be true, including the decision by Novo Nordisk to withdraw their porcine insulin from the UK market in late 2007. The backlash from the patient community was significant toward Novo, as patients who had been stabilized on the older porcine products for many years rebelled against a decision they saw as purely strategically and financially motivated. Their demand in the end was met by the Indian generic player Wockhardt who provided an alternative with their Hypurin® porcine insulin range, while Novo focused on switching patients from the older animal insulin to the more modern recombinant human insulins and insulin analogs.

The decision of Novo to withdraw their porcine insulin range was not necessarily the wrong decision, but it may have been the way in which the withdrawal was managed that left something to be desired. One company that has developed a complementary business model for these situations is Idis, a UK-based solution provider to the drug industry that specializes in the provision of named-patient programs (NPP). Such programs are most commonly used early in the product life cycle, as part of prelaunch activity where NPPs are used to provide access to unlicensed medicines to patients who do not fit the criteria for ongoing clinical studies, or who need continued access to the drugs once a clinical study has completed and before the drug is formally approved.

NPP programs can also form a valuable element of the geographic optimization process, either as a way of providing a route for patients to access a specific formulation of a drug in markets where it has never been launched, or where it has been withdrawn. Such a program typically works by centralizing the storage and distribution of the manufactured product, and delivering the drug direct to the physician who requires it for a specific named patient for whom the drug is intended. Such programs can function globally, allowing for rationalization programs to take place while leaving in place a system which enables any remaining global supply of the formulation to be distributed to the patients that need it most, wherever in the world they may be. By centralizing the distribution, efficiencies in the supply chain can be realized, while the ethical concerns of withdrawal can be managed. Or in reverse, the needs of patient access in new markets can be met without the need for full marketing infrastructure to be in place.

Fundamentally, the goal of any harmonization or rationalization program is to ensure that the global brand profitability can be optimized within the context of ethical patient access to medicines wherever possible. Moving forward, this is likely to become an increasing feature of the most successful established product and mature brand teams within the drug industry.

CHAPTER 21

OTC Switching

While geographic expansion is one way to drive greater access to patients, switching to "over-the-counter" (OTC) status is another option, essentially enabling the company to communicate directly with the patient and to drive the patient to make the final treatment choice. Now this strategy is rather obviously not open to all drugs. It would not make sense to allow a patient to walk into a pharmacy and buy whatever he wanted. But it has increasingly become an important consideration for the drug industry as it seeks both to establish a greater presence in growth markets and to shore up industry prospects in an increasingly generic Western market environment. Figure 21.1 highlights some of the drivers of Rx versus OTC strategy for different brands.

The best-known strategy here is the formal Rx to OTC switch. This is typically only applicable to drugs treating indications that can be self-diagnosed, self-treated, and self-monitored. The most common agents that meet these requirements are mild painkillers, allergy drugs, and treatments for gastrointestinal disorders such as heartburn, acid reflux, diarrhea, and constipation. There have been many successful OTC switches over the last 10 years, with well-known brands such as Pepcid®, Voltaren®, Zyrtec®, and Prilosec® all being switched in some form or another to OTC status.

Efforts have been made to extend the scope of agents that could be switched to OTC status, driven both by a push from the drug industry and by a pull from health authorities. Indeed, back in 2002, the United Kingdom Medicines and Healthcare Products Regulatory Agency (MHRA) released a position paper highlighting 12 potential drug classes that were considered at the time as viable for OTC switching, including antihypertensives, proton-pump inhibitors, and even Viagra®. This in part led to Merck & Co. experimenting with the OTC switch of a low-dose formulation of its blockbuster statin Zocor® (simvastatin), which it launched in the United Kingdom under the brand OTC

Pharmaceutical Lifecycle Management: Making the Most of Each and Every Brand, First Edition.
Tony Ellery and Neal Hansen.
© 2012 John Wiley & Sons, Inc. Published 2012 by John Wiley & Sons, Inc.

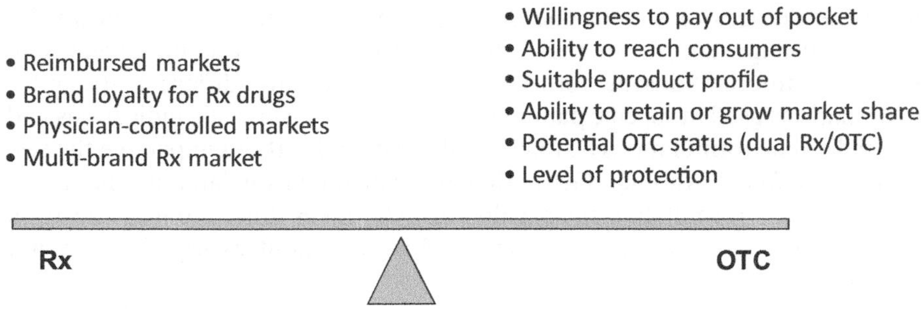

- Reimbursed markets
- Brand loyalty for Rx drugs
- Physician-controlled markets
- Multi-brand Rx market

- Willingness to pay out of pocket
- Ability to reach consumers
- Suitable product profile
- Ability to retain or grow market share
- Potential OTC status (dual Rx/OTC)
- Level of protection

Rx   OTC

FIGURE 21.1. Balance between Rx and OTC strategies. *Source:* Datamonitor.

Zocor HeartPro® in 2004. The success of this agent was limited (only taking 1% of the franchise within the first quarter), and the performance has not triggered a windfall of copycat OTC switches from the other statins. The primary reason for this is likely to be the challenge of encouraging a patient to continue to buy the drug OTC, when they have no real symptoms of the disease. Unlike pain, allergy, or gastrointestinal (GI) disorders, patients requiring statins do not immediately feel the benefits of their medication, nor do they feel the consequences of not taking it. As such, it is much more likely that patients will become noncompliant. Now some would argue that if people take vitamins and minerals on a daily basis to keep healthy, why not a statin? It is something of a quandary, but is most likely explained by the consumer believing that vitamins and minerals are "natural" therapies, and thus more acceptable, than something they see as more of an artificial drug. In addition, the costs of self-medicating with Zocor HeartPro were not attractive compared with taking the prescription drug. Indeed, at launch, a 1-month supply cost £12.99, compared with the prescription charge at the time of just £6.65.

The process by which a brand is switched can be complex and costly and is governed by the type of OTC status sought (which varies between markets) and the subsequent requirement (or not) of supportive clinical data and specific formulations to enter the market. Now the authors of this book are by no means experts in the regulatory technicalities of the OTC switch—that is best left to true specialists—but the success of an OTC strategy will be shaped by a number of factors, including choice of dosages to switch, geographic focus of strategy, timing of launch, and level of corporate support. Let us look at each of these in turn and assess how they have been used in the past to influence lifecycle management (LCM) strategy.

21.1 WHAT TO SWITCH: CHOOSING THE BEST APPROACH

The first critical factor to consider is what formulations or dosages to switch to OTC—should one just switch the entire brand franchise, selected commercially available dosages or should one develop a new formulation specifically for OTC? An important factor that will influence this choice is the diversity of usage of different dosage forms—in other words are different strengths/ formulations used in specific patient populations or for specific indications and can individual formulations be realistically switched without impacting the rest of the portfolio? Another factor that we will touch on later is timing—to develop a new formulation specifically for OTC takes time, and if the decision to switch is made late in the life cycle, close to patent expiry, this may not be viable.

The ability to gain regulatory exclusivity can also be a driver of choice in choosing what to switch. In many countries, periods of market exclusivity can be granted to OTC switches where significant new clinical data have been required to support the switch. In the United States, 3 years of OTC market exclusivity can be awarded in such a situation, while in Europe, an additional 1 year of exclusivity for the OTC form is possible. In many cases, the easiest way to gain this exclusivity is to develop specific formulations or dosage forms to switch which will be supported by their own clinical data package. This is obviously a more costly strategy, but the benefits of first-to-market advantage and exclusivity can outweigh the costs in many situations.

Another consideration is the company's future presence in the therapeutic category, which can play out in two key dimensions. On one side, switching an older franchise to OTC can create "space" for new drug classes to enter and allow the marketing organization to focus on the new agent. This works well if the new drug class is well differentiated from the switched class, so not threatened by a reinforced OTC market. On the flip side, an aggressive OTC switch of a full brand franchise could be detrimental to a company that has a less well-differentiated future portfolio, and in this case may benefit from a switch of only those elements of the brand franchise that targeted milder disease.

The case studies presented in the Appendix for Claritin®/Clarinex® from Schering-Plough (Case History 7) and Losec®/Nexium® from AstraZeneca (Case History 22) highlight how the decision to switch to OTC, and specifically what to switch, can have a major impact on portfolio success. On the positive side, the decision by AstraZeneca to develop a low-dose formulation of Losec to launch OTC in the United States demonstrated how to effectively use OTC as a pull-through for a future franchise. With 3 years of exclusivity on the OTC form, AstraZeneca was able to capture patients that would not typically present to a physician on the low-dose form while maintaining a therapeutic role in the more severe patients presenting to a physician with the standard Losec doses and more importantly, the more potent Nexium franchise. In an ideal situation, AstraZeneca could capture patients earlier in the disease with the OTC form and then, should their disease progress, transition them to the Nexium franchise in the physician's office, minimizing potential loss to standard omeprazole generics (after all, they had already failed on omeprazole, albeit the OTC form).

By contrast, Claritin's OTC switch in the United States essentially destroyed the Rx market for the entire class, significantly inhibiting the potential of the Rx follow-up agent Clarinex. In this case, the entire Claritin franchise was switched without the need for new studies, so no exclusivity was granted, and multiple OTC versions of the parent molecule were launched at the same time (at patent expiry of the Claritin brand). Clarinex was not deemed sufficiently differentiated by payers and prescribers to the now available OTC forms to resist negative class-level effects, and the decision of payer groups in the United States to drive patients to OTC led to a significant worsening of the reimbursement tier status of Clarinex, essentially killing the brand. Now hindsight is a wonderful thing, and the exact same situation may have played out with standard generic competition had Schering-Plough not decided to launch OTC; Clarinex's future was always on a knife-edge based on its failure to significantly differentiate. Indeed the decision to launch the OTC form at least secured a revenue stream in the consumer market from the franchise moving forward, which may not have been the case in the Rx market. However the comparison between the success of the AstraZeneca Losec/Nexium strategy and that of Schering-Plough does illustrate the critical issues of what to switch, how to benefit from switching, and what to try to avoid in terms of portfolio-wide impact.

21.2   WHERE TO SWITCH: DEALING WITH INTERMARKET VARIABILITY

The success of an OTC strategy is as much about where it is implemented as it is about what to switch—even the best thought-out strategy can flounder if it fails to align with local market dynamics in terms of OTC classifications, patient willingness to pay, and other critical stakeholder dynamics. The world is far from a uniform place when it comes to pharmaceuticals, and the OTC markets are no different, with significant variations in strategy required for any kind of pan-market roll-out plan.

The first factor that will shape strategy and approach is the OTC status that can be awarded in different markets. Most markets operate either a two- or a three-status system, with each having a full Rx status (prescription only) and a full OTC status (on the pharmacy shelf, no need for health-care professional input—known as general sales list in some markets such as the United Kingdom). The markets with the additional third tier tend to have an option for "behind-the-counter" (BTC) or pharmacy-only medicine where the patient must ask a pharmacist specifically for the drug and the pharmacist can use his or her judgment to determine if it is appropriate. The value of this third tier of OTC is that it enables a broader range of agents to be considered for switching, as it provides regulators with the reassurance of a health-care professional-controlled step in the patient acquisition process. Recent switches that have benefited from this form of classification in the United Kingdom include OTC Heart-Pro® from Merck as described earlier in this chapter, together with the antiobesity drug orlistat and the erectile dysfunction agent Viagra, all of which would have struggled to get approved as true OTC agents.

The debate over BTC versus OTC and Rx has raged for several years in the United States, where current legislation only supports a two-status model except in very rare occasions such as the BTC status awarded to the emergency contraceptive Plan B® for women over the age of 18. Proponents of BTC claim greater access to drugs and health-care system savings, while opponents focus on issues regarding patient safety and concerns that insurers may no longer cover certain medicines, raising the costs to consumers. In 2009, the U.S. Government Accountability Office (GAO) updated a 1995 study focused on exploring the potential of a formal BTC system in the United States, taking learnings from the United Kingdom, Australia, Italy, and the Netherlands as markets that had all implemented changes to their classification systems since the original 1995 report. The study not only acknowledged many benefits of the BTC classification, but also highlighted significant logistical, training, and implementation barriers to making it a reality in the United States. That said, the focus of the U.S. Health-Care system on finding ways to reduce health-care spending may well lead to further consideration of an expanded BTC system in the future, opening the U.S. market to a broader range of OTC options.

OTC status on its own is not the only factor that will influence in which markets a company may consider switching a formulation to OTC. A second key consideration is what happens to the Rx form once the OTC form is available. In many markets, a drug is either OTC or Rx, but cannot be both—as such, switching to OTC means the switched drug can no longer be prescribed by a physician, only recommended for purchase as an OTC. This can prove a significant challenge in markets where copy products or clones exist before patent expiry. In Spain for example, an OTC switch can be a disaster for a brand, as the prevalence of copy products which would still have Rx status enables physicians to continue prescribing competitor versions of the same molecule instead of recommending the OTC-switched brand (which they can no longer prescribe). By contrast, the UK system allows for dual Rx/OTC status, allowing physicians to still prescribe the drug even if it is available OTC. As such, the competitive risk of a Spanish OTC switch is considerably higher than a UK OTC switch for many agents.

Success in an OTC market rather obviously requires one key factor—a willingness of the patient to pay for an OTC medication, or more specifically, to pay the difference between an Rx and an OTC medicine. This willingness itself can also be a key shaping factor in the decision of where to switch. In the United States, the question is the difference in price between the full out-of-pocket cost of the OTC versus the co-pay for a similar Rx agent. In the United Kingdom, it may be the difference between the standard prescription charge for an Rx drug and the acquisition price of the OTC. In these markets, in many cases, the OTC form works out cheaper than the Rx and thus is supported by patients.

In markets where the provision of health-care services is fully state funded, patients are often unwilling to consider paying for their own medicines as the difference in out-of-pocket expenditure between an Rx medicine (which will often be free) and the OTC form can be significant. In France for example, the OTC market is very limited as the out-of-pocket expenditure of Rx medication is so small that patients are unwilling to switch to an OTC form. This is further compounded by a general perception in France that OTC agents are largely ineffective compared with Rx drugs. In markets such as France, the validity of an OTC switch is limited, and competing more effectively in the Rx market is often the best route.

A third category of markets that should be considered are the extensively self-pay markets, where patients are responsible for the costs of their own drugs even for Rx products. In these countries, the line between Rx and OTC is significantly blurred, particularly outside of the hospital sector, with retail pharmacies playing a much greater role in the dispensing decision for all drugs and patient choice carrying a greater influence. In these countries, many Rx drugs are handled more like BTC drugs in markets such as the United Kingdom, with the pharmacist dispensing therapies which officially require a prescription, but which in reality are deemed safe enough for a patient to buy direct. In these markets, the decision to formally switch a drug to OTC may not in reality make a significant difference to usage, and thus may not make sense. However, the OTC mentality of pharmacist focus, patient-centric packaging, and so on, may be more important to support the Rx brands, thus blurring the line between traditional pharmaceutical and consumer goods marketing approaches.

The bottom line regarding where to switch is simple—there is no such thing as a global OTC switch strategy—companies should instead focus on providing the tools and support to enable individual markets to determine the risk/reward profile of an OTC switch and develop a tailored approach to optimize value.

21.3   WHEN TO SWITCH: BALANCING THE PRODUCT LIFE CYCLE?

Choosing when to switch a brand to OTC can make the difference between a well-coordinated success, and a free-for-all with multiple players operating at the same time. Balancing the right point in the life cycle to switch can be a real challenge, with the goal of minimizing impact on the value of the Rx market while maximizing the opportunity to create a sustainable long-term OTC offering. Switching earlier in the life cycle gives time to build a sustainable uptake before competition arrives, but at the cost of lower revenue and

profits (as OTC products typically command lower prices with increased promotion costs). Switching later can minimize impact on the Rx market before
patent expiry, but can also lead to a more competitive landscape at launch.

Two primary influencing factors in the timing of switch relate to what is
being switched and any regulatory exclusivities that can be gained. If the entire
franchise is being switched, and there is no exclusivity to be gained, the only
way to get any form of first-to-market advantage will be to launch ahead of
patent expiry—sacrificing some of the Rx value to gain a head start in the
OTC market. Alternatively, launching OTC at the point of patent expiry and
taking on whatever competition arrives from the start can be a viable strategy
if the company has a well-structured OTC business and is likely to succeed in
the face of competition. By contrast, if only certain dosage forms are to be
launched OTC, the flexibility of timing is greater with earlier launching now
viable without impacting the full Rx market. If an exclusivity period is also
awarded, then launching close to, or even after patent expiry can be managed
without the concern over immediate competition—that way, full revenues
from the Rx market can be reaped ahead of a period of exclusive life for the
OTC brand as well.

In reality, the decision of when to switch will also be influenced by competition. If the opportunity to be the first-in-class OTC is open, but only if switching ahead of patent expiry, a company must weigh up the benefits of OTC class
leadership versus lost Rx revenue. By contrast, if a company knows it will be
a late entrant in the OTC market, it can wait to the last minute to launch an
OTC version knowing that others have already built OTC demand that they
may be able to capitalize on.

21.4   HOW TO MAKE THE SWITCH SUCCESSFUL: WHAT CORPORATE SUPPORT IS REQUIRED?

Just reclassifying a brand's status to OTC is not sufficient to drive success. It
is also essential that the appropriate organizational structure is put behind the
new brand to drive consumer interest. Companies driving success in OTC
typically have dedicated consumer health-care businesses that can support an
OTC franchise with complementary product lines. These businesses typically
need access to different marketing channels, including direct-to-consumer
advertising outside of the United States, in-store promotions, and strong pharmacy relationships. For many companies, this does not come naturally, so the
best route to an effective OTC launch is to partner with an established player.
A good example of this was the OTC launch of Roche's orlistat, a weight-loss
agent sold as Xenical® in the Rx market and as Alli® in the OTC market. To
support effective commercialization of the consumer version of the drug,
Roche granted exclusive worldwide rights excluding Japan to GlaxoSmithKline
(GSK) Consumer Healthcare, recognizing the value in using an established
player to drive greater reach.

In summary, the OTC switch strategy can be effective for selected brands in specific markets, provided the corporate structure is present to support the launch. Driving a long-term opportunity in the consumer market can be an effective way to extend a product's value-generating life cycle, but the reality is that it is simply not a feasible strategy for many brands in indications that cannot be self-managed.

CHAPTER 22

Brand Loyalty and Service Programs

The concept of "brand loyalty" is something that some parts of the drug industry believe they have mastered in that they are able to drive preferential use of their brand over that of a rival, even at times when their own brand is at best similar, and occasionally slightly inferior, on a purely clinical basis. However, we would challenge that what the drug industry has in the most part achieved is "molecular loyalty" as opposed to true brand loyalty. Stakeholders may indeed be committed to the value of the molecular entity (i.e., the drug itself), but their true loyalty to the brand (i.e., what else the company provides) is less strong, as witnessed by the often very aggressive generic erosion of what had previously been a very brand-loyal product.

The value of specific brand loyalty programs changes at different stages of the product life cycle, primarily on the basis of different stakeholder influence in the pre- and postpatent expiry phases. In the prepatent expiry phase, the physician remains the key stakeholder, with the payer and patient as the primary influencers. Schemes targeted to these three will be the focus for success. Once generic competition is available, the pharmacist gains in importance, as do the payer and patient, while in many markets the influence of the physician is significantly reduced in the final dispensing decisions.

In the early launch stages of a brand, support programs are likely to focus on one or more of three drivers of growth—education, logistical support, and reimbursement/payer support. Physician-targeted continuing medical education (CME) schemes and patient-targeted disease awareness sites are common programs put in place for launch brands, with the goal of increasing diagnosis rates for the targeted disease and early adoption of the new molecule. The services can be provided directly by the promoting company, or in partnership with one of the large number of specialist medical education providers, and typically form a core part of the launch marketing plan.

Pharmaceutical Lifecycle Management: Making the Most of Each and Every Brand, First Edition.
Tony Ellery and Neal Hansen.
© 2012 John Wiley & Sons, Inc. Published 2012 by John Wiley & Sons, Inc.

Logistical support services are less common, and tend to focus on drugs with specific logistical challenges in getting the drug to the patient—or the patient to the drug. When Eli Lilly first launched the antisepsis drug Xigris® in the United States, they faced a timing challenge—on the one side, the drug needed to be administered within a very tight treatment window after the diagnosis of severe sepsis, but on the other side, hospital pharmacists did not want to stock such an expensive drug that would only be required on very rare occasions. To deal with this challenge, Lilly partnered with logistics provider Syncor International in 2001 to ensure that the drug could be delivered anywhere in the United States within 3 h, ensuring that pharmacies that did not, or could not, stock the drug were still able to meet patient and physician need.

For Novartis's osteoporosis agent Aclasta®, the challenge was/is to get the patient to the drug, not so much the other way around. Unlike its oral rivals, which could be simply collected from the nearest pharmacy, Aclasta needed to be administered as a 15-min infusion, which in many cases could not be handled in the doctor's office. In Canada, Novartis developed the "For My Bones" program to include patient and physician tools to enable easy identification of infusion centers where Aclasta could be administered. The goal of the program was to make the process as smooth and as hassle-free as possible, partnering the logistical support with other patient education materials to ease the overall management of osteoporosis. By ensuring patients could only access the site if enrolled in the physician's office, Novartis could also ensure the program was specific to Aclasta patients, creating a tailored community for its patients that it hoped could help drive compliance with the once-yearly treatment plan.

The third challenge many brands face at launch is reimbursement support, so a further focus for support services can be in the provision of reimbursement assistance or support programs, targeted both to physicians and patients. For physicians, services include support with paperwork processing and support in communications with payer authorities on behalf of individual patients. Depending on the national reimbursement system and the status of the individual drug (e.g., if prior authorization is required or specific diagnostic testing before a treatment is approved for reimbursement), such paperwork challenges can be significant for physicians, and any support provided by the drug company can be highly beneficial. For patients, the programs can include call centers to advise on reimbursement support, specific patient assistance programs for people with inadequate coverage, and starter pack/bridging programs to enable patient access while insurance coverage is under negotiation. One such example is the Lundbeck SHARE® program, which supports patients and caregivers in the epilepsy market. Sabril® (vigabatrin) is indicated as adjunctive therapy for patients with refractory complex partial seizures (CPS) who have inadequately responded to several alternative treatments and for whom the potential benefits outweigh the risk of vision loss. As the drug carries a significant risk of permanent vision loss, Sabril is available only through a special restricted distribution program called SHARE (http://www.lundbeckshare.com). For health-care professionals, the SHARE program provides a registration process to enable them to prescribe the drug, education materials, and support services for patient access and reimbursement. For patients, the site provides a reimbursement support service, co-pay assistance, and a patient starter Rx program to cover delays in insurance approval (where permitted). The site also provides information of patient assistance programs for uninsured patients. By providing these support resources, Lundbeck aims to ease what would otherwise be a very complex prescription and approval process while providing the regulators with the oversight required to ensure the drug can only be used in patients with the appropriate risk/benefit profile.

The launch phase is not the only point in the life cycle where support and service programs can play a valuable role. Throughout the on-patent life, service programs can be put in place to ease drug access, enhance patient experience, and improve outcomes, both in terms of patient health and utilization of health-care resources. The competitive environment in the growth hormone sector, which saw five key players compete for many years, led to the evolution of well-developed service and support programs as all of the players sought to differentiate their brands (which were medically almost identical) from their rivals. Pfizer's Genotropin® brand has been supported by numerous programs including disease awareness, physician and nurse support programs, multiple delivery devices (including a Pen delivery system, a disposable pre-filled device, and flexible dosing through a traditional syringe), and reimbursement support, including the Pfizer BRIDGE Program® which provides families with patient care consultants to support through the treatment and reimbursement process.

In the later stages of the product's life cycle, when a brand is facing up to competition either for new agents entering the market or from impending or direct generic competition, it can be very easy for companies to make the decision to withdraw support programs, focusing on cost reduction to improve profitability. Indeed, when facing generic competition, it can be a major challenge to justify spending on support programs when health-care systems seem to be driven more by cost than by value. In these stages of the life cycle, the critical balance that must be struck is to invest in programs targeted toward stakeholders that can actually influence the *dispensing* decision, not just the prescription process. As such, in many markets, the physician is no longer a valuable target for support programs, as pharmacist substitution rules will often negate their influence. In general, at this point in the life cycle, four main clusters of country can be identified, largely based on the balance of power of stakeholders, and as such, the mix of programs should be varied accordingly:

- Payer-controlled markets (including Germany, the United States): In these countries, payer policy is strictly enforced, with physicians and pharmacists having limited power to significantly influence choice of brand once a generic is available. In such markets, patients are often forced to pay more if they want the brand, so programs targeted to the payer should be the focus, with the goal of limiting additional cost to the patient where possible if they stick with the brand. The case study illustrating the support programs put in place for Enbrel® in Germany, included in the Appendix, details how Wyeth partnered with one of the largest sick funds to deliver programs that ensured greater compliance for Enbrel, driving enhanced value to the payer (improved outcome, better utilization of resources) while securing a better working relationship with Wyeth at a time of significantly increasing competition, and potential future generic/biosimilar competition.

- Pharmacist-controlled markets (including the United Kingdom, Norway): In these countries, pharmacists are the primary stakeholder driving generic switching and as such, pharmacist-targeted programs may be required. A key challenge here is that for the most part, brand companies have traditionally ignored the pharmacist as a key stakeholder, so implementing programs for the pharmacist is often challenging. In addition, the generics industry has by contrast focused heavily on the pharmacist as an influential customer, making the job even harder for brand companies. Beyond financial deals (covered in the next chapter), the opportunities for pharmacist-targeted services may be limited.

- Physician-influenced markets (including Japan, France, Spain, and Italy): In these countries, physicians still have significant control over the final dispensing decisions, and brand loyalty programs targeted toward physicians will still carry value.

- Patient-driven markets (self-pay markets including most of the BRICT [Brazil, Russia, India, China, and Turkey] countries and many growth markets): In these countries, patients are the final decision makers and pay out of pocket, so programs must be targeted to their needs and the needs of those who can influence their spending (e.g., physicians), irrespective of lifecycle stage.

As highlighted at the start of this chapter, the goal of brand loyalty and support/service programs is to build added value beyond the molecule itself, which is realized as a perceived, or ideally proven, outcome benefit for the health-care system, either in terms of patient outcome benefit or an improvement in health-care utilization. The overall goal should be to prove that the support services ensure better "value" for money from treating with the brand than with a competitor, generic or otherwise. As such, it is difficult to talk about service programs independently of one key area of focus in improving this perception of value—namely acquisition price. This is the focus of the next chapter, and in many cases, it is the interplay of value-added services with strategic pricing programs that will lead to sustainable success.

CHAPTER 23

Strategic Pricing Strategies

While pricing is not traditionally seen as one of the pillars of lifecycle management (LCM), the reality of the drug industry world today is such that the balance between clinical (efficacy, safety, outcomes) and commercial (price, access) value propositions is so important that both principles must be interlinked. Understanding the forces that impact pricing strategy throughout the product life cycle is essential for effective LCM planning, while exploring the tools available to enhance the overall value proposition at different stages can make the difference between success and failure.

The interplay between three key factors will traditionally influence the pricing strategy for a brand family:

- The stage of the product life cycle—launch, growth, or expiry
- The geographical focus of the brand and the influence of different stakeholders within each country
- The level of competitive differentiation and competitor strategy

23.1 PRICING STRATEGY AND TACTICS IN THE LAUNCH AND GROWTH PHASES

During the development phase, one of the most important factors that influence the choice of first indication will be the expected market access environment—which option will provide the best chance of achieving a price that provides the greatest chance of strong return of investment (ROI) from the full development plan? For many companies, this leads to a search for a niche indication that could potentially carry an orphan drug designation, providing extended regulatory exclusivity and the greater chance of premium

Pharmaceutical Lifecycle Management: Making the Most of Each and Every Brand, First Edition.
Tony Ellery and Neal Hansen.
© 2012 John Wiley & Sons, Inc. Published 2012 by John Wiley & Sons, Inc.

pricing. However, while niche indications may provide for a high price at launch, such a price would not be sustainable if the brand is targeted for mass market indications later in the life cycle. Indeed, starting the regulatory "clock" with a niche indication may limit the ability to generate the full returns from a larger target population that launches later with a reduced exclusivity window, even if the first indication carries an orphan designation.

In general, the goal should be to select an indication and a target population within that indication that allows for the optimum balance between maximizing return with one that will provide the greatest market access. But what happens if the market access story is not strong enough to convince payers and providers to reimburse and/or use the drug at the desired price? Is dropping the price to the "desired" level the only way forward? Now we have discussed earlier in this book the option of patient selection—using prognostic criteria to help select which patients are most likely to respond to the drug or which patients are likely to have an adverse reaction to the drug. By selecting the patients with the most favorable risk/benefit profile, a stronger pharmaco-economic argument can be built to help sustain the desired launch price. But again, what happens if a company cannot predict who will respond well and who will respond badly? What are the pricing options available then to support launch at a sustainable price?

At its most basic level, the only way forward is to reduce the cost to the health-care system, typically in one of two ways—drop the list price or rebate the system for failures. The first is the easiest to implement but potentially the most negatively impactful. By reducing the list price, the pharmacoeconomic argument can obviously be improved, but at what cost to the brand? If the price needs to be reduced in one country to ensure reimbursement, it may lead to broader price reductions in countries that reference the initial target market, leading to an overall price reduction simply to keep one country happy. Additionally, dropping the price at launch might negatively impact the future potential of the brand, if subsequent indications would be able to gain strong market access with the initial target price. In reality, it is very difficult for companies in most markets to raise the price significantly after launch, even with new indications. The general rule is that the price can easily come down, but list price increases will typically only be reserved for cases where a significant new formulation has launched which cannot be interchanged with the original dosage forms—for example, the launch of a patch formulation compared with a base oral. Back in 2006, Andrew Witty, then Head of European Pharmaceuticals at GlaxoSmithKline (GSK), announced the company was exploring novel pricing models with two European countries whereby the company would be allowed to increase or reduce the list price of its drugs *after* launch based on the outcome of critical Phase IV clinical trials. This would therefore allow GSK to consider launching at a lower price to attract reimbursement with a limited launch data package, with the reassurance that the price could be increased at a later date should the broader Phase IV data prove to be of greater value. Alternatively, it could allow the health authorities to accept a higher price with the reassurance that prices would be dropped if the follow-on data were not as robust as the company expected. Whether GSK moved closer to agreement with these discussions or not, this has not been seen as a widely accepted approach with payers, particularly in Europe, where the list price is not often the tool used for negotiation.

What has increased in prevalence is the risk share/rebate deal, whereby the company agrees to accept some of the financial risk of nonperformance of the brand to allow access to the drug at the desired price. Typically, such deals revolve around the drug company rebating the cost of "failed" patients to the health authority, thus reducing the overall cost of drug use. This is essentially a retrospective personalized medicine approach—in the end, the health-care system only pays for the patients who respond to the therapy. This tactic has been commonly applied in the United Kingdom for high-priced biologics in the oncology market, where the standard cost-effectiveness argument would not stand up to National Institute for Health and Clinical Excellence (NICE) scrutiny. Famously in 2007, NICE endorsed a proposed risk-sharing deal put forward by Janssen-Cilag for the multiple myeloma agent Velcade®, which would see patients who demonstrated full or partial response to therapy after a maximum of four treatment cycles being kept on therapy, fully reimbursed by the National Health Service (NHS). By contrast, anyone showing a minimal or no response would be taken off the drug and the costs of the drug reimbursed by the manufacturer. This allowed Janssen to maintain a desired price in the United Kingdom, while still maintaining a good market access position.

Rebating the system the costs of drug failure is not the only option available for companies seeking to enhance their launch market access position. Following on from the Velcade deal in the United Kingdom, the launch of Revlimid® (lenalidomide) by Celgene, also for multiple myeloma, was supported by a deal that would see the NHS pick up the costs of the first 2 years of treatment, while Celgene would bear the costs for any patient requiring therapy beyond the 2 years. At an annual cost of therapy of around £36,000, the deal ensured that the NHS could effectively predict the maximum cost per patient with the reassurance of not having to restrict supply to patients requiring longer term therapy.

When faced with the challenges of launching Aclasta® as a once-yearly therapy for osteoporosis, Novartis had to overcome the challenge of a very high upfront cost to payers compared with the more traditional weekly oral therapies. In Germany and several other countries, Novartis developed innovative risk-sharing deals that would essentially insure the payer against drug failure, which for an osteoporosis drug means a fracture, during the first 12 months of therapy. In an excerpt from the company's 6-K filing in February 2008, Novartis highlighted that this helped to speed up reimbursement negotiations for Aclasta with German authorities and that such novel commercial models would become increasingly common. Joe Jiminez, then Head of the Pharmaceutical division was quoted as saying:

Payers obviously want fair value for their investment and if we offer them guaranteed value for their money, very often they will accept our prices. I think you can offer an attractive proposition if you have differentiated products in a specialty category. We start to reflect on the payer's value proposition very early in our development process and the end point is reflected in our clinical and marketing plans. This will become an integral part of our marketing strategy.

So a company has its brand on the market, with favorable pricing and good market access . . . all is well with the world and they can sit back and relax, right? Sadly, this is most certainly not the case for most brands in today's world—as the product moves through its on-patent life cycle, its pricing strategy will be challenged with both opportunities and threats that must be effectively managed. In terms of opportunities, companies need to explore how brand-value arguments (in terms of either pricing or formulary position) can be enhanced by further LCM efforts—where can premium prices be achieved? How can preferential tier status or formulary positioning be achieved? By contrast, threats are primarily the result of changes in an ever-evolving competitive landscape, be it from a new competitor launch, head-to-head data, the patent expiry of a class leader, or even a competitor pricing play.

The case study highlighting the challenges faced by Pfizer/Eisai's Aricept® (Case History 3 in the Appendix) shows how some companies are striving to engage actively with payers to provide the evidence from the real world that a drug class has a meaningful and cost-effective place in the treatment paradigm later in the product life cycle. The adoption of a very similar risk-sharing deal to that developed for Novartis's Aclasta at launch was adopted by Procter and Gamble (P&G) in the United States for Actonel® after the launch of generic competitors to key rival Fosamax®. In April 2009, P&G rolled out a pay for nonperformance risk-sharing scheme for Actonel in the United States. If a patient insured by insurance company Health Alliance suffered any fracture (except a spinal cord fracture) despite faithfully taking Actonel, P&G agreed to pay for the required medical care. This type of plan penalizes poor therapeutic responses and lowers the cost for payers. In Actonel's case, Health Alliance members would receive a rebate for the average cost of a small fracture (US$6000) and up to US$30,000 for a hip fracture from P&G, while the insurer would reimburse co-payments made and any cost sharing the patient incurred related to the fracture, from prescriptions to hospital stays.

23.2 PRICING STRATEGY AND TACTICS FOLLOWING PATENT EXPIRY

As discussed in the previous section, pricing strategies and tactics play a key role in the prepatent expiry phases of the life cycle to ensure the brand has favorable access when compared with other competitor brands, where a clinical differentiation story (effectiveness) may need to be bolstered with strong value arguments (cost). In the postpatent expiry world, once generic rivals are available, the biggest challenge is that the effectiveness arguments have essentially been nullified—rivals with exactly the same molecule are available so cost, and any other value-adding services the companies can provide, become the only points of competition. At this stage, companies have to make a decision—do we reduce our acquisition prices to compete with generics, or do we maintain a premium and hope that the additional costs can be offset by the perceived additional "value" our brand can deliver, at least for a proportion of users?

Consider the following hypothetical situation. A brand sells for US$10 per day before patent expiry. At patent expiry, generic rivals launch at a price of US$2 per day and steal 90% of the brand share. If this could be predicted in advance, should the brand company reduce their price to compete with the generic? If the company dropped its price to US$2 per day, and could therefore negate any cost benefit for the generic, it could afford to lose 50% of its business and still generate the same top-line return as by keeping its price at the full US$10. This argument holds true until the company starts to look below the top line. If we assume that the brand operates at a 90% profit margin at its branded price, thus carries a cost to the company of US$1 per day of treatment to offset the US$10 price, the argument now starts to fall apart. The reduced-price scenario cannot match the price-maintained scenario unless the reduced-price brand can retain 90% of patients on the brand, which is unlikely.

So does this mean companies should not bother to compete on price with generics? Absolutely not—it just means that companies need to consider both where and when to compete, and through what mechanism such price competition is most effective. Essentially, the decision to compete on price should be considered based on the interplay between three main factors:

- The complexity of the product, and thus the expected degree of generic competition
- The individual country dynamics, and thus the different stakeholders that carry the greatest influence
- The phase of generic competition, and thus the intensity of focus for generic players

Product complexity will influence the decision to compete on price, as it will influence the intensity of generic competition, and thus the need for generic companies themselves to lower their prices—after all, it is not in the interest of a generic player to lower the price more than absolutely necessary, as they will make less profit! For a simple-to-manufacture, mass-market product, as highlighted earlier in this book, generic competition can be very intense, pushing prices in some markets to extremely low levels—in these situations, there is little point in a branded player competing on price as they will never be able to make a return comparable to that achieved by maintaining a high price and accepting the standard erosion. By contrast, for a product that is difficult to manufacture and thus may only face generic competition from one or two generics, competing on price is a valid option, as the generic company may only reduce their price by 20–30% of that of the brand. For the generic company these "barriers to entry" products are identified in advance as targets to generate maximum profit, so intense price competition is not desirable from their side, so they are less likely to react aggressively to a brand price reduction. This has played out in recent years with the launch of the first biosimilars, as described in the biologics chapter of this book, where list price reductions for the branded players have been used to even the playing field for new entrants.

Individual country dynamics have a significant impact in the decision to compete on price, and in the selection of the most effective process through which such competition is most effectively played out. This topic most probably warrants an entire book of its own, so we will not try to pull out all of the details here! However, three core principles of country dynamics should be highlighted when choosing whether to compete on price—what might a company be forced to do, what happens if they do not compete on price, and who actually is the primary decision maker influenced by price?

In terms of what a company might be forced to do, some countries such as France and Austria impose price cuts on branded agents once generics reach the market, or once a certain volume of generics hits the market. In these situations, price competition is inevitable, and in some cases can automatically level the playing field. More frequently, the key factor for consideration is what happens if you do not compete on price. For many countries, reference pricing systems will kick in once a generic competitor reaches the market. In Spain and Italy, the introduction of reference pricing systems for generics was seen as a tool to stimulate greater levels of generic competition, by limiting reimbursement levels to the generic price. For the most part, what actually transpired is that branded companies chose instead to drop their price to remain in the reference price bracket, thus ensuring patients would not have to pay out of pocket for the more expensive brand. In such markets, companies must decide whether to drop the price, and face the consequences elsewhere in the world where that price is referenced, or accept the premium that will have to be paid by patients and the limitations that might result.

Stakeholder balance of power and influence at patent expiry is a key factor in determining which route to choose when looking to reduce price. As highlighted in the chapter focused on brand loyalty and service, there are essentially four market types—payer-controlled, pharmacist-controlled, physician-influenced, and patient-driven. Different approaches to price competition will play out in different ways depending on the type of market under consideration.

List Price Reduction. This tactic can be considered for payer-controlled markets, where the list price influences reimbursement policy and in patient-driven markets where the ultimate price is a key deciding factor for patients.

Volume-Based Discounting. This tactic can be employed in markets where the key decision makers are buying large volumes of drug, including the payer- and pharmacist-controlled markets, and thus the ability to negotiate attractive discounts on larger volumes can help to influence final dispensing decisions. Such discounts can be provided at the wholesaler or pharmacy level, with the key challenge in ensuring that the discount is still felt by the ultimate decision maker.

Volume-Based Rebating. This tactic, which essentially plays on the reverse of the discounting approach, will see a buyer rebated an agreed percentage of the list price based on different volume levels attained. This allows the end buyer to see the value of the deal without having to commit up front to buying the stock. This is often a tactic employed with payers in the United States throughout the product life cycle to drive preferential formulary position and is used extensively throughout the world to incentivize local payers, including hospital and retail pharmacies to drive usage.

Co-Payment Support. This tactic focuses on the patient, and their out-of-pocket costs associated with a brand, either by topping up a limited reimbursement situation or in providing some support to total out-of-pocket costs. Such tactics are obviously focused on markets where patients carry the burden of out-of-pocket costs based on their brand choice, and thus are most relevant to patient-driven and some payer-controlled markets, where the difference in price between the brand and a generic rival is significant enough to deter spending, but not so high as to make any contribution to the costs meaningless.

The third factor that can be considered in terms of decision to compete on price is time—should a company compete with generics from the moment of launch, or should they only compete once generic competition has stabilized? In many countries, the most intense period of generic competition will be within the first 6–12 months. In the United States and the United Kingdom, it is not uncommon to see more than 10 generic players gaining approval and launching within the first few days of patent expiry. Part of the reason this happens is that the price reduction is not instantaneous, and generic players can make good money as the price drops. For example in the United Kingdom, the drug tariff price, which represents the price at which a pharmacist will be reimbursed for a generic, resets typically every 3 months, so any price reductions during that 3-month period will allow the pharmacist to make more money—it also means that the generic players do not need to drop their prices quite as low to ensure a strong pull from the customer base. All of this leads to many companies entering at launch, potentially reducing the attractiveness of competition from the incumbent branded payer. By contrast, once the level of competition has stabilized, and reimbursement prices have leveled off, many generic players will withdraw from the market, focusing their efforts on new opportunities. As such, it is not uncommon to see a stable competition from only two or three generic players in a market that saw 10–15 generic competitors at launch, often at a significantly higher price point than the lows seen when the generic competition was most intense. In this situation, it may be viable for the branded player to consider price competition several years after patent expiry, when the stable environment is less likely to result in dramatic actions by the competition.

A final factor that must be considered when deciding whether or not to compete on price with a generic is the potential impact on the broader portfolio. Now we will discuss the broader concepts of portfolio management and its impact on individual brand LCM later in this book, but when it comes to pricing, the arguments are pretty simple. If reducing the price of the brand to compete with a generic drives the overall pricing in the branded market to a very low level, this may be detrimental to the fortunes of future brand launches in the market. Consider a company that has a patent expiry coming up for a key brand, together with the impending launch of two new pipeline products. If one of the two new products is to be used in combination with the older brand, a list-price reduction for the core brand could be welcomed, as it would allow a reduction in overall cost of therapy for the new agent. This could be seen with the pricing of the fixed-dose combination (FDC) Vytorin® from Merck/Schering-Plough in the United States. The pricing of the FDC essentially threw in the older simvastatin component for free, allowing the new agent to enter the market at a low additional cost to current standards of care. However, if the second of the two new agents was designed to replace the older agent, then a list-price reduction for the core drug could damage the overall cost effectiveness argument for the new drug, making the barrier to entry higher. Some might say that the entry of generics in the first place would make this decision a moot point, but still a company trying to push a new replacement product at a significant premium to its own older brand will likely struggle!

Once we get into the challenges of portfolio dynamics, particularly with regard to pricing, we start to open a new set of tactics which will be considered in the next chapter—if a company decides that it cannot, or should not, compete on price with generics, does that mean it has to give up on all the switched or switchable patients? Alternatively, can the company look at other ways to compete directly in this space with its own generics—after all, if you can't beat them, should you consider joining them?

CHAPTER 24

Generic Strategies and Tactics

This chapter will focus on one of the more controversial, but increasingly common tactics that can be adopted by the branded drug industry—the development of own generic strategies to enable more effective competition in the patent-expired world. Such tactics have come under intense scrutiny over the last 10–15 years, as competition authorities seek to unravel certain deals undertaken between brand and generic companies which are deemed to be anticompetitive and against the best interest of the public. The authors of this book wholeheartedly support these investigations, and the focus of this chapter will be to examine how generic strategies can work in a competitive universe, thus excluding any focus on deals that seek to disrupt or delay the arrival of other generics on the market. As such, we will also focus on generic strategies that result from a free choice of the branded company, not simply as a result of a settlement of ongoing patent litigation with a generic firm.

The first question that needs to be asked is why would a company consider its own generic strategy in the first place? After all, if they have spent the previous 15–20 years focused on their brand, why would they want to introduce another generic competitor, rather than focusing on competing head-on with the generics? The answer to this question really stems from the efforts health authorities have made to promote and drive generic competition, and the success that these efforts have had. In many countries, including the United States and most northern European markets, it is simply not possible for a brand to compete in a generic world and still be profitable. As such, the only option to play in this space is to consider a generic strategy by which you can play with a second brand and have the flexibility to drive a different pricing policy. By using two different approaches, the brand company can maximize the value of the parent brand at full price for those patients that will not be switched, while taking as much share as possible of the generic market for those patients that would be lost anyway. Figure 24.1 highlights the concept of "ideal" brand/generic strategies.

Pharmaceutical Lifecycle Management: Making the Most of Each and Every Brand, First Edition.
Tony Ellery and Neal Hansen.
© 2012 John Wiley & Sons, Inc. Published 2012 by John Wiley & Sons, Inc.

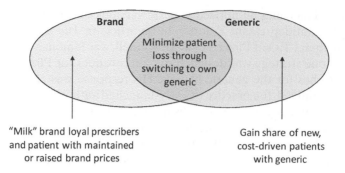

FIGURE 24.1. Goals of generic strategies. *Source:* Datamonitor.

So should a generic strategy always be adopted in every country? Again, the answer to that question is absolutely not, with the interplay between expected competitive dynamics and the validity of competing with the brand being the driving factor. In those markets identified in the previous section where competing on list price with generics is viable for the brand (e.g., some of the reference priced markets such as Spain and Italy), launching a generic makes no sense. By contrast, in both the United Kingdom and the United States, the expected price erosion due to generic competition will be so high that an own generic strategy might be worthwhile. From a competitive standpoint, the expected number of generic competitors will also have a shaping impact on the decision to pursue an own generic strategy. If the number of generics expected to reach the market is very low, say only one or two, and launching an own generic is expected to materially increase the overall impact on the brand, then the strategy may not make sense. Similarly, if there are expected to be 15–20 competitors on the market, there would be little reason to believe that an own generic would be able to capture a meaningful share of the generic market. The most successful generic strategies play in the middle ground, working in the zone where adding another generic will not significantly change the overall level of erosion, but where the own generic itself is in a position to take a competitive piece of the generic pie.

Let us consider three examples. In the first scenario, Brand X is facing patent expiry in the United States, and generic company Y has the first-to-file status on the brand and thus will have 180 days of exclusivity before other generics hit the market. Should the brand company launch its own generic? On the one side, increasing the competition from one to two generics might materially increase the overall generic competition, while on the other hand, a second generic could absolutely aim to capture at least 50% of the overall generic market. This very situation has played out a number of times in the United States in recent years, with the end result being a similar overall level of generic competition to the brand (where erosion of 90% of volume can be expected even with just one generic), and some useful additional revenue for the brand company from its generic. Pfizer has led the way with its Greenstone generic arm, launching authorized generic versions of a number of its drugs, including the antidepressant Zoloft®. In an article in *The Wall Street Journal* in 2006, the then CEO of Pfizer, Hank McKinnell, was famously asked whether the Greenstone strategy was designed to gain revenues for Pfizer or simply to cause headaches for the generic players. His response was clear—"Both are good things." Indeed, the practice of early-launched authorized generics, where the branded company essentially sells a license to their drug during the 180-day exclusivity period, is coming under increasing scrutiny by competition authorities. Detractors argue that this practice stifles the generic industry by reducing the value of one of their key incentives to challenge patents. The proponents simply argue that they are giving the public access to a more competitive generic market, which typically sees prices drop quicker than they would without the authorized generic, thus saving money.

In a second scenario, let us consider the potential to launch the first generic in a country ahead of other players in an effort to create a sustainable first-to-market advantage. This is a strategy which is very geographically dependent—in some countries, such as France, traditionally, the first generic to market commands some first-launch loyalty and has maintained the greatest share, while in many other countries, the first generic can launch at a higher price than subsequent rivals. In these environments, launching an own generic slightly before patent expiry might give a sustained advantage in the generic space that could outweigh any lost revenues from a generic launching a few weeks earlier than expected. This has been one of the key contributing factors to the success of Sanofi-Aventis's authorized generic strategies in France, where it has used its well-reputed Winthrop generic business to launch early-moving generics for many years. However, in a market like the United States, where first-mover generic advantage is wiped out within days if cheaper generic rivals appear, such a strategic goal is unlikely to be achievable.

A final example can play out in potentially the most severe generic environment of all—the introduction of tender contracts for generic drugs. In this environment, companies are asked to submit bids for an exclusive contract to supply a generic for a defined period of time, essentially removing all other players from the reimbursed coverage of that provider. Such deals are becoming increasingly common with German sick funds and in selected other markets, including Canada. In this situation, a branded company will have the opportunity to use an own generic strategy to compete within the tendering process (provided it can make and sell the drug cheaply enough), while maintaining its core brand price for people not covered by the relevant insurance scheme. Indeed, in Canada, Pfizer successfully won an exclusive tender contract in Saskatchewan for amlodipine, which it had previously sold in the branded space as Norvasc®, through its own Gen-Med generic business. This allowed Pfizer to maintain its dominance of the sector in both the patent-protected and the patent-expired worlds.

So a brand company has decided that it could be beneficial to play in the generic arena as part of its brand lifecycle management (LCM) strategy—what are the options available to it to execute the strategy? Essentially, the company has three choices—a true "own" generic, where the drug is sold by the company itself as a low-priced generic; a licensed generic, where the company sells the drug on to a third party, usually a generic player to market under that company's brand; or an authorized generic where the brand company simply allows, or authorizes, a partner generic company to launch its own version without claiming infringement of the patent.

The first two of these options involve the company's own product being sold as a generic, and as such, the strategy carries not only several benefits, but also some key requirements. On the benefits front, these strategies help utilize existing manufacturing capacity that might otherwise be surplus to requirements in a highly competitive world, and these strategies also ensure a continued return on investment, albeit at a lower profitability, for an extended period of time. To make such a strategy work, however, the cost of manufacturing must be comparable to that of the generic rivals—often something that is not the case in today's world. If generic rivals can make the drug significantly more cheaply than the branded player, any strategy that relies on using the branded player's supply will not be as price competitive and thus less likely to succeed.

Assuming the cost of manufacturing is competitive, the next question is who markets the generic—the company itself, or a third party licensee? In reality, there are actually three options here—the company itself, the company's own generic subsidiary (if it has one), or a third party. If the company does have its own generic subsidiary, such as Novartis with Sandoz, Pfizer with Greenstone, and Sanofi-Aventis with Winthrop, the decision is simple. If, however, the company does not have an in-house generic business, the decision is a little trickier. Many companies feel they could market their own generic and thus maximize the profitability from the generic drug. However, they tend to forget one critical factor—for a generic company, each individual drug benefits from being part of a massive portfolio, and the cost benefits of inclusion in large generic bundles most often outweigh any individual drug cost benefits that a branded company could offer. In the simplest terms, generic companies are the best at selling generic drugs—they have the right relationships, the right portfolios, the right selling structures and mind-sets for the job. On this basis, in the majority of cases, the licensed generic strategy, where the company chooses to out-license its own product to a generic marketer, is the best route to success.

The third approach—the authorized generic—is a little more complicated. Such deals have a lot of public visibility, mainly as many of them result from patent settlements between branded and generic players and are thus under scrutiny for anticompetitiveness. When not resulting from a legal settlement, such deals revolve around one factor—how much is a generic company willing to pay the brand company to get a first-to-market advantage? From the branded company perspective, the question is how much has to be paid to compensate for giving up a few weeks or months of patent life. Given these situations, it is unsurprising that such deals are most prevalent in markets where a first-to-market advantage can be sustained (such as France), or where competition will be forcibly limited (such as during a 180-day exclusivity period in the United States). These are often the simplest deals to negotiate as they revolve around the branded company agreeing to do nothing in response to an aggressive launch, provided they are paid upfront.

BUILDING A GENERIC PORTFOLIO: OLD VERSUS NEW THINKING

Now all of the options described so far focus on the specific brand that is being managed, but the generic strategies of brand companies are now starting to look more expansively at the development or acquisition of full generic portfolios. Having one's own generic business is nothing new—in the 1990s, many companies had built their own generic arms to compete in the rapidly growing U.S. and European generic market. However, as the decade closed, many of the major players sold off their generic businesses as the market became more competitive and the challenges of running two very different operations under the same roof became unmanageable. A few companies kept their businesses running, with Sandoz and Winthrop the most notable successes, and over the last few years, the interest in having a generic portfolio has increased, but for very different reasons.

The initial interest was indeed focused on major markets for some—Pfizer's Greenstone grew in stature as a result of Pfizer's internal authorized generic strategies, highlighting a renewed value of the in-house generic business. However, the primary driver of renewed interest in generic portfolios has come from the need to build more competitive propositions in growth markets. In markets such as India, Latin America, Central and Eastern Europe, and North Africa, local players sell broad portfolios of drugs, both branded and generic, and garner success through much more diverse deals, more closely resembling those of a generic business in the traditional Western markets. As such, major Western players are often at a disadvantage in the local market, given that they only sell a small range of drugs in any therapeutic category, and cannot offer a competitive portfolio. Given this scenario, many players have been looking to bolster their portfolios with selected generic drugs to give a more competitive total offering. In 2010, AstraZeneca signed three deals with Indian generic players to gain access to a broad portfolio of agents to sell as branded generics alongside the AstraZeneca portfolio in key emerging growth markets. The first deal, signed in March 2010, was with Torrent Pharmaceuticals and focused on 18 products in 9 unspecified markets, while follow-up deals with Aurobindo Pharma and Intas Pharmaceuticals followed in September 2010. The AstraZeneca approach followed actions by GlaxoSmithKline (GSK) in 2009 to license a generic portfolio from Dr. Reddy's to support the Aspen generic business they acquired in South Africa.

So, can we expect more companies to follow suit and blend the borders between the branded and generic worlds? The answer to that question must be yes—the blending of the traditional branded drug and generic models is essential to compete in many of the growth markets that the drug industry will be reliant on for survival over the coming years. Daiichi-Sankyo's acquisition of Ranbaxy, and the subsequent reorganization of the company into a "hybrid" business model that blends the strengths of the two organizations, will be of significant interest to watch. If the combined company can successfully develop the most effective portfolio approach for each market globally, then it stands a strong chance of evolving into a model for the future of the pharmaceutical industry. The challenges of integrating a Japanese and an Indian company will no doubt be momentous, but if the strategy works, it may be the best deal ever made for either player.

CHAPTER 25

Exit Strategies

The final chapter in our coverage of commercial lifecycle management (LCM) focuses on the most decisive tactic of them all, namely the decision to exit the market. For some this may seem like an insane idea. After all, why not just keep the drug on the market with minimum sales and marketing support and just reap the profits? There is something to be said for this viewpoint, as the mature phase is often the most profitable, and as we will see later in the chapters focusing on portfolio management, Established Brands businesses are increasingly driving the cash flow for new product development. However, there are at least four valid reasons why a company should seriously consider exiting a market, and this chapter will focus both on the rationale and the approaches to market exit.

Exit Driver 1—Patient Safety. The first, and most obvious, reason to exit a market is a forced withdrawal, typically as a result of concerns over patient safety. As this is most commonly not a strategic decision, but instead a reaction to market events, we will not focus on this topic other than to say all companies should develop effective contingency strategies to ensure any product can be swiftly and effectively withdrawn without compromising patient care. Such withdrawals can be permanent or temporary (e.g., if there is a problem with a batch of drug), and effective contingency strategies should include both removal of the contested product from the market and ideally support in transitioning patients to a suitable alternative.

Exit Driver 2—Change in Strategy. A more common rationale for exiting a market is a change in strategy that leaves certain products within the portfolio out of focus. This can be at the therapeutic level, where a company chooses to exit a complete therapy area, or at a brand level, where a company elects to stay in the therapy area, but with a slimmed down portfolio. A good example of a therapeutic exit was seen in 2011,

Pharmaceutical Lifecycle Management: Making the Most of Each and Every Brand, First Edition.
Tony Ellery and Neal Hansen.
© 2012 John Wiley & Sons, Inc. Published 2012 by John Wiley & Sons, Inc.

with the decision of Sanofi-Aventis to sell its U.S. dermatology business. The business had been described by chief executive Chris Viehbacher as "too small" in 2009, and in a company statement in April 2011, Sanofi-Aventis highlighted it was "exploring strategic alternatives for the US dermatology business in keeping with its strategy to reallocate resources to high growth areas." At the product level, strategic withdrawals can be seen as one approach to drive uptake of a new brand. When Novo Nordisk made the decision to withdraw its older porcine insulin range from the UK market, part of the goal was to transition patients onto the newer and safer human and modern recombinant insulins. Unfortunately, the withdrawal had something of a backlash, as patients stabilized on the porcine insulin range did not want to be forcibly switched, and the company came under fire for the decision.

Exit Driver 3—Failing Profitability. While in general mature product portfolios deliver strong profit margins, this is not always the case at the individual brand or at the individual stock keeping unit (SKU) level. There are many reasons that could contribute to falling profitability for a brand, including generic competition, failing market share in the face of newer competition, and price erosion. All of these factors will impact the top-line performance and may reduce the relative profitability of the brand or SKU, but many other factors impacting the cost line could also impact profitability. Changes in the availability of raw materials, upgrades to older manufacturing facilities, or increases in outsourced supply costs can all drive a previously profitable product into loss-making territory.

As highlighted above, two options for product withdrawal can play out in this environment. First, the decision could be made to just withdraw the full brand portfolio, for example, if the raw material costs become prohibitive or the core manufacturing plant for the formulated drug needs significant investment. Alternatively, a company could look to rationalize its SKU range, removing from the market the less profitable formulations and dosage forms, keeping a minimum number of active formulations that between them generate the maximum profit. For example, one pharmaceutical company realized that for one of its key products more than 15 different bottle designs existed across the world for the same dosage form. As you can imagine, this was not the most cost-efficient situation, so significant supply chain cost savings could be made by removing 14 from the market. This approach resonates well with geographic optimization strategies discussed earlier in the book.

Exit Driver 4—Opportunity Cash. The final driver for considering exiting a market would be to generate a one-off cash injection to the business. Brands that may seem undesirable to a parent company based on their size and strategic value may represent a significant opportunity to smaller companies who can play a different game. In many cases, a smaller company may be able to buy an older brand, invest carefully, and increase prices to drive an improved overall performance. As such, the smaller company may be willing to pay an attractive sum to the branded player for the rights to the drug, giving the parent company the opportunity to trade off long-term declining revenues against a one-off cash injection.

EXECUTING THE EXIT STRATEGY

Whatever the driver of exiting the market, companies essentially have two options to execute the strategy—sell or withdraw. Selling the drug is often the simplest option, provided a suitable acquirer can be found. The advantage of this approach is that the parent company can pull out of the market without impacting patient access to the brand. By contrast, withdrawing the agent completely requires a focused and responsible approach from the entire organization, coordinating the supply chain and logistics tactics with appropriate communication to health-care professions, regulators, and patients. Brand companies must ensure that patients have access to an appropriate alternative therapeutic option, either a generic or a comparable brand, or that supply can be met on an as-needed basis from other markets. This latter approach, typically adopting a named-patient program (NPP), can be an effective way of responsibly managing withdrawal from one or many markets. By leaving in place such a program, any patient who really needs access to the drug will be able to get it even without a commercially available drug in that country. The NPP approach can also be used to manage a final manufacturing batch for a product that is being completely withdrawn, ensuring that any last remaining stocks of the drug are supplied only to the patients that need it the most on a specific physician request basis. This process can either be managed by the company itself or by specialist companies such as Idis, who will support companies by taking on the final batch themselves and managing the remaining demand.

BIOLOGICS AND BIOSIMILARS

CHAPTER 26

Biologics and LCM

The next two chapters focus on the changing role of lifecycle management (LCM) in the biologics arena, and how the advent and increasing acceptance of biosimilars will shape the focus of LCM activities moving forward.

Until comparatively recently, Big Pharma's success in maintaining strong growth in the highly profitable branded drug industry was based on its ability to discover, develop, and market drugs containing small and usually easily synthesized molecules as active substances. As we have seen, the basis of this success was patent protection of the structure of these small molecules, which enabled premium prices to be maintained despite the relatively low production costs.

Despite controls on drug prices and increasingly aggressive generic competition, this business model continued to prove highly successful until a hitherto unexpected problem emerged in the mid-1990s; the R&D pipelines of patented new small molecules dried up.

26.1 EMERGENCE OF BIOTECH

Parallel to this trend, however, genetic engineering was starting to create the first drugs based on proteins from genetically engineered cells. The infant biotech industry was entering a phase of rapid growth. In 1988, only five proteins from genetically engineered cells had been approved as drugs by the Food and Drug Administration (FDA); 12 years later, this number had soared to nearly a hundred and fifty.

As so often happens when industry life cycles go through a paradigm shift, it was not the established "small-molecule" players of Big Pharma that led the biotech revolution in medicine but rather it was small, young organizations with names like Amgen, Biogen, Celgene, Chiron, Genentech, Genzyme, and Immunex.

Pharmaceutical Lifecycle Management: Making the Most of Each and Every Brand, First Edition.
Tony Ellery and Neal Hansen.
© 2012 John Wiley & Sons, Inc. Published 2012 by John Wiley & Sons, Inc.

Big Pharma hung on to its R&D focus on small molecules to well past its sell-by date, and only gradually accepted that biologics offered the growth opportunities that small molecules seemed to be no longer able to provide. Tentative attempts to build in-house biotech units were often hampered by a lack of expertise in the new skills required to research and develop proteins, as well as by internal resistance to the paradigm change by scientists who had made their names—and grown their companies—by bringing small molecules to market.

This situation triggered a wave of deal making between Big Pharma and biotech companies, initially mainly as licensing and codevelopment deals but then increasingly as acquisitions. Roche swallowed Genentech, Amgen grabbed Immunex, Abbott took CAT via Knoll, and Novartis acquired Chiron.

The business vision of biotech companies changed. For many years, they had followed the same script—go public as early as possible, keep raising money for as long as it takes to get their products to market, and thus evolve into the next Amgen or Genentech or—better still—the next Pfizer or Merck. But as the new millennium began, this vision started to become more pragmatic. Seeing the plight in which Big Pharma found itself, and also driven by a level of skepticism among investors concerning the long-term future of biotech, more and more biotechs looked for the "get rich quick" option of selling out to Big Pharma as early as possible. Between 2003 and 2006, the number of biotech acquisitions by large pharmaceutical companies exceeded the number of initial public offerings by biotechs by a factor of six.

26.2 SOME DEFINITIONS

Before we consider LCM of biologics, it will be helpful to consider some definitions, especially as they are used by regulatory authorities.

26.2.1 Biologics

Different authorities define the term "biologic" in different ways. The FDA bases its very broad definition on the traditional view of what biotechnology is, while the European Union (EU) prefers a narrower and more modern perspective. The FDA definition comprises

- Allergenics (Allergen Patch Tests, Allergenic Extracts)
- Blood and Blood Products (Blood, Blood Components, Blood Bank Devices, Blood Donor Screening Tests)
- Cellular and Gene Therapy Products (Gene-Based Treatments, Cell-Based Treatments, Cloning)
- Tissue and Tissue Products (Bone, Skin, Corneas, Ligaments, Tendons, Stem Cells, Sperm, Heart Valves)

- Vaccines (Vaccines for Use in Children and Adults, Tuberculin Testing)
- Xenotransplantation (Transplantation of Nonhuman Cells, Tissues, or Organs into a Human)

The full FDA definition of biologics is to be found in 21 CFR 600.3. Despite the somewhat antiquated language, most of the products that we now think of as biologics, or biopharmaceuticals, are covered by the FDA definition. Exceptions are some simple products such as insulin and other recombinant hormones which the FDA regulates as drugs. Biologics are regulated by the Center for Biologics Evaluation and Research (CBER) branch of FDA while drugs are regulated by the Center for Drug Evaluation and Research (CDER) branch. This difference is critically important when we address the issue of generic biologics and biosimilars in the United States in the next chapter.

The EU definition is much tighter than the FDA definition. The EU considers a "biological medicinal product" to be "a protein or nucleic acid-based pharmaceutical substance used for therapeutic or in vivo diagnostic purposes, which is produced by means other than direct extraction from a native (nonengineered) biological source." The EU definition thus really only covers genetically engineered products and products based on monoclonal antibodies (mAbs).

26.3 UPTAKE AND VALUE OF BIOLOGICS

Biologics have become a more attractive area for R&D investment by pharmaceutical companies during recent years for a variety of reasons. First, as we have discussed, they were the only real alternative as small-molecule pipelines started to fail.

But there were also positive reasons that drew more and more companies into the biotechnology arena. The biggest initial attraction was that the rapidly accelerating understanding of the genes involved in diseases, disease pathways, and drug-response sites was leading to the discovery of hundreds of new targets in the body. As new biologic drugs capable of interacting with these targets were discovered and moved into development, it emerged that biologics showed lower attrition rates during development. Biologics are much less likely to produce unexpected off-target activities than small organic molecules of xenobiotic origin. Moreover, they tend to have simpler and more predictable metabolic pathways and pharmacokinetic properties. As a result, the failure rate of biologics in animal toxicity studies is lower than that of small molecules. With only 1 in 10,000 of small molecules synthesized actually ever making it to market, this is a huge benefit. Although it has sometimes been claimed that the development costs are lower for a biologic than for a small molecule, this has not been generally confirmed.

One disadvantage of biologics is the high investments required for their technical development and manufacturing in these times of health-care cost containment. Producing biologics is a complicated and time-intensive process. It may take years just to identify the therapeutic protein, determine its gene sequence, and design the process for making the molecule. Once the process has been scaled up, host cells that have been transformed to produce the gene of interest must be manufactured under tightly controlled environmental conditions in large stainless-steel tanks. The cells are maintained and stimulated to produce the target proteins under precise culture conditions that include an optimal and often cell-specific balance of temperature, oxygen, acidity, and other variables. The proteins are then isolated from the cultures, stringently tested at every step of purification, and formulated into the drug products. Every step of the manufacturing process requires parameters to be kept within very narrow tolerances. The manufacturing processes are thus very expensive, and often require additional investments in new equipment or even new plants.

This disadvantage is compensated for by the fact that biologics generally command much higher prices than do small-molecule pharmaceuticals. Biologics mostly target difficult-to-treat diseases like specific cancers and auto-immune disease, and because the patient populations are rather small, payers accept higher prices. For example, a course of treatment with bevacizumab (Avastin®, marketed by Roche) in the United Kingdom to treat colorectal cancer costs £21,000 per patient. Other therapies used to treat rare, genetic diseases such as Pompe's disease cost in excess of £230,000 per year to treat an adult. As we shall see in a moment, another reason for the high prices is the absence of generic competition.

Commercially, the biologics market has emerged as a critical growth driver of the pharmaceutical industry over the last few decades and displays some unique characteristics compared to the small-molecule market:

- High historic sales growth, in a short space of time: According to Datamonitor, global sales of biologics (excluding vaccines) reached US$116 billion in 2010, up 7% on 2009 sales and accounting for 20% of total pharmaceutical sales. Moreover, between 2004 and 2010, the biologics market grew at a compound annual growth rate (CAGR) of 12.8%.
- A large proportion of the market is concentrated in a small number of products: Unlike the small molecule market, where the value of the market is spread across a large number of products, more than 50% of the biologics market in revenue terms is concentrated in just 20 products (in a market of over 250 products). Key drivers of this performance are the mAbs, a class of product that generated sales of US$47 billion in 2010.
- Strong future performance is predicted: Sales growth of the biologics market is set to maintain a robust trajectory, averaging 5% year-on-year growth through to 2015 to reach US$145 billion. Comparing this to the small-molecule segment, where sales growth is expected to remain flat between 2010 and 2015, it is easy to see the importance of biologics to current and future strategy.

Unsurprisingly, there has been significant effort put into controlling the costs associated with biologic prescribing and use. One of the more controversial ways of doing this has been the establishment of legislation that allows companies to develop and commercialize "generic" or similar versions of biologics with the goal of stimulating price competition in the same way that classic generics do in the small-molecule world. The last decade has seen the emergence of biosimilar approval guidelines, and it has been market forces that have influenced their arrival. At one end, there was, and continues to be, a push from the generic industry to develop alternatives to current agents due to the significant value present in the biologics space. Moreover, the impending patent cliff, access to low-cost manufacturing in India and China, and an improved technology base are all contributing to this market push.

Additionally, there is a market pull for access to cheaper biologic therapies, with the cost of health care, in particular spending on biologics, becoming a major issue for developed and developing nations. As lobbying efforts increase, as payers demand more value for money, and as patients themselves push for access to cheaper medications, lower cost options are being seen as a much-needed "safety valve," through which much of the pent-up pressure of health-care spending can be released.

26.4 LCM OF BIOLOGICS

Before we get to the question of "genericization" of biologics, let us look at differences between LCM of small molecules and of biologics earlier in the life cycle. The first biologics, like insulin, growth hormone, erythropoietin, and granulocyte colony-stimulating factor (G-CSF) relied heavily on classic LCM approaches to drive differentiation, as the base molecules themselves were rather undifferentiated. Examples would include device differentiation in insulin and growth hormone, and second-generation molecules in the insulin class, moving from animal insulin to recombinant insulin, and then to analogs.

Driven by an overarching desire to innovate and launch new products, biologics companies strived to improve currently marketed products, either by making them easier to use, gaining new indications, or by developing and launching devices that would allow patients to self-administer. A brief overview of how some of these tactics have been used by innovator companies is provided below.

26.4.1 Next-Generation Biologics

Developed by Amgen and Kirin in a joint venture, Epogen® (EPO-alfa) was the first recombinant version of EPO to reach the market. It was launched in the United States in 1989 for the treatment of chronic kidney disease (CKD)-related anemia. Approval for the treatment of chemotherapy-related anemia was granted in 1993 in the United States and in 1994 in the EU and Japan. The joint venture through which Epogen was developed resulted in segmentation of the market by geography and indication.

Aranesp® (darbepoetin-alfa) is Amgen's second-generation recombinant human EPO. A follow-on to Epogen, it has as a single difference in the glycosylation pattern. Aranesp has one more sialic acid residue than Epogen, and it was found that this one difference increased Aranesp's half-life by up to three times. This extended half-life enables Aranesp to be administered less frequently than Epogen (in addition to other competing EPO products), thereby improving patient convenience and side effects linked to the infusion/injection of biologic products.

Despite this innovative approach to extending the half-life of human EPO, and potentially delivering benefits to patients and other key stakeholders, a pharmacoeconomic analysis of the use of first-generation EPO-alfa versus darbepoetin-alfa came out in favor of first-generation EPO. The authors stated that ". . . based on all available data and current average wholesale pricing (AWP) of these agents, the pharmacoeconomic advantage appears to favour EPO-alfa." What this analysis did not take into account was the amount of deep discount Amgen is able to do in order to drive uptake of Aranesp, but the clinical message is clear: innovation for the sake of it has limited impact on clinical outcomes.

26.4.2 Reformulation

Neupogen® (filgrastim) is a granulocyte colony stimulating factor (G-CSF) which was first launched in the United States in 1997 and in Europe in 1998. The product is indicated for the treatment of neutropenia (i.e., a low number of neutrophils) associated with chemotherapy and bone marrow transplantation.

Developed in-house, Neulasta® (polyethylene glycol [PEG]-filgrastim) is a longer-acting version of Neupogen, manufactured by covalently binding it with PEG. Neulasta was launched in 2002 in the United States and Europe, and a Phase III breast cancer trial showed that it offered the advantage of once-weekly dosing, as opposed to the once-a-day dosing that is required for Neupogen. A further advantage of Neulasta is that it is cleared by neutrophils, not by the kidneys. This promotes a self-regulating cycle (i.e., it is increasingly metabolized as a patient's neutrophil count increases in response to the drug).

Interestingly, from a cost-effectiveness perspective, PEG-filgrastim has been shown to be better than filgrastim. In a study published in 2010, the authors demonstrated that primary prophylaxis of febrile neutropenia in Germany breast cancer patients using a single dose of PEG-filgrastim is cost saving compared to 11-day use of filgrastim, and cost-effective compared to 6-day use of filgrastim in patients with breast cancer. Clinically, the jury is still out. A study published in 2011 showed that prophylaxis of febrile neutropenia with PEG-filgrastim in Asian lymphoma patients did not show a therapeutic advantage for preventing neutropenic outcomes compared with daily filgrastim prophylaxis.

26.4.3 Indication Expansion

As discussed already in this book, indication expansion is a very common LCM strategy, with more than 75% of the 50 top-selling brands in 2006 having had at least one additional indication approved since their initial launch in the United States. Indication expansion is just as valid a strategy for biologics, with many diseases particularly in the inflammatory and oncology segments sharing common pathways through which biologic agents can exert their effects. Within the biologics market, a good example of how indication expansion has been used as an LCM strategy is Humira®.

Originally developed by Cambridge Antibody Technology and subsequently licensed to Knoll (which was acquired by Abbott in 2001), Humira (adalimumab) is a self-injectable fully human mAb targeted against tumor necrosis factor-alfa (TNF-alfa), a potent proinflammatory mediator that plays a pivotal role in a wide range of human inflammatory diseases.

Humira was first launched in the United States in January 2003 for adults with moderately to severely active rheumatoid arthritis (RA) and has since made rapid clinical progress, gaining authorization for a much wider range of immunological diseases in the United States, Europe, and Rest of World (RoW) territories. Humira is now indicated for psoriatic arthritis (PsA), ankylosing spondylitis (AS), Crohn's disease (CD), psoriasis, ulcerative colitis (UC), and juvenile rheumatoid arthritis (JRA), a comprehensive range of autoimmune disorder approvals.

26.4.4 Self-Injection Devices

The market for self-injection devices started back in 1984 with the launch of the first insulin pens. Today's insulin pens (e.g., the Lantus Solostar®) have enabled innovator companies to drive market share and create significant brand loyalty by providing real-life benefits to patients in terms of disease self-management. Subsequent self-injection device launches have been seen for somatropin (e.g., Pfizer's Genotropin® Pen), the anti-TNFs (e.g., Enbrel's SureClick® Self-Injector), interferon-beta (e.g., Rebif's RebiJect® II Pen), and follicle-stimulating hormone (e.g., Follistim's AQ Cartridge®). Interestingly, the SureClick® system used for Enbrel® is also used for Aranesp and Neulasta.

Across many therapy areas, a simple prefilled syringe can bring immediate and much-needed patient convenience to an injection therapy. It empowers the patient and provides him or her with a huge sense of freedom, thereby improving quality of life. This has been well illustrated over the last few years following the successful launch of all of the self-injection devices mentioned previously. Patients become emotionally attached to their devices, seeing them as an integral part of their therapeutic regimen. Brand loyalty ensues, and patients become very hard to convince that they should be switched to another brand, unless there is a compelling clinical or financial argument.

More recently, Roche has stepped up LCM activity on Herceptin® (trastuzumab), a mAb treatment for breast cancer. Roche has invested close to CHF190 m (US$183 m) at two production sites to manufacture devices that will allow patients to self-administer a subcutaneous formulation of Herceptin. One site will supply the devices for a Phase III study which could support approval of the subcutaneous formulation. In this study, 552 patients with Stages I–IIIc breast cancer will receive chemotherapy in combination with either subcutaneous or intravenous Herceptin before surgery, followed by 10 three-weekly infusions of subcutaneous or intravenous Herceptin.

Herceptin's current intravenous formulation requires patients to receive the drug in hospital via a 1-hour infusion. The subcutaneous formulation (developed in partnership with Halozyme Therapeutics) should increase convenience, allowing patients to self-administer the drug at home via a 5-min infusion. This is important given that Herceptin is administered for up to a year in early-stage breast cancer. Additionally, this would help to reduce costs associated with patient hospitalization and could improve the drug's side-effect profile by reducing infusion reactions. Many challenges still exist, not least being able to ensure patient compliance with self-injections. However, the improved patient convenience is likely to be hugely attractive to patients and caregivers.

CHAPTER 27

Biosimilars and Their Impact on Biologic LCM

The emergence of biosimilars as a nascent segment of the biopharmaceutical market has prompted branded biologic players to reassess how to effectively manage pipelines and on-market biologic portfolios. Unlike small-molecule focused pharmaceutical companies, which have been competing with generics since the mid-1980s, biologics companies have been comparatively immune to nonbranded competition, until now. Gone are the days when branded biologic companies can act as if the only competition that exists is from other branded biologic companies. Biosimilars have been called the most disruptive technology of the decade. As such, robust and effective lifecycle management (LCM) of branded biologic assets has now become a highly important activity for branded biopharmaceutical companies.

Before we continue to examine biosimilars in depth, we should first clarify what we mean by a biosimilar, and how this terminology fits with other terms such as biogenerics and follow-on biologics (FOBs).

27.1 CHANGING TERMINOLOGY: BIOGENERICS, BIOSIMILARS, AND FOBs

Within the small-molecule (chemical) pharmaceuticals market, the concept of an identical copy of a brand is relatively simple: generic equivalents can be created provided the same chemical syntheses can be mimicked, with straightforward chemical testing needed to prove identity. The critical challenge with products derived from biotechnology is first the ability to copy the manufacturing process, a process which is heavily reliant on either raw materials being obtained from biologic sources, or biological synthesis in natural cells, which are both many times more complex than chemical processes. Unlike

Pharmaceutical Lifecycle Management: Making the Most of Each and Every Brand, First Edition.
Tony Ellery and Neal Hansen.
© 2012 John Wiley & Sons, Inc. Published 2012 by John Wiley & Sons, Inc.

small-molecule drugs, biologics are usually very complex molecules which can be susceptible to even minor changes in the manufacturing process. The generic manufacturer is unlikely to have access to the originator's molecular clone or cell bank, nor know details of the fermentation and purification processes. It is therefore not possible for generic manufacturers to precisely reproduce the chemical composition and impurity profile of a brand the way they can with small-molecule pharmaceuticals.

The ability of a generic company to prove that its product is the "same" as the reference product is also significantly more challenging, with existing techniques unable to truly prove identity without high levels of investments in clinical trials (which themselves would normally support a New Drug Application (NDA) or biologics license application (BLA) filing for a novel therapeutic product). Indeed, these clinical trials would still not be able to categorically prove identity, rather similarity between two biologic products. These are costs not borne by chemical generics, which benefit from an abbreviated process that draws on the original product's filing.

The term "biogeneric" is therefore considered by many to be misleading, as the copy product can rarely be a true copy in the small-molecule sense. For this reason, the terms "biosimilars" or "follow-on biologics" are preferred for such copy products.

As we have seen, the term "biologic" means different things to different people, and the situation is just as inconsistent when we come to "generic biologics." Again, there are no widely recognized or simple definitions for these complex products.

In a regulatory context, "biosimilars" are biologics which have obtained market approval by submitting an abbreviated application in which adequate similarity to an approved reference product has been demonstrated. Terminology across markets and regulatory bodies varies, but there is fundamental agreement on the definition of a biosimilar as being a biological product that is similar, not the same, as a currently marketed reference product. The European Medicines Agency (EMA) defines a biosimilar as follows: ". . . where a biological medicinal product which is similar to a reference biological product does not meet the conditions in the definition of generic medicinal products, owing to, in particular, differences relating to raw materials or differences in manufacturing processes of the biological medicinal product and the reference biological medicinal product." Using this definition, there are several biosimilars on the European Union (EU) market and in a few other countries, but none yet in the United States where the legislation necessary to allow the approval of biosimilars was only enacted in March 2010.

Confusingly, the term "biosimilar" is sometimes also used in nonregulatory context to describe products that contain similar active agents which were approved based on full registration dossiers.

The term "follow-on biologic" is also controversial. To some it seems to imply that the product is an improved, next-generation drug when it is often simply a more-or-less accurate attempt to copy a successful brand.

Pragmatically, it seems appropriate to restrict the term "biogeneric" to products made by exactly the same process, manufactured using consistent biological sources (e.g., genes, cell lines), consistent processes and process conditions, and utilizing consistent in-process and end-product controls and assays to produce a product with a consistent set of final specifications. In other words, the process is the product! In practice, a biogeneric can only be made by the innovator or its licensor which has access to all of the above biological sources and information.

It would be sensible to restrict the term "follow-on biologics" to protein and peptide products that are so similar to a product that has already been granted marketing approval that the applicant should be allowed to rely on some form of abbreviated application for approval, leaning heavily on the existing documentation and knowledge regarding the safety and effectiveness of the approved product. These FOBs could be produced by biotech processes or even derived from natural sources. Were this definition to gain general usage, then only simple biological molecules could be included, largely the same group of molecules that the Food and Drug Administration (FDA) already regulates as drugs rather than as biologics (including, for example, insulin, growth hormones, and calcitonin).

The term "biosimilar" could then be reserved for the biologics that are of the greatest concern to regulatory authorities today, namely copy products of complex proteins and especially monoclonal antibodies (mAbs).

Others are better qualified than we are to decide whether our definitions are the most suitable, but we would strongly plead for a series of definitions that mean the same thing to people in different geographies and in different functions in the industry (e.g., scientists, marketers, payers, and regulators).

27.2 WHY ARE BIOSIMILARS A BIG DEAL?

As outlined previously, the global biologics market reached US$116 billion in 2009, and is predicted to reach US$145 billion by 2015. In contrast to the much-vaunted "small-molecule" patent cliff that arrived in 2011, patent expiries in the biologics sector are not expected to reach critical levels and outpace those in the small-molecule sector until 2013. By then, biosimilar legislation will be in place—and working—across all developed markets, allowing biosimilar developers to launch biosimilar versions of several biologic products.

According to recent analysis by Ameet Mallik, Global Head of Sandoz Biopharmaceuticals, quoted in *MedAdNews* in October 2011, an estimated US$63 billion (~40%) in global biologic sales will lose patent protection by 2016, creating a significant pot of money for biosimilar manufacturers to target. Analysis by Datamonitor suggests that the biosimilars market is set to reach US$3.7 billion by 2015, driven by rapid uptake of biosimilars in several classes.

While these figures sound like significant opportunities, the relative success of biosimilars is likely to vary by product and therapy area. The role played by the doctor or nurse, how influential the payer is, the influence of manufacturing capacity, and the importance of a device to the delivery of the product are just some of the key influences on biosimilar success.

27.3 HOW ARE BIOSIMILARS DIFFERENT?

While biosimilars now form part of the wider pharmaceutical and biotechnology market, the skill set required for effective manufacture, development, and commercialization of biosimilars is different when compared to conventional "small-molecule" generics. Comparing some key characteristics of generic, biosimilar and biologic manufacturing, development and regulation, it can be seen that biosimilars have more in common with innovative biologics than with small-molecule generics.

Most critically, developing a small-molecule generic only requires Phase I bioequivalence testing, costs around US$2 million, takes between 18 and 24 months, and requires only a small number of patients (20–100, depending on the product). Biosimilar development invariably requires multiple Phase III clinical trials involving hundreds of patients, costs US$80–$120 million, and takes 6–8 years to complete. Despite the obvious challenges involved in the development of biosimilars, multiple companies have entered into the biosimilars market, investing significant resources in establishing a robust biosimilar presence.

27.4 BIOSIMILAR APPROVAL PATHWAYS

Similar to small-molecule generics, governments around the world are developing biosimilar legislation in order to promote the development and commercialization of cheaper versions of branded biologics. It is essential, therefore, that the reader understands how biosimilars are approved. This section provides a very brief overview of key regulatory issues in a selection of markets. For additional information, the reader is urged to seek additional sources of information for a more detailed review.

27.4.1 Biosimilars in Europe

A legal pathway for the approval of similar biological medicinal products (biosimilars) has existed in the EU since 2005, following the release of guideline CHMP/437/04, a document which provided guidance to manufacturers interested in "develop[ing] a new biological medicinal product claimed to be "similar" to a reference medicinal product which has been granted a marketing authorization in the Community. . . ." The approval pathway for biosimilars in Europe contains much higher regulatory requirements compared to small-molecule generic drugs, or for a change in the production process by the originator company. The EMA has issued a number of guidelines that detail the requirements for market approval. In addition to these general guidelines, the EMA has published a number of class-specific guidelines, including guidelines for human insulin, low-molecular weight heparin (LMWH), erythropoietin (EPO), somatropin, granulocyte colony-stimulating factor (G-CSF; filgrastim), and interferon-alfa (IFN-alfa). Additionally, draft guidance is currently being reviewed for interferon-beta (IFN-beta), follicle-stimulating hormone (FSH), and mAbs. The regulatory requirements vary by class of product, but invariably, Phase III clinical trials are required before any marketing authorizations can be allowed.

27.4.2 Biosimilars in the United States

With the enactment of The Patient Protection and Affordable Care Act (PPACA) in the United States in March 2010 by President Barack Obama, and amendment of The Public Health Services Act (PHSA), the United States now has a pathway for the approval of applications for biological products shown to be biosimilar to a licensed reference product. This is possible via the inclusion of The Biologics Price Competition and Innovation Act (BPCIA) of 2009 within the PPACA, which among other things adds three new sections to the PHSA—351(k), 351(l), and 351(m)—allowing licensure of biosimilars on the U.S. market. However, at the time of writing this book, the FDA had still not published any clear guidance on what the requirements are for gaining a biosimilar approval in the United States.

In summary, the BPCIA creates standards for biological products to be licensed as either biosimilar or interchangeable. A biosimilar product is one that, as compared to the originally approved reference product, (1) is used in the same manner and treatment, (2) is manufactured in a facility and through a process that meets standards for safety, purity, and potency, and (3) has data based on testing supporting its high similarity. An interchangeable product is a biosimilar product that meets additional standards so that it can be substituted for the reference product without the intervention of the health-care provider who prescribed the reference product.

Innovators are still protected under the BPCIA. Even if patents have expired on the innovator product, no biosimilar product can be granted a market authorization by the FDA until the reference product has been licensed for 12 years. The length of this market exclusivity period was the most contentious aspect of the biosimilar pathway negotiations. Despite the generics lobby in the United States asking for 5 years, and President Obama asking for 7 years, the award of 12 years can be seen as nothing else other than a victory for innovator companies.

In terms of making an application for a biosimilar approval (termed a 351k application), biosimilar companies must submit a large amount of data that demonstrate (1) the biological product that is the subject of the application is "biosimilar" to a single reference product; (2) the biological product and reference product use the same mechanism(s) of action for the condition(s) of use prescribed, recommended, or suggested in the proposed labeling, but only to the extent the mechanism(s) of action are known for the reference product; (3) the condition(s) of use prescribed, recommended, or suggested in the labeling proposed for the biological product have been previously approved for the reference product within the U.S. market; (4) the biological product has the same route of administration, dosage form, and strength as the reference product; (5) the facility in which the biological product is manufactured, processed, packed, or held meets standards designed to assure that the biological product continues to be safe, pure, and potent (essentially meaning that the facility needs to be FDA approved).

Despite this progress, many questions still remain. Will the FDA be accepting biosimilar applications immediately? Can the applications be submitted before the user fees are established? What will the data requirements be to establish "high similarity" and "interchangeability?" How will applicants demonstrate there are no "clinically meaningful differences" between the biosimilar and reference product in terms of safety, efficacy, purity, and potency, without doing extensive clinical trials?

To provide a forum where these and many other questions related to the approval of biosimilars in the United States could be addressed, the FDA held in November 2010 a 2-day public hearing to obtain input on specific issues and challenges associated with the implementation of the BPCIA of 2009. The FDA recently announced that over 800 participants registered to attend the meeting in person, and over 40 presentations were made on subjects including patient safety, clinical trials, interchangeability, and substitution.

In February 2011, the FDA's Commissioner, Dr. Margaret Hamburg, stated that more details on the biosimilar development pathway were coming "very soon." As of December 2011, no announcements had been made.

27.4.3 Biosimilars around the World

Since the EMA published its biosimilar legislation in 2005, biosimilar development guidance has emerged in several other markets, with other markets either slow, or unwilling, to follow the EMA's lead.

- *Australia*: In June 2006, the Australian government's Department of Health and Ageing Therapeutic Goods Administration (TGA) adopted EMA's biosimilar development guidelines "en-bloc" (including European Commission (EC) Directives and Regulations). Since that time, biosimilar somatropin (Omnitrope®; Sandoz) and filgrastim (Nivestim; Hospira) have been approved in Australia.
- *Canada*: Health Canada released final guidance on the development of biosimilar products in May 2010; the guidance document outlines the regulatory review process that Health Canada will implement for a so-called Subsequent Entry Biologic (SEB). It is noteworthy that SEB

regulation will take place entirely through guidance documents, not through any amendments to the Food and Drug Regulations or to the Patented Medicines (Notice of Compliance) Regulations (PM-NOC Regulations). In April 2009, Sandoz received Health Canada approval for Omnitrope, the first SEB approval despite the final guidance not being in place for another year.

• *Japan*: The Ministry of Health, Labor and Wealth (MHLW) in Japan has also published a guideline to allow the approval of biosimilars. Similar to Australia, the Japanese system is based on the EMA biosimilar pathway. Following the publication of this guidance, two biosimilars were approved; Somatropin BS SC injection 5 mg and 10 mg (recombinant somatropin) from Sandoz KK, and Epogen (EPO-alfa) BS Injection from JCR Pharma and Kissei Pharma.

• *Less Regulated Markets*: The regulatory barriers to market entry are not as strict in various developing markets, such as India, China, and Russia. The focus is on improving patient access and managing health-care costs. As a result, a wide range of products are available in these markets where formal biosimilar legislation has yet to be introduced. As such, so-called copy biologics available in these markets cannot be called biosimilars as they have not been approved by a formal development pathway. Biosimilar development legislation is emerging in these markets, but it will take time before products developed and approved in these markets will be approvable in markets such as the EU, United States, Japan, and other developed, Western markets.

27.5 SUBSTITUTION OF BIOSIMILARS

The biosimilars market is very new, and as such, there are a number of critical, market-shaping uncertainties that exist. Potentially the most critical is substitution, either automatic or therapeutic.

27.5.1 Automatic Substitution

Substitution by pharmacists of one product with another that has the same International Nonproprietary Name (INN) is common practice with generic drugs in many EU countries. But is substitution appropriate for biologics? Unlike more common small-molecule drugs, biologics generally exhibit high molecular complexity and microheterogeneity. Biologicals are also very sensitive to manufacturing process changes, including the choice of the cell type, along with production, purification, and formulation processes. In view of the complexity and sensitivity of biologics to the manufacturing process, no two biotech medicines can be exactly the same, hence the term biosimilar.

It is argued that as a direct consequence of their complexity, automatic substitution of biologics for a biosimilar could give rise to different clinical consequences and therefore, many believe that this should be ruled out for reasons of patient safety. Several EU agencies, including the EMA, have advised that the decision to treat a patient with a biosimilar medicine should be taken following the opinion of a qualified health-care professional.

Measures to prevent automatic substitution of biosimilars are already in place in several EU member states, and others have taken steps to limit the practice. Substitution is also on the agenda in other regions, such as Canada, where automatic substitution is not recommended, and in the Middle East, where it has been recommended that products should be clearly identified as biosimilar on the label. What happens in the United States on this front is likely to be driven by payer involvement in the biosimilars market.

One specific case where automatic substitution has been put forward, and then challenged has been Norway. Following on from its progeneric position, the Norwegian government has become supporters of biosimilars. Although Norway is not part of the EU, the process for pharmaceutical registration has been aligned to EU regulations. The 2004 regulatory reforms within the country made the centralized procedure mandatory for all new active substances and all drugs in a number of drug categories, including all biotech and biosimilar products.

Norway's most recent attempt to support the use of biosimilars came in June 2010 when the Norwegian Medicines Agency (NoMA; Statens Legemiddelverk) stated that it was going to add two biosimilar filgrastim products—specifically TevaGrastim® and RatioGrastim®—to its substitution list (byttelisten) for recently approved drugs. This move would have provided physicians and pharmacists with a clear incentive to use biosimilar filgrastim in situations where otherwise only the branded product—Amgen's Neupogen®—was available. However, no sooner had NoMA published its plans, the Oslo City Court made a ruling which prohibited the implementation of NoMA's planned listing, prompted by a lawsuit submitted to the courts by Amgen. In March 2011, the Oslo District Court in Norway concluded that the Norwegian Medicines Agency's attempt to include TevaGrastim® and RatioGrastim® on the country's substitution list is invalid. The Norwegian Pharmacy Act, therefore, does not authorize substitution of these biological medicines for biosimilar versions.

27.5.2 Therapeutic Substitution

As described earlier in the book, therapeutic substitution is the interchange of a less costly drug in place of another (usually more expensive branded) treatment, based on the premise that the cheaper version has the same therapeutic effect. Therapeutic substitution can take place at many levels within the health-care system (e.g., a decision made by a prescribing physician or dispensing pharmacist, an amendment to a hospital formulary, or a policy decision made by a health-care provider). It is a valid goal, but only when certain key assumptions are met: first, that there is true equivalence of the substituted product (in terms of overall patient outcomes), and second, that any such substitution has been achieved via a partnership between payer, prescribing physician, and patient.

Therapeutic substitution has been used by payers in the past to cut costs of drug budgets. For example, therapeutic substitution happened much earlier than patent expiry in the angiotensin receptor blocker (ARB) market in the United Kingdom, with companies pregenericizing their own class. Takeda reduced the price of candesartan (marketed as Amias®) by 40% and cut its physician sales force to offer a more attractive proposition to payers in a market where they were one of seven competing products. Merck Sharpe & Dohme (MSD) followed suit in the summer of 2007, reducing their prices substantially (2 years ahead of patent expiry) to create a low-price market. What followed was a period of intense pricing competition among ARB manufacturers up until September 2009 when Cozaar® (losartan) lost patent protection, and generic ARBs reached the market.

In settings where there is high degree of comfort with the interchangeable use of biologic therapies, therapeutic substitution has the potential to significantly impact branded market share. For example, in the renal dialysis market, physicians at the Virginia Commonwealth University Health System (VCUHS) developed and implemented a therapeutic interchange program to convert therapy for all in-patients undergoing dialysis from EPO-alfa to darbepoetin-alfa for treatment of chronic kidney disease-related anemia. Preliminary evaluation of the program demonstrated cost savings and reduced drug utilization of erythropoiesis-stimulating proteins in hospitalized dialysis patients. With biosimilar EPO-alfa now available across Europe, therapeutic substitution of branded EPO-alfa is a significant concern for innovator companies.

27.6 INNOVATOR RESPONSES TO BIOSIMILAR THREATS

Since the first approval of Omnitrope in 2006, to date another 13 biosimilars have been approved in Europe (based on four reference products). In the face of this new threat within the biologics market, various innovator companies have reacted very differently to biosimilars. Some reactions have been based on sound commercial logic, while others have attempted to call into question the safety and efficacy of biosimilars.

Challenging Biosimilar Safety. The EC was compelled to release a statement in May 2008 to defend its position on biosimilar approvals. On the back of criticism from innovator industry personnel, specifically Amgen, during various conferences, Nicolas Rossignol, head of the EC's pharmaceuticals unit, stated that "... I have seen arguments put on the table calling their safety into question, but I have a message: we have promoted and developed with the European Medicines Agency (EMA) a special biosimilars framework. So we are confident that if a product meets all the requirements and gets a marketing authorization from the commission, it means that the product is as safe and effective as any other product authorized by the commission." While biosimilar manufacturers were also warned about concerns regarding biosimilar quality in certain Central and Eastern European (CEE) markets, the message from the EC was clear; do not question the safety of biosimilars if EMA approves them.

Competing on Price. Within the EPO market, the pricing of EPOs has been forced down dramatically by the regional contract tenders that operate across many European markets, including the United Kingdom and Germany. Within the United Kingdom, each tender specifically seeks the supply and delivery of EPO and the associated nursing services. These tendering arrangements generate huge decreases in EPO drug costs. Pharmacists in the United Kingdom have commented that branded EPO manufacturers are able to offer discounts of up to 70% in order to secure the business.

Exiting the Market. In the face of biosimilar competition within the EPO market, and an uncertain future, Shire announced that it was exiting the EPO market in August 2008 with the withdrawal of Dynepo® (EPO-delta). When the product was launched in March 2007, Shire had great hopes for Dynepo, but Q2 2008 results were poor, with the product earning just US$7 million. Total 2007 sales were also lower than expected, at just US$14 million. Shire attributed the discontinuation to significant reductions in prices, across the EPO market, following the entry of biosimilars. The company recorded charges of US$150 million as a result of the move, but said that it would redirect its resources to the launches of products within its CNS portfolio.

27.7 THE FUTURE FOR BIOLOGICS LCM

Key stakeholders and competitors are becoming increasingly comfortable with the approval and use of biosimilars in key markets. On that basis, future LCM activities from innovator companies need to be based on an understanding of how the markets are evolving and how the initial biosimilars have been perceived. Innovator companies need to be able to handle uncertainty, potentially using scenario-based analyses to drive LCM decision making in the face of not knowing exactly how the market is going to evolve.

This is not to say that previous and current activities need to be stopped and/or reconsidered. Innovative ways of differentiating a brand in the biosimilar age can still include previously discussed tactics. What must be emphasized, however, is that new LCM strategies must be identified to complement current activities for biologics brands to remain competitive.

The following sections highlight how some of the changes in biosimilar development are shaping three of the key LCM approaches for biologics.

27.7.1 Legal Strategies in the United States

In addition to outlining issues in relation to the biosimilar and interchangeability determination, along with information on data exclusivity, the BPCIA in the United States also contains a preapproval patent litigation framework that could significantly influence a biosimilar development company from pursuing a biosimilar application under the Act.

Under the terms of the Act, there is a special prelitigation procedure requiring (1) the biosimilar applicant formally communicating to the innovator product owner its intention to seek marketing approval for a biosimilar version of its product; (2) exchange of lists of patents between the biosimilar and innovator companies where a claim of patent infringement could reasonably be asserted by the reference product sponsor; (3) exchange of infringement claims and defenses; and (4) dispute resolution negotiations before an infringement suit can be filed.

From beginning to end, approximately 250–300 days are likely to elapse between acceptance of the biosimilar application by the FDA and filing of any patent infringement lawsuit. In addition to this delay, the FDA is likely to take much longer to review biosimilar applications compared to generics, thereby significantly delaying any biosimilar launches in the United States.

In comparison, there is no special prelitigation procedure in Europe. No notice by the biosimilar applicant is required to the reference product sponsor. That said, notice is sometimes given by biosimilar manufacturers in order to allow patent issues to be addressed, thereby minimizing the chance for an injunction inherent in an at-risk launch. Unless the prelitigation provisions of the Act are modified, there is a significant risk that the biosimilars pathway in the United States will not be used, with companies instead selecting the BLA route.

Teva chose such a strategy for its biosimilar filgrastim, Neutroval® (previously called XM02), and submitted a BLA in November 2009. However, despite an assertion at the time that this was the best course of action for the company, Teva announced in September 2010 that the FDA had been unable to approve the product based on the data package submitted. While no specifics were given by Teva in relation to what the FDA has requested, anecdotal data from industry sources suggest that product quality and efficacy were key concerns.

All of this seems academic now, as new information on Teva's submission and data package for Neutroval emerged in July 2011. Around the same time that Teva submitted its BLA to the FDA, Amgen filed a patent infringement claim in federal court to block Teva's attempt to sell Neutroval, should the FDA approve the product. In July 2011, the U.S. District Court in Pennsylvania entered final judgment and a permanent injunction against Teva prohibiting them from infringing Amgen's patents relating to human G-CSF and methods for its use. Moreover, Teva admitted that its Neutroval product infringed two Amgen patents at issue in the litigation (US 5,580,755 and US 5,582,823) and that those patents were valid and enforceable. The Court's injunction extends until November 10, 2013, after which date Teva may sell Neutroval in the United States. Regarding Neugranin®, Teva's pegylated G-CSF product, Teva also agreed not to sell Neugranin until November 10, 2013 unless it first obtains a final court decision that Amgen's patents are not infringed by Neugranin. Whether this issue changes the way in which Teva and other biosimilar players approach market entry in the United States remains to be seen. It does highlight, however, that robust IP due diligence in the United States is critical for any biosimilar company to be successful in getting products approved.

27.7.2 Indication Expansion in Europe

The EMA's guideline on Similar Biological Medicinal Products containing Biotechnology-Derived Proteins as Active Substance: Non-Clinical and Clinical Issues states that "... in case the originally authorised medicinal product has more than one indication, the efficacy and safety of the medicinal product claimed to be similar has to be justified or, if necessary, demonstrated separately for each of the claimed indications. However, in certain cases it may be possible to extrapolate therapeutic similarity shown in one indication to other indications of the reference medicinal product."

Justification for extrapolation will depend on clinical experience, available literature data, and whether or not the same mechanisms of action or the same receptor(s) are involved in all indications. As such, extrapolation is not automatic; rather, it needs to be earned and justified by the company developing the biosimilar. Extrapolation of indications was allowed for somatropins and filgrastims, but subcutaneous administration was not approved for biosimilar EPO-alfa, even after the reference product regained approval for this route.

The issue of extrapolation has been debated more in recent months after the EMA published its draft guideline for the development of biosimilar mAbs. The overarching aim of the guideline is to prove biosimilarity of biosimilar mAbs, not clinical benefit per se. The argument is that the innovator company has already established this. On the subject of extrapolation, the guideline states that "extrapolation of clinical efficacy and safety data to other indications of the reference mAb, not specifically studied during the clinical development of the drug, is possible, based on the results of the overall evidence provided." However, the guidance does state that "if a reference mAb is licensed both as an immunomodulator and as an anticancer antibody, the scientific justification as regards extrapolation between the two (or more) indications is more challenging."

Based on the position of the EMA, indication expansion strategies for innovative biologics could potentially lose some of their impact for future biologics LCM activities. Before products lose patent protection, indication expansion remains a critical strategy for improving market share and gaining access to new patients. However, once products lose patent protection (and data exclusivity periods expire), biosimilar companies have the potential to gain all of the innovator product's indications by simply proving biosimilarity to the reference product.

Granted, extrapolation of indications across therapy areas remains a huge challenge. Sandoz and Teva, both developing a biosimilar version of rituximab (Rituxan®/MabThera®; Roche), are conducting clinical development programs in both of rituximab's indications, namely oncology and inflammation. However, across other classes of product, outside of the mAbs, extrapolation of indications has been seen. As such, innovator strategies will need to take this into account when planning LCM activities for their brands.

27.7.3 Brand Loyalty Programs and Services

Both now and in the future, brand and corporate-level differentiation will become critical for innovative biologic manufacturers. In a market where biosimilars are competing for the same patients, the ability to differentiate at the molecule level (i.e., branded EPO-alfa vs. biosimilar EPO-alfa) will become very challenging. As such, companies will need to develop strategies to differentiate products on the basis of branding and corporate identity.

One such way of doing this is by providing key stakeholders with products and services associated with the brand. Critically, these services should either not be offered by other companies, or must be superior to similar services offered by competing brands and biosimilars. Moreover, these services must be linked extensively to the brand identity of the product, rather than the molecule in question, thereby creating a perception in the mind of stakeholders that choosing (or staying with) a particular brand will provide them with benefits outside of clinical benefits provided by the molecule. As with small molecules, the challenge is to move from molecular loyalty to brand loyalty.

27.8 THE EMERGENCE OF THE "INNOVASIMILAR" BIOPHARMA COMPANY

When biosimilars first emerged, and stakeholders began to understand the attractions of taking part in the biosimilars market, it became a question of when, not if, innovative biopharma companies would get involved. Following a model similar to Novartis/Sandoz, companies have either made significant investments in the space or made firm commitments to explore opportunities within the biosimilars market in the future:

- *AstraZeneca*: Newly appointed CEO, David Brennan, commented at a company meeting that he was studying the launch of biosimilars to build on AstraZeneca's existing operations in biological medicines. "A company like ours with the capability like ours has capacity to do that . . . ," he informed journalists.

- *Pfizer*: Former CEO, Jeff Kindler, stated in December 2009 that the company was looking into opportunities within the "generic biotechnology medicines" market, a strategy the company has followed through on with its US$350 million biosimilar insulin deal with Indian biosimilar manufacturer, Biocon.
- *Amgen*: Amgen has come under significant commercial pressure from the launch of biosimilars in Europe. Biosimilar versions of filgrastim have been launched in Europe and continue to have an impact on Neupogen and Neulasta®. It is interesting, therefore, that the company has expressed an interest in taking part in the biosimilars market. In January 2011, Amgen's CEO stated at the JPMorgan Healthcare Conference in San Francisco that the company was "…expressing interest in the biosimilars space, largely led by market structure of high entry barriers to the biosimilars market and availability of required infrastructure with it." At the same conference, Biogen Idec announced it was considering its options in the biosimilars market.

Perhaps the most high-profile move into the biosimilars market by an innovative biopharma company is that of Merck & Co. Merck began laying the foundations of its foray into the biosimilars market in 2006, when it acquired glycol-engineering specialist GlycoFi for US$400 million. Then in December 2008, a formal announcement of the establishment of Merck BioVentures (MBV) came, supported by a cash injection of US$1.5 billion to support clinical development, regulatory submissions, and commercialization. Moreover, GlycoFi's platform technology was put front and center of the new unit's strategy for manufacturing cost-effective biosimilar versions of complex biosimilars, including EPO-alfa, filgrastim, and mAbs.

Since the announcement, much information has emerged. There have been acquisitions. In February 2009, MBV announced the purchase of certain biosimilar assets from Insmed. In a deal valued at US$130 million, MBV acquired Insmed's products, INS-19 (filgrastim) and INS-20 (pegylated filgrastim), as well as control of Insmed's manufacturing facility in Boulder, Colorado. There have also been some challenges and issues. MBV announced in May 2010 that due to increased regulatory requirements from the FDA for one of its pipeline products, MK-2578 (a pegylated version of EPO-alfa), MBV were discontinuing the product's development. MBV has announced a strategic alliance with clinical research organization (CRO), Parexel, focused on the clinical development of biosimilars, indicating that perhaps MBV's internal capabilities in this regard are not at the necessary level. And most recently, Merck announced that it had licensed global rights (excluding Korea and Turkey) to HD-203, a biosimilar version of etanercept (Enbrel®; Pfizer/Amgen), for US$720 million.

Why has Merck decided to invest so heavily in the biosimilars market, considering the company is at the leading edge of biologics innovation across a number of therapy areas? Perhaps the answer lies in a presentation given by Merck at a recent biosimilars conference, at which two critical issues emerged. First, across the biologics market, there seems to be a perceived decline in the return on investment in relation to biologics LCM. Innovation is becoming harder to achieve, and payers are becoming more demanding in terms of what they expect from new therapies. Second, within a number of biopharmaceutical companies, including Merck, a balancing act between driving improved access to biologics and maintaining shareholder value has emerged, with investments in the biosimilars market seen as a way of ensuring both.

27.9 FINAL WORDS

Biosimilars are here to stay. More approvals are expected in markets where formal biosimilar legislation has been enacted. In the face of biosimilar competition, the tactical responses of innovative biopharmaceutical companies must be to remain ethical and stick to the facts. Questioning the safety of biosimilars, and spreading myths about biosimilars, will no longer be accepted.

Therefore, innovative biopharmaceutical companies must continue to innovate (where possible), strive to differentiate portfolios at the molecular, brand, and corporate level, and be prepared to compete with biosimilars. Strategies in this regard include creative pricing strategies, innovative forms of promotion, or by getting involved in the biosimilars market directly, either via internal development or by acquiring biosimilar assets from other companies . . . a strategy that is set to become a lot more popular in the future.

THE INTEGRATED BRAND LCM STRATEGY AND ITS IMPLEMENTATION

CHAPTER 28

Strategic Goals of LCM Brand Plans

Decision making in lifecycle management (LCM) is not a simple process. The range of options available to each potential molecule can be vast, and it is essential that the measures selected for a particular brand are mutually compatible, and ideally that they reinforce and support one another to give the best possible return on investment. Life is made more complicated by the fact that hard investment decisions often need to be made more than 5 years before any such option would reach the market. Choosing the best combination of LCM tactics is thus a choice wrought with risk.

The key step in ensuring that the brand LCM plan has a chance of representing the optimal constellation of LCM strategies and tactics is to first decide on the overall strategy for the brand.

This involves considering a number of key dimensions relating to both the product itself and the market into which it is being launched. Three of these key factors are

- Position to market
- Comparative clinical profile versus current gold standard
- Level of market unmet need

Let us look at these factors one at a time.

28.1 POSITION TO MARKET

Whether a product is first to class, a fast follower (second or third in class) or a me-too has a dramatic effect on the potential choice of LCM approach. For a first-in-class drug, the onus of LCM is on validation, expansion, and rearguard defense. Class-level validation requires the leading agent to prove

---

Pharmaceutical Lifecycle Management: Making the Most of Each and Every Brand, First Edition.
Tony Ellery and Neal Hansen.
© 2012 John Wiley & Sons, Inc. Published 2012 by John Wiley & Sons, Inc.

clinical superiority to existing gold standards, so Phase IV trial programs are often a critical focus. Indication expansion is in many cases a key driving factor for first-in-class LCM, as the new class has to establish the potential universe of patients, without the advantage of previous physician history with the class or mechanism of action. Finally, being first in class is great for class market share, but there is subsequently only one way that market share can go, and that is downwards! As such, mounting a rearguard defense to ensure the first in class remains the market leader is an essential part of LCM planning. The focus is on understanding where and how new products will seek to differentiate and minimizing the advantage (or at least the importance of that advantage) through effective brand management.

For fast-following drugs, the goals of LCM can be split, with expansion, differentiation, and defense the likely key goals. For many drug classes, the role of the second- and third-to-market drugs is to further expand the indication base for the class, rather than to extensively compete with the first-in-class agent. As an example, the launch of the second-in-class tumor necrosis factor-alpha (TNF-alpha) inhibitor Remicade® in Crohn's disease allowed it to gain a "first-in-market" positioning in this disease, although it had been beaten to market in its lead indication, rheumatoid arthritis, by Enbrel® from Immunex (now Amgen) and Wyeth. Remicade thus expanded the overall usability of the class of drugs in a broader range of immune diseases.

However, expansion is not the only goal of LCM for fast followers. Many products have the ambition to overcome the first-in-class agent and to take the market leadership. In this case, they target their LCM activities to drive competitive differentiation within the class. Within the erectile dysfunction market, for example, Pfizer's Viagra® was the first-in-class phosphodiesterase type-5 (PDE-V) inhibitor, and essentially was responsible for the creation of a treatable population for this previously untreated condition. When the fast following agents Cialis® (Eli Lilly) and Levitra® (Bayer) were launched, their primary goals were to displace Viagra and to ride the overall market growth already created by Pfizer, rather than to use LCM to expand the potential treatable population further.

For me-too products, the key challenge for LCM is to make the drug relevant. With potentially anywhere from three to ten products already approved in the class, establishing a valid real-world differentiation is critical to driving success for late class entrants. For many successful late market entrants, the drivers of success can be linked to basic clinical profile. Pfizer's Lipitor®, for example, and indeed Merck's Zocor® before that, clearly differentiated from previous class entrants based on their efficacy at reducing low-density lipoprotein (LDL) levels, the key measure of success for a dyslipidemia drug at the time.

For other late entrant successes, alternative approaches to differentiation have led to class leadership. Merck's Fosamax® is well known as the market leader in the bisphosphonate class, generating peak global sales of over US$3 billion. However, it was only the fourth bisphosphonate to market, launching

16 years after the first class entrant, Procter and Gamble's Didronel®. The secret to the Fosamax success was in indication selection. Rather than following the previous class entrants into the hypercalcemia of malignancy and Paget's disease markets, Merck developed the market for the treatment of osteoporosis. By inventive use of diagnostic tools (bone mineral density measurements) to define a new treatable population, Merck was able to be first to market in the new indication, and rapidly established a market leadership position that has never been effectively challenged since.

28.2 COMPARATIVE CLINICAL PROFILE VERSUS GOLD STANDARD

As touched on in the case of Lipitor cited above, the base clinical profile that a product has at launch versus its key rivals is a critical factor in shaping the form of LCM required. If a drug is clearly differentiated from its main rivals on purely clinical measures (efficacy and safety), the goals of LCM will be different than for a product that needs more "creativity" in its approach to competition. This is well illustrated by the description of angiotensin-2 receptor blockers (ARBs) in Case History 9 in the Appendix.

28.3 LEVEL OF MARKET UNMET NEED

A third factor that will shape the approach to LCM is the innate level of unmet need within a therapeutic market. Fundamentally, to what extent will the simple availability of a new drug be sufficient to drive growth, at least during the launch phase? Historically, launching a first-in-class drug was relatively easy, as the improvements over existing therapies tended to be step changes, and the level of unmet medical need was a lot higher than in many of today's markets. In today's world, the success of the drug industry of the past few decades has led to a decrease in real unmet need, with cost containment exercises increasingly focusing on what is acceptable satisfaction of medical need as opposed to what provides the best possible outcome, irrespective of cost.

For a new drug launching in today's world, a critical element of effective LCM is the ability to profoundly understand the dimensions of real unmet need in the target indication. If efficacy is not really an unmet need, can an improvement in side effects make a real difference? If efficacy and safety are already a given, what new improvement (guaranteed compliance, truly improved convenience, reduced hospital costs, etc.) can be found to align a new drug with a communicable and relevant unmet need?

CHAPTER 29

Ten Keys to Successful LCM

We could no doubt expand the number 10 to 20 or more, or condense it down to 4 or 5. Ten seems about the right number to provide sufficient granularity to what we have to say without overcomplicating matters unnecessarily. So, these are the 10 factors as we see them.

1. Excellent functional expertise
2. Visible management support
3. Unambiguous ownership
4. An early start
5. A robust "broad to bespoke" process
6. Focus on "high-LCM value" brands
7. Adequate resources
8. Measurements and rewards
9. Training and support
10. Realism

29.1 EXCELLENT FUNCTIONAL EXPERTISE

Let us start off with a success factor which at first sight seems banal. Obviously, any company must have employees who know their jobs. The problem within the brand drug industry is that job requirements have changed considerably over the past 10 years or so, and not every employee—or every company—has been able to adapt to these new requirements.

In the good old days, the brand drug industry was a machine for creating and developing a reliable succession of new molecules, ticking the boxes that health authorities required to grant marketing approval, and then promoting

Pharmaceutical Lifecycle Management: Making the Most of Each and Every Brand, First Edition.
Tony Ellery and Neal Hansen.
© 2012 John Wiley & Sons, Inc. Published 2012 by John Wiley & Sons, Inc.

the new brands heavily to doctors using huge sales forces to get the drug prescribed. Manufacturing costs were not of much concern because the reimbursed prices of the brands were so high that companies were easily able to attain profit margins of 30% or more without worrying too much about the cost of goods sold or the efficiency of sales forces. Composition-of-matter patents were pretty much invulnerable, and even when those annoying little generic companies did bring their copies to market, there was little pressure to prescribe them, and the brand companies had in any case probably already created new formulations that provided more convenient dosing, and would thus be preferred by doctors and patients over the generic. A job in Big Pharma was pretty much a job for life, with a healthy base salary and not much of one's total income exposed to the vagaries of "management by objectives." This, then, is the environment in which many of today's brand drug industry employees grew up. And "employees" includes managers and executives!

Let us look at some of the key functions involved in lifecycle management (LCM) to see how these requirements have changed. We are going to indulge in a bit of black-and-white stereotyping to hammer our message home!

29.1.1   Patent Attorneys

Not so many years ago, the quiet guy in the corner at the project team meetings was probably the patent attorney. Mostly he got involved in team discussions only when asked his opinion on a specific patent issue, and then he often hedged and avoided committing himself to a clear—and helpful—answer. One true story serves to illustrate this. A few years ago, one of the authors was leading a project team meeting when a question was raised concerning the robustness of a key patent. "What are the chances that this patent will withstand challenge?" the patent attorney was asked. After a long pause, he timidly replied "I think it's about 50/50." Somewhat irritated, the project leader pointed out that important development decisions were dependent upon his answer and asked him to return to the patent department and come back to next month's project team meeting with a more helpful answer. Back he came, one month later, to deliver the statement "We have thoroughly analyzed the situation in the patent department and now we are certain that the chances are 50/50!"

Today, the job requirements are much higher. A patent attorney is expected to design integrated patent strategies in close collaboration with researchers and developers, and to be accountable for them. As generic companies grow more skilled, richer, and more aggressive, the patent attorney must be continuously reassessing the IP protecting the brand in the light of new legislation and new case rulings that might create new precedents. Today, brand company patent attorneys may find themselves in court facing brash young generic company patent attorneys with good business minds and well-honed debating skills. And the court is likely to be siding with the generic company from the start, for the reasons that we discussed under reputational issues in Chapter 1.

The brand company patent attorney of today needs just as much technical expertise as in the past, but today a different personality is often required— extroverted, self-confident, proactive, and a good negotiator.

29.1.2   Regulatory Affairs

The evolution of the role of regulatory affairs has been no less dramatic than that of the patent department. In many ways, the two functions have evolved along very similar lines. The stereotype picture of a traditional DRA person was of an introvert, locked away in his office, hidden behind huge stacks of regulatory files, assembling documents provided by other functions into regulatory submissions. He was a bit like a cross between a clerk and a librarian. Certainly, the collation of gigantic regulatory filings is still an important task in every DRA department, but the electronic age has resulted in electronic filings which take a lot of the drudgery out of DRA operations. This frees up more time for regulatory staff to concentrate on the more interesting, and more demanding, aspects of their job. Unfortunately, not all are capable of making that transition.

Today's DRA expert will be expected to negotiate with health authorities in new areas like biosimilars, biomarkers, companion diagnostics, and seamless, adaptive clinical trial designs. It is no longer enough to tick the boxes provided by the health authorities. Some of those boxes do not even exist yet, and industry and health authorities are working together to decide how best to address new questions, to decide what it is feasible for industry to provide, and how this matches what health authorities believe they require to ensure that safety, efficacy, and quality standards are satisfied.

A DRA expert of the old school once said to one of the authors, "My job is to represent the health authorities within the company." Oh no, it's not! This statement sounds too much like quality control—checking the output of the individual departments and rejecting it if it is not up to scratch. Rather, think quality assurance. It is the DRA expert's role to work together with the functions to ensure that their output does meet health authority requirements in the first place; and sometimes even to work together with the health authorities to define exactly what those requirements should be.

29.1.3   Clinical Development

We need to mention clinical development as it usually represents by far the biggest investment in any development project. However, we would argue that the job requirements have probably changed least in this function. The ability to design appropriate clinical trials, to motivate the best centers to participate in them, to recruit patients within the required timelines, and to correctly interpret the trial results were and remain the key skills that the clinical development function must master. Of course there have been changes here too, with seamless, adaptive designs and biomarkers, for example, but these have been evolutionary changes rather than the disruptive changes that we have described for patent attorneys and DRA experts.

29.1.4   Formulation Scientists

In the past, even some large, brand companies had formulation departments which were not very innovative and not very capable of thinking out of the box regarding new delivery technologies and systems. The reason for this lies in the very nature of the branded drug industry. When you bring an innovative new molecule to market, the reason it will be prescribed is primarily its efficacy and its safety, or rather the relationship between the two. The first-in-class molecule that addresses a disease with significant unmet needs does not require an elegant formulation to win prescriptions. Furthermore, probably the single most important success factor in the development of a new molecule was speed to market, for three main reasons:

1. Delays heavily impact net present value (NPV), all other things being equal.
2. Competitors in the same class might get to market first.
3. The patent clock is ticking.

Obviously, companies did not want to spend extra time in development tweaking formulations. The result was that new molecules tended to get launched first in simple, proven, low-risk formulations. And as a new crop of innovative molecules was already in the pipeline, there was often comparatively little motivation to improve the formulation following launch. Perhaps a capsule would be replaced by a tablet or extra dosages added, but—once again—well-established, low-risk technologies were likely to be preferred. Probably the first occasion when brand companies consistently sought to adopt new technologies was when the winners and losers in a drug class started to be influenced by whether the drug was administered three times, twice, or once daily.

Another important aspect in formulation departments was the "not invented here" syndrome. Companies tended to stick with their old tried-and-tested in-house delivery technologies rather than looking outside to see what third parties could offer. Again, this behavior is in the very nature of the brand industry, where proprietary chemistry and knowledge constitutes the high ground. Compare this to generics, where the whole foundation of the industry is the ability to copy something that was invented by somebody else. As an aside, which is not really related only to LCM, we would mention that some brand companies today seem to have overcompensated by acquiring a "not invented *there*" mind-set, where disillusionment with the output of their own research labs has tended to make them look more favorably upon product acquisitions and in-licensing deals than on their own in-house projects.

Generic companies are much more ready to accept that specialized drug delivery players may have superior knowledge and technologies in their own particular areas of expertise, and to work with them in creating supergenerics which are not merely copies of the original brand and therefore can confer a competitive advantage within the crowded generics market.

Today's formulation departments in the branded drug industry also need to be more open to the idea that third parties may be better able to create value-adding new formulations than they are themselves. In some cases, it may make sense to try to internalize this expertise, by acquiring the third party or by obtaining exclusivity for a specific technology either totally or for a particular indication or drug class. But this usually only makes sense as an investment when the technology is applicable to several in-house projects. In most cases, it will be enough to gain access to the technology only for the individual molecule or substance class that will benefit from its usage.

29.1.5   Marketing and Sales

We will not go into the changes in the marketing and sales model for branded pharmaceuticals in depth here as they are already well documented elsewhere, and broadly recognized. For decades, the branded drug model was based primarily on convincing physicians to prescribe specific drugs by filling their waiting rooms with huge numbers of sales representatives ready to present their glossy brochures and sales pitches as to why their drug was preferable to the offerings of competitors. These sales pitches were supported by different incentives to the doctors to prescribe certain drugs; the incentives included direct payments, large numbers of free samples, sponsoring in the form of consultancy contracts, donations to clinics, invitations to conferences, luxury cruises, presents for the spouse, meals in luxury restaurants, and much else besides. Although many of these physician incentives have since been made illegal in many countries, there can be little doubt that the model worked! Companies found that physicians were really not that much different from housewives buying washing powders. Lots of promotion, advertising, and incentives led to higher sales. However, many physicians started complaining bitterly about this behavior, pointing out that all these visits were taking away the time that they should be spending with patients. But the statistics still showed that the more representatives you could afford to send calling on physicians, the more drug you would sell. At its peak in 2005, Pfizer employed 38,000 sales representatives worldwide, the equivalent of three U.S. Army Divisions. The numbers have decreased somewhat in recent years, with an industry total of around 75,000 sales representatives employed in the United States in mid-2011 compared to over 100,000 in mid-2006.

Managed care started to take the decision as to which drugs could be prescribed away from the physician and put it into the hands of the third-party payers, who were only interested in the real-life economics of new drug offerings. The traditional marketing and sales model was put into question. As a consequence, companies started to downsize their sales forces, although the paradigm change to a new selling model has not yet really established itself, and Big Pharma companies are still waiting anxiously to see which of their peers blinks first in eliminating its conventional sales forces, at least in the United States, before committing themselves fully to the new paradigm.

The game in the future will be won and lost according to which companies are best able to get their drugs reimbursed by medical insurance institutions, government or private, at an acceptable price. Excellent relationships with wholesalers and pharmacists will also become ever more crucial. Patients, increasingly knowledgeable about their diseases, thanks to the Internet, will challenge physicians more frequently instead of blindly accepting their pronouncements. The physician is still a key part of the equation, but he is no longer the whole equation. Generic companies are better placed to thrive in the new environment in that their marketing and sales employees are already operating under what is likely to become the new model in more and more countries. The payers obviously prefer generics, and patients will move increasingly in this direction as well as co-pays increase. Moreover, the acceptance that generics are just as good as the original brands will grow, thanks to government propaganda and the greater professionalism and quality standards of the generics industry.

29.1.6 Manufacturing

The cost of goods of virtually every patented small-molecular drug product is only a tiny fraction of the selling price, much lower than in most other manufactured goods industries. For many years there was therefore little motivation to reduce the cost of goods. However, with price pressures increasing and product portfolios aging, cost consciousness in drug manufacturing became more of an issue as brand companies strove to maintain both their R&D and marketing and sales spends without damaging the traditionally high profit margins of around 30% that investors had come to expect. In a way, this was a little unfair on manufacturing departments, as there were far higher potential savings in R&D, and particularly in marketing and sales. In a typical Big Pharma company, manufacturing costs are only about 10% of brand sales while R&D costs are nearer to 20% and marketing and sales costs are nearer to 35%. Today, while it is hard to justify a lower spend than 20% of sales for R&D, especially in view of the fact that even this investment is not producing the required steady stream of new molecules, it is obvious from what was written above that marketing and sales spending could be considerably reduced if they were to be redirected to the new decision makers, the payers.

Still, in many companies it was manufacturing costs that first came under the microscope, with the result that this function has already gone a long way to adjust to the new industry model. Principles of lean manufacturing and a willingness to move production into cheaper countries, or even to outsource it, are well established in most Big Pharma companies, so that although generic companies still have a lower cost base than the brand industry, the gap has been partially closed. And it is more important now that brand companies maintain pressure to keep manufacturing costs down as the cost of goods of many of the new sophisticated biologics will be much higher than for small-molecular drugs, and in tomorrow's environment this will not be fully compensated for by higher prices.

One could consider other functions too, but these are the ones where a lack of the right kind of expertise can damage LCM efforts most. In other functions involved in LCM, it is important to increase the sensitivity to specific issues. To take one concrete example of this, the legal department needs to be acutely aware of the issue of anticompetitive behavior, and to ensure that LCM efforts are conducted within the limits of what is allowed. A little while ago, a company that was setting up an LCM website on its intranet asked representatives of various functions to contribute text regarding the different LCM strategies. A marketer described in writing the process of "stuffing channels just before patent expiry to deny generics access to the market." Fortunately the legal department spotted this description of flagrant anticompetitive behavior just one day before it went live on the intranet, accessible to tens of thousands of employees. As the website purported to be a training instrument for LCM teams, there would have been some very red faces and a significant exposure of the company to litigation had the website gone live with this sentence in it! The fact that the marketer was a fairly junior member of his department suggested that the marketing department needed to look harder at its understanding of "empowerment" and that the legal team needed to instigate appropriate training programs with a minimum of delay.

29.2   VISIBLE MANAGEMENT SUPPORT

As we saw right back in the Introduction to this book, most pharmaceutical executives felt in 2005 that their companies should be doing a better job on LCM. One can hope that the situation has improved, but evolution is a slow process and anecdotal evidence—for example Q + As and discussions with senior executives at LCM conferences and seminars—suggests that there is still concern in many companies that LCM could be better. As we have already seen, one issue is that the main purpose of brand companies is to discover new medicines and bring them to market. Contrast this with large parts of the branded consumer goods industry. At Coca Cola, for example, the brand directors do not have to push uphill against a mind-set that believes that the main purpose of the company is to invent new soft drinks. Maintaining and optimizing the existing brands is obviously job number one, and everybody in the organization knows and accepts it. But in the branded drug industry LCM efforts, which are aimed at maintaining existing assets, are predestined to take a back seat unless management expends significant energy in promoting their importance.

As is so often the case, it all comes down to the question of whether management is walking the talk. Of course it is perfectly possible for a company with a healthy R&D pipeline of new molecules to look at LCM, and especially late-stage lifecycle management (LLCM), and to decide not to give it high priority. LCM involves a lot of work, often only with modest returns and increasingly high barriers to commercial success. "Lots of shearing and not much wool," as the Australians say. The problem is to be found in companies which claim that LCM is an important part of their overall strategy, and then neglect it.

It is understandable that companies do not shout too loudly about their LCM efforts in their press conferences and public statements. Some aspects of LCM, and especially LLCM, have got a bad name, and in any case, an overemphasis of LCM projects looks like a confession that the new molecular entity (NME) pipeline really is not quite as robust as the company would like the analysts and investors to believe.

But internally, if a company truly believes that LCM is important, then its behavior should match its aspiration and that is in our experience often not the case. Here are a few questions that such a company should be asking itself:

- Where does LCM figure in the list of company priorities for the year?
- When was the last time that the CEO used the term LCM in a major presentation to staff?
- At what level in the company is LCM sponsored?
- What is the rank of the highest executive with responsibility for LCM?
- Are some of the annual awards going to employees and teams who have demonstrated excellent LCM, for example, by minimizing sales erosion after patent expiry, or only to those working on new products?
- When development resources get tight, is it always the LCM projects that are put on the back burner?
- What type of employee is being selected for the LCM positions? Are these top performers and future stars, or are they rather the folk who did not quite make the grade in their functions, for example, marketers who did a poor job on a launch product? Are they the employees who nobody is quite sure what to do with in the couple of years before they can be early retired?
- What are the next positions of employees in LCM positions? Are they getting promoted into more senior roles?

Whatever management is saying, it is the answers to these questions and others like them which will determine whether the company is really taking LCM seriously or just paying it lip service.

29.3 UNAMBIGUOUS OWNERSHIP

This success factor is often closely related to the lack of management support, but it is sufficiently important to warrant its own bullet point. It is very revealing to ask participants at conferences questions along the following lines. "Who is responsible at your company for manufacturing? And who is responsible for drug development? And who is responsible for LCM?"

Invariably, the first two questions get an unambiguous answer—Fred Smith or Wendy Jones. But that is decidedly not what happens when the third question is posed. Typical answers include "Nobody," "Everybody," "I don't know," "Marketing," "the Brand Director," "the Project Leader."

A generation ago, the question "Who is responsible for quality?" would likely have provoked the same response, but then hard lessons were learned from the success of Japanese manufacturing companies, especially in consumer electronics and later automobiles, so that Western companies enthusiastically, if belatedly, climbed onto the Total Quality Management (TQM) bandwagon. Today, every company will have senior executives who have the word "Quality" in their job titles.

But this is still the exception rather than the rule in the case of LCM. Where a specific individual does have the words "lifecycle management" in his job title, this is likely to be a rather junior person in a staff position who advises and supports development and/or marketing functions.

Even at the brand or project team level, the question as to who is responsible for LCM frequently provokes blank looks. The answer "Everybody" can reliably be interpreted to mean "Nobody." Sometimes a team member will be named, but additional questions tend to reveal a less than ideal situation. In one case, the person responsible was the formulations chemist. Now that may be a good solution for some aspects of LCM, but this individual is unlikely to be the right person when it comes to indication expansion or defense of the primary patent. With brands that have been on the market for a while, it is often a more junior brand manager who is made responsible for LCM. Unfortunately, it is likely to be low on his list of priorities and his prior experience of LCM is often zero.

We would argue that things only get done well if a named person with experience and seniority is made responsible and accountable for the activities and their results. We will be looking at how to achieve this in the next chapter.

29.4   AN EARLY START

We are often asked "When is the right time to start LCM of a brand?" The invariable answer is "Earlier than you think" or "Earlier than you are doing it in your company at present," but the "right time" is going to depend on what you include in your definition of LCM.

Back in the Introduction to this book we stated that we would be defining LCM as "all of the measures taken to grow, maintain, and defend the sales and profits of a pharmaceutical brand following its development, launch, marketing, and sales in its first formulation and its first indication," so let us stick with that definition here.

What is the earliest point of time at which one has both the need and the necessary information to make decisions that will impact LCM? Well, let us take just one example—indication sequencing—to illustrate how very early this is.

LCM involves deciding which indications should be developed for a new drug, and in which order. One could argue that LCM should therefore begin even before the patients are selected for proof-of-concept (PoC) clinical trials. We would argue that this is too early, for at least three reasons.

First, scientific considerations should predominate when the patient populations for PoC trials are being selected. The new molecule must be given the best possible chance of being able to show what effects it can have in the body, for example, how it interacts with biological targets or how it influences a biomarker or disease end point. It is not wise to endanger the chances of getting a relevant and accurate PoC readout by making compromises with the selection of patients. And until one is sure that the molecule is worth developing, it really does not make a whole lot of sense to consider how one will optimize it over the coming years; one is reminded of the first step in the recipe for cooking grizzly bear steaks, "First catch your grizzly!"

Second, LCM expertise and resources are always at a premium in a company and they must be used wisely. Most of the pre-PoC compounds will not make it to market, and it is therefore not good economics to unleash the full spectrum of LCM analyses and planning instruments on a molecule too early in its development.

Third, and very pragmatically, in many companies, PoC trials are likely to lie within the responsibility of the research (rather than development) function, or in a separate early development department. These are unlikely to have either the knowledge or team structure that is needed to accommodate full LCM.

We would argue that LCM should formally be started once the PoC has proven positive and before the compound has been accepted into the development portfolio. Ideally in fact, the first LCM Plan should be part of the post-PoC documentation provided to justify that the compound be moved into development. After all, the value of many compounds to the company is not represented only by their first indications. We will look later and in depth at what aspects of LCM should be addressed in this very first LCM Plan. Certainly, the whole question of indication selection and sequencing must be analyzed before any decision can be taken as to which the initial indication should be.

Independently of when the formal LCM process is initiated with an individual compound, we would emphasize that an "LCM mind-set" is needed throughout the company. As an example, even before PoCs are being considered, a researcher talking with a patent attorney should be considering not just how robustly a new compound can be patented, but also how broadly the class can be protected, what additional aspects of the compound can be protected, and what investigations should be started, and when, with a view to generating secondary patents later which may help to protect the future brand for longer (e.g., a chemical intermediate produced during an improved synthesis). Consideration needs to be given to the precise language of each patent so as to facilitate future line extensions of the brand. Poor wording in a patent can block the subsequent granting of secondary patents which would have a later expiry date than the composition of matter patent.

We are often asked when late LCM (LLCM) efforts should commence. We view this as a rhetorical question, as LCM and LLCM planning should mesh seamlessly together, and there should not really even be a separate LLCM entity. If we rephrase the question to ask when LCM planning should begin for those activities that are aimed at either prolonging exclusivity or at retaining more postexclusivity market share, then we would say not less than 5 years before patent expiry. But even this answer needs to be interpreted carefully, as the main instrument for ensuring exclusivity is the composition-of-matter patent, and this will already have been written well, or badly, more than 20 years before it expires!

It is a source of amazement to us how late some brand teams—and even some companies—react to impending patent expiry, panicking a year or less before exclusivity is due to be lost and only then intensively seeking ways to withstand the generic onslaught. Recently, one of us was approached by a Top Ten branded drug company to support the creation of the very first LCM plan for a particular brand. When we asked when the protecting patent was due to expire, we were told it had expired 2 years ago! On the day a patent is issued, one already knows the day it will expire, 20 years or so in the future, so there is absolutely no excuse for not being prepared for that sad event well in advance. The earlier in the life cycle that LLCM planning is started, the more likely it is that the molecule can be improved upon, or value-added and patent-protected line extensions can be developed. A new product can then be introduced that really does offer more value than a generic, instead of the company having to resort to the kind of last-ditch delaying tactics which merely deny patients access to a generic which is the exact equivalent of the brand.

29.5 A ROBUST "BROAD TO BESPOKE" PROCESS

This point ties in with the previous one. LCM planning should not be a knee-jerk reaction to impending disaster just before patent expiry.

Instead, it should be a proactive and strategic process. The initial LCM Plan which is initiated early in development is expanded and modified as needs arise throughout the life cycle. Updated versions of the plan will be required at important development milestones, and in response to major changes in the environment in which the brand will be expected to perform (e.g., if a competitor drug performs much better than anticipated, or if a new regulatory hurdle is introduced in a major market). We will be examining the process in detail in the next chapter.

The first version of the LCM Plan will have lots of gaps, as the molecule is not yet well characterized, and the company may not yet really know what it has on its hands. However, as we have already seen, some decisions just have to made even at this early stage, and it is clearly preferable to do this based on a careful evaluation of the information that one does have available rather than procrastinating and losing an opportunity, or proceeding based only on gut feeling. A good example of an early decision that must be taken is whether or not the initial indication should be an orphan disease. An example of an LCM strategy that would certainly not be a topic early in the life cycle is whether to shift a low dose of the brand to over-the-counter (OTC) status.

As more information is gained about the molecule, the LCM Plan may change considerably if there are unexpected findings. In any case, the plan is likely to get more specific and perhaps to narrow its focus based on a more realistic expectation of what the molecule can achieve; the opposite is, of course, also possible, when emerging preclinical or clinical results suggest that additional indications could be feasible.

At any stage of the life cycle, the LCM Plan should be the basis for all of the functional activities. In other words, every element of the LCM Plan must be supported by the necessary development work at the appropriate time. Equally important in these times of cost consciousness and limited resources, the functions should not be wasting their time on work that does not support elements of the LCM Plan.

What do we mean by "broad to bespoke?" Again, we will be going into more detail in the next chapter, but we mean that all possible LCM measures should first be considered, and then a tailored portfolio of measures which is specific for each brand should be created. The best LCM plans are to be found when different LCM measures synergize and reinforce one another—for example, when a new dosage regimen in a new formulation delivered by a different route of administration is selected for a new indication.

When creating an LCM Plan, never underestimate the importance of the process itself and not just of its end product. Bringing together different functions to brainstorm and discuss LCM options will promote understanding for the risks and opportunities that the brand will face, and will improve buy-in to the activities defined in the plan. And better buy-in means faster and more enthusiastic implementation once the plan has been approved.

29.6 FOCUS ON "HIGH LCM VALUE BRANDS"

As companies get more sensitized to the need for and potential of brand LCM, some have started to allocate resources to brands using the watering-can principle. For example, each brand director may be told that he can spend X% of sales on LCM measures (new indications, line extensions, and the like). This is a superficially attractive alternative as it reinforces the empowerment of the brand directors. But we do not like the approach and believe that it is usually just an easy way out rather than a considered strategy. The fact is that some brands offer huge opportunities for LCM and others do not, and resources should be allocated on the basis of these opportunities. Now some LCM measures are universal, and should be applied to every brand and every development project. Examples would include patents and regulatory exclusivities. But in other cases, where the measures are more complicated and more expensive, one must be more selective. An easily formulated active substance in a convenient once-daily tablet formulation, where the active substance can only be used for one disease, is likely to hold less potential for line extensions than a hard-to-formulate, three-times daily capsule with potentially multiple indications. Each LCM project should be judged on its own merits and rated accordingly in the portfolio prioritization process.

A case can be made for deciding "top-down" what percentage of the overall development budget should be spent on NME projects and what percentage on LCM projects, and there may be further subdivisions in larger companies, for example, between therapeutic areas, but within its own pool, each LCM project should be judged individually on its own merits. We will be coming back to this topic in Part H.

29.7   ADEQUATE RESOURCES

This point is really applicable to any project, but it is included here as it is often the LCM projects which suffer first when the development budget is under fire and costs have to be cut. In most companies, preference tends to be given to late-stage Phase III NME projects and first-in-class NMEs anywhere in the pipeline. This is not wrong, but it does mean that LCM projects are often under-resourced and timelines start to slip. The problem here is that LCM projects are very frequently time critical. We are not necessarily looking for higher prioritization of LCM projects in such a situation, but we would suggest that the project leader or brand director makes it very clear to his management what the implications of the resource reduction will be. Often, there is no justification in proceeding with the project if it is to be significantly delayed, and this needs to be communicated. An excellent LCM Plan, with time horizons specified for each of the LCM measures, helps to get the message across and may even result in resources being reallocated. If the resources are not forthcoming, then it may be necessary to cancel the LCM project or to seek an external partner who will resource the project and share in the rewards.

29.8   MEASUREMENTS AND REWARDS

We have all heard the saying "You get what you measure," and it is very applicable to LCM. We would add ". . . so be very careful what you measure." In both cases, you can replace the word "measure" with "reward!"

Selecting the right parameters to measure and to reward is actually rather difficult in LCM, because activities performed and decisions taken today will probably only pay off in several years' time. What one requires is reliable "lead indicators" that predict whether a secondary patent will prove to be robust or whether an LCM decision will turn out to have been the correct one, rather than a "lag indicator" which only tells you much later whether it has led to success or not. Let us take an example. The decision to invest in a reformulation of a brand to retain market share after patent expiry will have to be taken at least 4, better 5 years before the patent is due to expire. One must calculate that it will take about 2 years to develop and test the formulation (and this assumes that the technology is readily available), a year to get it approved, and then 2 years to obtain pricing and reimbursement and to allow the marketing function enough time to convert physicians and patients to the new formulation in preference to the old formulation that is about to be genericized. If it is to be successful and recover the investment in its development, then the new formulation must retain sufficiently more market share than was predicted for the old formulation. Payers, physicians, and patients must all acknowledge that the new formulation is an advance over the old one. Moreover, the intellectual property protecting the formulation patent must be strong enough to resist challenge by generic companies and broad enough to prevent a bioequivalent formulation to be achieved without infringing the patent or patents. Not until about a year after patent expiry can one make the call as to whether the market share of the brand really is higher than it would have been without the new formulation. In other words, the final deliverable, the better market share, will not be apparent until 6 years after the decision was taken to develop the new formulation. Only then will it be possible to measure directly whether the decision was a good one.

In many other areas of the company, the time interval between a decision or action and the measurable final deliverable is much shorter. Thus, one can measure the performance of sales representatives by measuring whether they reach quarterly sales targets, or weekly, or even daily targets for the numbers of physicians visited. Manufacturing can be judged on whether it fills its orders without delays, or on the percentage of batches passing quality control testing, and so on. In some areas of development, there are also excellent surrogate end points for predicting whether an ongoing activity, and therefore also the underlying decisions, will lead to ultimate success. Examples would include the rate of patient recruitment in clinical trials or the accelerated stability results for a new formulation.

So what can we use as the lead indicator that an LCM decision or a whole LCM Plan will lead to success, probably years down the road? The only one we have identified that seems to have any real value is a numerical evaluation of the LCM Plan and the decisions contained therein by an experienced group of senior managers.

Such an evaluation is also the only practical way we have identified of rewarding short term the strategic performance of the members of LCM teams. By the time the deliverables of the LCM Plan can be directly measured, the members of the LCM team that made that decision are likely to be in completely new positions in the company. This is especially true for members from the marketing function as these tend to change their jobs more often than, say, patent attorneys or formulation chemists. It is, of course, theoretically possible to defer rewards until the deliverables have been measured, but few companies have tried to do this in practice as it would involve a large administrative effort and would be a very difficult internal selling job. Imagine telling the head of your Swedish affiliate that despite his impressive sales growth last year his bonus will be reduced because of a wrong decision made by his LCM team 5 years earlier!

As an aside, some skeptics doubt the effectiveness of reward schemes, as they believe that money is a poor motivator. While we would accept that money is sometimes overrated as a motivator, we would still urge these skeptics to try a little experiment in their companies. Inform all employees that next year's bonus will be increased by 10% for anyone wearing a green hat to the office on St. Patrick's Day, and then watch what happens!

Finally, never confuse the terms "reward" and "recognition." An anecdote from early in the career of one of the authors should suffice to illustrate this. When your manager comes to you with a brown envelope containing US$500 and says: "Great job at last week's project review. This is for you but don't tell anyone you got it!" that is "reward" but not "recognition." Do not underestimate the motivational power of recognition either. Giving an LCM team a major company award will considerably increase the number of employees asking to be considered for inclusion on an LCM team.

29.9 TRAINING AND SUPPORT

Many of the employees who work on LCM teams will do so only once or twice in their whole careers. It is unreasonable to expect them to master the whole gamut of potential LCM strategies and individual measures without providing them with expert training and support. We will be looking more closely at training when we consider the benefits of an LCM Centre of Excellence in the next chapter.

29.10 REALISM

Time and time again we see LCM plans that are based on unrealistically optimistic assumptions about how the future will look. This may involve wishful thinking about the brand itself, for example, its ability to address additional diseases or the robustness of its secondary patents, or regarding the future environment in which the brand will be expected to perform. Examples of the latter would be underestimating the effects of cost containment measures such as price or reimbursement parameters, or assuming that generic erosion rates will be lower than they in reality are likely to be. This tendency to be overly optimistic is one reason why it is so important that every LCM Plan contains a list of all of the key assumptions underlying the plan. We will be looking at this in Chapter 31.

This, then, completes the list of the 10 key factors that will determine the success of your LCM efforts.

CHAPTER 30

Organizational Structures and Systems for Ensuring Successful LCM

How should companies organize themselves to ensure that their lifecycle management (LCM) efforts are successful? There are several alternative structures, each with its own pros and cons, and we will give an overview here and discuss the criteria for deciding which organizational structure may be most appropriate for your company.

LCM is a highly cross-functional effort, and the LCM program for a brand—as described in the LCM Plan—requires the coordinated collaboration of a wide range of functions from different parts of the organization. This will include research, clinical development, regulatory affairs, formulations, marketing, competitive intelligence, patents, legal, pricing and reimbursement, business development, manufacturing, and others besides. The LCM program for each brand is likely to comprise several distinct development projects (e.g., new formulations, new indications) and a range of other intra- and interfunctional cooperative efforts (e.g., designing patent strategies, indication sequencing, and market segmentation between different formulations). The entire LCM program for a brand is thus comparable to a very complex project with a variety of dependent subprojects, and the factors determining the optimal organizational structure are thus similar to those for determining the best project management structure.

30.1 ORGANIZATION OF PROJECT AND BRAND MANAGEMENT

At the most basic level, there are three possible project management structures:

- Functional structure
- Project structure
- Matrix structure

Pharmaceutical Lifecycle Management: Making the Most of Each and Every Brand, First Edition.
Tony Ellery and Neal Hansen.
© 2012 John Wiley & Sons, Inc. Published 2012 by John Wiley & Sons, Inc.

30.1.1   Functional Structure

In this form it is better to speak of a project coordinator rather than a project leader as there is little opportunity for this person to function as a true leader. The power lies within the functions, and a project coordinator is chosen who tries to coordinate cross-functional activities while remaining within his function, reporting to his functional head. Often, this individual has little or no experience of leading a cross-functional team and has poor knowledge of the work that is actually performed in the other functions. As an example, a clinician from clinical development may be asked to serve as a project coordinator and is expected to "lead" a team consisting of representatives of all of the other functions involved in the project. In reality, the power remains with the function, and the project is likely to be conducted in the way that the head of clinical development feels is best as he remains the supervisor of the project coordinator, determining this individual's objectives and deciding how well he has achieved them. Other members of the team, for example, the marketing representative, are in a weak position. Work tends to get done sequentially, function by function, with each function unable to start work until the preceding function has finished its job. Infinite time is lost at functional interfaces as most issues have to get elevated to the heads of the respective functions for resolution. Often, because the supervisor of the project coordinators has his own functional priorities, he is unlikely to give the project coordinator job to his best people, and this compounds the problem further as the team has weak leadership. The advantages of the functional structure in project management are twofold. First, it is cheap, because the project coordinator role is taken by existing staff, usually without any additional training, and second, because there is no real challenge to the authority of functional heads. The downsides are a lack of expertise, unclear leadership on the team, no accountability, and inevitable project delays and reworks. However, this structure can work well when there is a low level of cross-functional coordination (e.g., when few functions are involved or when there is no opportunity to overlap activities to win time) or when the project work in each function is very routine, and everybody knows exactly what they have to do, and when.

30.1.2   Project Structure

In a project structure, a project leader is named for the duration of the project, and most or all of the functions involved in the project delegate team members or whole sections of their departments who will report solid-line to the project leader for the duration of the project. The project leader role is obviously an attractive and demanding one in this case, and can be staffed with high performers who are being developed for general management roles. The project leader really does act as the CEO of the project, with full accountability for the results. He holds the project budget, which is not the case with the functional structure, and "he who pays the piper calls the tune." Problems can arise at the interface between the team members and the line functions that they represent. On the one hand, the supervisor is often uncomfortable with the concept of somebody other than himself holding the budget (internal and external) for work done in his function. And the team member himself may be in a difficult position, because his functional colleagues may resent the fact that he has been given what is often perceived as a preferred position, and this means he may have problems during the project and even more so when he has to reintegrate into his "home" function once the project has been completed. His career development may be favored by the fact that he has served in this important position, but all too often, the opposite is the case and his career development is interrupted, and his functional development (e.g., training) put on hold for as long as he works on the project, which can be a matter of years. Often, at the conclusion of such a "heavyweight project," the project leader and key team members leave the company as they are unwilling to return to a less visible and less prestigious role within their functions, or because they have such bad relationships with their functional colleagues that they can no longer be assimilated. This can be an acceptable price to pay, as a project structure is only ever chosen for major projects that are of key strategic importance for the company, and typically those where there are major skill or knowledge gaps in the functions that must be built up for the future. By far the biggest disadvantage of a project structure is that it is very expensive in manpower. In the functional structure, where team members report to their functional heads, they can be employed on multiple projects and their capacity juggled by their supervisors according to the needs of these projects and also of nonproject activities within the function. This flexibility is lost in a project structure. A project team member only works on that one project, reporting to the project leader, regardless of whether his capacity is being fully utilized or not at any one time. Invariably, the creation of a project structure therefore requires higher staff numbers than a functional structure.

We have had direct experience of just one example of a true, uncompromising project structure in a pharmaceutical company, and that was for a nondrug project. In the mid-1990s, the shape of the contact lens industry was going through a huge, disruptive paradigm change. Up until that date, a contact-lens wearer bought two contact lenses per year, washing and disinfecting them every night and putting them back into his eyes in the morning. And then Johnson & Johnson (J&J) introduced the first daily-disposable contact lenses. Suddenly, wearers needed 730 lenses per year instead of two! And the whole business of washing and disinfecting contact lenses disappeared. Ciba Vision (a Novartis company) was manufacturing the traditional contact lenses, but with an unprofitably high cost of goods, and they were making their profits from the saline and disinfectant solutions. Unless Ciba Vision could move its business to disposable contact lenses extremely quickly, it was going to go out of business. Everything would have to change—the cost of goods would have to drop from several dollars to a few cents per lens, completely new polymers would have to be found or invented. New machines for manufacturing contact lenses would have to be designed and built. Massive changes would be needed in quality control (each lens manufactured was checked manually under the old paradigm), warehousing, distribution, and marketing. The existing staff in the functions would have to forget most of what they knew and learn completely new skills. Ciba Vision decided that the only solution in this existence-threatening situation was to create a heavyweight project team. A suitable person was identified as project leader, and a heavyweight team was recruited, mostly but not exclusively from existing staff. For the duration of the project, the team members—and in some functions, whole sections of employees—would report to the project leader. This involved not just the developers and marketers, but research, engineering, manufacturing, finance, human resources, supply chain, and so on. Wherever feasible, the team members and the sections of employees working on the project were physically taken out of their functional environment and moved into separate offices and labs dedicated only to the project. This colocating of all project staff was an important element in underlining that they were now virtually part of a largely independent, stand-alone venture within the company. The only tangible difference between the project and a separate business unit was that the project was a temporary structure, designed to disappear once the new type of contact lens had been delivered to the market; at that stage everybody would be returned to their original functions. The costs were high, but it did not matter—the alternative was oblivion. The project was a success, and Ciba Vision succeeded in launching its own excellent daily-disposable contact lens before J&J's lead in the market became too big to handle.

30.1.3 Matrix Structure

The matrix structure was an attempt to combine the advantages of the functional structure and the project structure while avoiding the problems of both. As with all compromises, it is not a perfect solution, but it has worked rather well and is still today the dominant form for managing projects in many industries, including the drug industry. A well-known statement of Winston Churchill concerning democracy can be purloined to summarize why matrix management is so widely used: "No one pretends that 'matrix management' is perfect or all-wise. Indeed it has been said that it is the worst form of government—except all those other forms that have been tried from time to time."

A matrix structure balances authority and accountability between the functions and the project leaders. Typically, although this varies according to the size of the organization, the project leaders are grouped together in a project management department, which is itself structured like a function. There is a very wide range of possible matrix structures, all the way from nearly-functional to nearly-project structures. The nearly-functional variant is often called a "weak matrix" and the nearly-project organization a "strong matrix." It seems to be a characteristic of many companies that they like to believe that their matrix is stronger than it really is. The reason for this is that management knows that a near-project structure is desirable, but none of the functions really want to sacrifice any of their power. Let us look at the weak matrix first.

In a weak matrix the project leader reports in to a project management function. Team members are nominated by the functions to join his project team, but continue to report solid-line to the function. The project team elaborates a project plan, with the project team members negotiating with their respective functions for the resources needed to complete their part of the work. The functions hold the internal and external budgets for this work. Each functional head determines how well project objectives have been met in his department and conducts the performance evaluation of his team members.

In a strong matrix, the project leader may report in to a project management organization, but may alternatively report to a more senior person, for example, the head of a therapeutic area or, in smaller companies, to the CEO. The project leader selects which team members he wants from the respective line functions, negotiating with them if that person is not available. The project leader has a veto if the functional head nominates somebody who the project leader considers to be unsuited for the task. Key team members may even be given a direct reporting line to the project leader, as in a project structure. While the internal budget continues to be held by the functions, the external budget is held by the project leader. The performance evaluation of team members as it relates to project work is conducted by the project leader, while the function evaluates the performance on nonproject tasks.

Between these two extremes, there is any number of alternatives. For example, the functions may retain the right to evaluate performance, but the project leader may be given the external budget, or vice versa.

The advantages of the matrix structure are self-evident. It is less expensive than a project structure, but it brings a stronger project focus than a functional structure. The main disadvantage is an ambiguity about who is accountable for what, and a comprehensive set of rules is essential to make the matrix structure work well and avoid endless discussions between the functions and the project leader regarding who is responsible for what. As a general guideline, the project leader should, via the approved project plan, determine what work is done, what it may cost to perform, and by when it must be delivered (what, how much, and when?) while the function determines who in the department actually performs the work and is responsible that the work is done to the required quality (who and how?). This sounds neat, but it does not prevent all such discussions. Deciding whether something is a "what" or a "how" is the commonest area of dispute, for example, when the project leader sees the choice of a comparator in a clinical trial as a "what" is being done while the function sees it as a "how" the clinical trial should be run. The "what/how" discussion between project leader and function head tends to take place most frequently in the function from which the project leader originally came.

These, then are the alternative structures for managing projects, and all that we have written in the last few pages should be kept in mind as we proceed to look at the different structures for managing LCM.

30.2 PROJECT AND BRAND LCM STRUCTURES

The first question to ask is whether LCM can be managed successfully by the existing organization. Let us make some assumptions as to what that is. Most companies utilize project teams to bring drugs to market, and then brand teams to manage the marketed drugs. The project team will be dominated by R&D functions, like research, preclinical safety, clinical development, regulatory affairs, and formulations. Marketing will also be represented, possibly by a member of an early commercialization function or by the future brand director, perhaps supported by members of the competitive intelligence and/or pricing and reimbursement functions. There is probably a patent attorney on the team. In large organizations, with many functional units, there may be a core project team, supported by an extended project team whose members are only called upon when their special expertise is required. The core team members should consist at the very least of the project leader, clinical development, marketing, and regulatory affairs. Overall operational responsibility for the project probably lies with the head of development of the company or therapeutic area, although approval of the project objectives plan is likely to be within the remit of a cross-functional decision board of senior managers including research, development, marketing, finances, and possibly country or regional representation.

Following the first approval of the new drug, or shortly before, overall responsibility for the brand is usually transferred to the marketing department. The project leader is succeeded by a brand director, although the project leader may stay on as a brand team member to ensure continuity. Some R&D functions, for example, research, formulations, and preclinical safety, are likely to withdraw from the core brand team and be replaced by additional members of marketing and other commercial functions. The brand team is likely to retain clinical and regulatory members. In many companies, the marketing members of the brand team report solid-line to the brand director, but not usually the development members. In project teams, on the other hand, the reporting relationships to the project leader are usually all dotted lines.

To what extent can LCM be integrated into this structure as it already exists in many companies? The first question to answer is whether LCM can simply be added to the duties of the existing project and brand teams. This was the normal approach in the past, and still has much to recommend it. Advantages include clear ownership of the LCM planning and execution by the project or brand team, plus the fact that most of the project/brand knowledge resides in these teams, and LCM Plans do need to be tailored to each individual project/brand according to its own special requirements. There are two main disadvantages. First, many if not most members of the project/brand team may have very little experience of LCM. We have often seen the results of this in practice. For example, an LCM Plan may contain a really well conceived indication expansion strategy, but this is not tied in with an accompanying new formulation strategy, or the pricing or regulatory consequences of the indication sequence have not been thought through. Closer examination of the team members may then reveal that only the clinical development team member has prior experience of LCM. The second disadvantage results from how the project/brand team sets its priorities. The project team's main focus will be hitting the next project milestones, such as the start and completion of Phase IIb or III clinical trials for the lead indication, or regulatory submission, or approval. In particular, as these important deadlines approach, there is little time or motivation in the team to consider the longer term future and health of the brand. However much senior management does try to "walk the talk" of LCM, their main focus and thus the key objectives which the team are set and incentivized to achieve will inevitably focus on these short-term elements. Often it is the marketing representative on the team who raises his hand at this stage to point out that LCM is being neglected, but the development team members and the project leader are likely to be too busy concentrating in the short term. Later, once responsibility for the brand has been transferred to marketing at or shortly before launch, the main priority of the team shifts to short-term, commercial objectives such as getting the right price, reimbursement, and growing sales. LCM is still being neglected, but this time, it may be the development members of the team who are getting a bit frustrated, because they have ideas for new formulations or combinations, but it is difficult to get a place on the team meeting agenda because the focus is elsewhere.

How can these two issues be addressed without changing the basic project team/brand team structure that the company depends upon?

Let us look first at the issue of a lack of LCM experience on the team. To some extent, this can be improved by selecting the team members more carefully, but experience shows that it will only be possible to give a minority of the teams a full range of experienced members. Most teams will be populated by functional representatives with little or no experience of LCM. Bearing in mind that LCM was undervalued by companies until comparatively recently, a project leader/brand director may well not even want the people with LCM experience on the team as these are unlikely to be the stars in their functions. We believe the best way of addressing the issue is to create an LCM Center of Excellence (LCM CoE) in the company, a cross-functional group of people with deep experience of LCM who advise and support the different project/brand teams. We will be looking at concept of an LCM CoE later in the chapter.

The second issue, the fact that teams are likely to concentrate their efforts on the short-term needs of the project/brand and neglect planning for its long-term health, is more difficult to address, and is in fact one of the root problems that have to be solved if LCM is to be consistently and successfully conducted in a company. As an example, let us take a future brand that is in the middle of Phase III trials for its first indication. The team's main objectives are likely to be completion of Phase III recruiting, completion of the study report, and assembly and filing of the regulatory dossier. There may be a secondary objective on their incentive sheets, something about completing an LCM Plan for the next 5 or 10 years, but this is unlikely to hold the team's attention for long. After all, if the trials are not successful or the dossier is not approved, then there will not even be a brand in 5 years! So the team moves from short-term goal to short-term goal without spending enough time on the longer term priorities. Management may be a bit unhappy if the LCM Plan is delivered late or has poor quality, but the team knows that failure to hit the development milestones—or in the case of a brand team, the sales figures—will make them more than just a bit unhappy. Obviously, senior management can improve the situation by giving the LCM objectives a higher weighting, and the project leader/brand director can decide to dedicate whole team meetings just to LCM when there is a lull in the need to focus on the short-term issues (e.g., immediately after dossier submission), but this is only likely to provide a partial solution and is certainly not the route to ensuring excellence.

It is possible to solve the problem if management is willing to give the team more resources so that they can address both the short- and long-term future, but experience shows that the extra resources are frequently just sucked in to reduce the risk of missing the short-term objectives unless other measures are taken too.

One such measure is to create a subteam of the main project/brand team consisting of extra team members whose sole responsibility is LCM. A minimum core subteam size of one dedicated development and one dedicated marketing person seems to be necessary, the development representative probably coming from clinical development, and other members of the project/ brand team may be included in these subteam meetings (e.g., formulations, regulatory, or patents) as required, and especially when their contributions are not required for the overall team's short-term objectives. The subteam should be responsible to the project/brand team, just as the clinical, marketing, or regulatory subteam would be. We strongly believe that the LCM aspects of the brand should be handled by a subteam rather than by a separate team with a separate team leader as this latter solution causes confusion and endless discussions concerning territory, responsibility, and accountability. Each brand should have just one project team, which later mutates into just one brand team.

Everything we have written so far on this subject assumes the simplest case, that a drug is destined for use in only one indication, or in closely related indications within the same therapeutic area (e.g., hypertension and cardiac failure). Life gets rather more complicated when the same molecule is to be used for multiple indications in different therapeutic areas (e.g., psoriasis and rheumatoid arthritis), and this is the case with many biologics which represent an ever-increasing proportion of the R&D pipeline. But we believe that the same basic principles of clear leadership and accountability apply. In such a situation, it is therefore advisable to create an overarching "molecule project team" during development which oversees the individual projects and individual project teams which are responsible for the single indications. Each of these subsidiary project teams may also have LCM responsibilities, and could therefore also have their own LCM subteams. The guiding principle should always be that there is ultimately only one person and one team with overall responsibility for development of the molecule, with all other project teams, and their subsidiary subteams reporting, within the framework of the matrix structure, to that person/that team. The "molecule project team" may be specially created for the purpose if sufficient resources are available, or the role may be awarded to the project team that will bring the first indication to market, or to the project team responsible for the biggest, potentially most profitable indication.

After the initial approval, LCM efforts may spawn multiple brands, such as indication-specific brands and fixed-dose combinations. At that stage, each brand will probably be entrusted to different brand directors and brand teams, possibly even in different therapeutic areas. And there may be one or more project teams working concurrently on additional indications in still other therapeutic areas. This is obviously very tricky to manage, and the last word has probably not been spoken on how best to organize in this situation, but the basis for success lies in frequent and open communications between the different brand and project teams, to discuss their respective plans to ensure that synergies are being exploited and problems avoided. This is crucial, because actions taken by one brand team or project team may have effects on the others. As an example, a decision to go into a new indication with very sick patients could result in clinical trials with a plethora of side effects which then might have to appear in the label of an earlier, already approved indication where these side effects would not be acceptable. Or the price that the drug would receive in a new indication would endanger the price structure in existing indications. Senior management can help to keep the communication channels open, and prevent one team or therapeutic area from damaging the overall value of the molecule to the company, by incentivizing key players on the total performance of the various brands rather than just on the performance in the individual therapeutic areas.

The question arises as to where in the organizational chart the project leaders and brand directors can best be placed. Often, project leaders report in to development and brand directors to marketing. We believe there are two good alternative structures, which are actually not that much different from each other, and it is largely a question of company culture which would work best. In the first variant, all project leaders report into a centralized project management function, the head of this function being at more or less the same hierarchical level as the heads of development and marketing. We believe this is preferable to having the project management function reporting to either development or marketing, as it ensures a better balance of the sometimes conflicting interests of these two departments. Each project leader has a dotted-line relationship to the management of the relevant therapeutic area. In the second variant, the project leaders report solid-line to their respective therapeutic area management. But in this second situation, too, there must be a forum where all the project leaders of the company can meet and share experiences, and a centralized support organization which provides resource planning and tracking tools and support personnel for creating project plans, reports, and so on. It is wasteful of resources to decentralize these project support functions which do not need to have specialized knowledge and skills in a particular therapeutic area.

30.3 LCM CENTER OF EXCELLENCE

If the company is big enough to justify the effort, it is very beneficial to create an LCM CoE to support project and brand teams. This group of experts should not be making project and brand decisions, as these are best made by the people that know the molecule and its market best, but rather supporting the project and brand teams in making those decisions and in creating their LCM Plans. This support can take many forms, and the composition of the LCM CoE will largely depend on the extent of the services offered, so let us look at the options for different services before talking about team composition:

Raising Awareness of LCM. The creation of an LCM CoE is an excellent way for management to show that it is walking the talk and to underline its commitment to improving LCM. Once management has broadcast the existence of the LCM CoE and expressed its support of it, the CoE can start to raise the awareness level of LCM and what it can achieve. All available internal communication media should be utilized for this, including internal company announcements, presentations to management boards and teams, articles on the intranet and in in-company magazines and letters, flyers, giveaways like LCM mouse pads, and so on. Stories of individuals or teams in the company who have had notable LCM successes are very effective, and especially so if the success has been recognized by management in the form of awards or job promotions. The CoE should create and disseminate a wide range of information sources including third-party articles and reports on LCM, case histories of successful and unsuccessful LCM (internal and external), links to external LCM courses and conferences, and so on. Do not underestimate the importance of also raising awareness to the very existence of the CoE team. We recently learned of a company with an excellent section on LCM on its intranet, but most teams did not even know of its existence as the company had over half a million pages on its intranet and less than one in ten of these was being visited.

"Raising awareness" can evolve into an ongoing process of "maintaining awareness." The magazine articles and flyers can develop into a regular LCM Newsletter which will contain new case histories, explanations of new legislative changes regarding LCM, results of court decisions that could impact LCM strategies, and so on. This newsletter can be either a hard copy or intranet based.

LCM Training. The LCM CoE may be asked to create and conduct internal training courses on LCM, very much along the lines of this book. Utilizing speakers from the line functions involved in LCM will ensure that the courses are relevant for the teams and also help to increase buy-in for LCM within the functions. However, it is also valuable to include sessions with consultants who have worked with other companies both to introduce new ideas and perspectives, but also to underline that the new emphasis is not just an internal fad but a part of an industry-wide trend that needs to be taken very seriously. These courses are a good venue for the legal department to explain what one can and cannot do and say regarding competition with generic companies. The training can be "live," or intranet based, or a combination of the two. Companies that really want to improve LCM may decide to make the courses compulsory. Using a senior manager to introduce training sessions is another good way of visibly confirming the company's commitment to LCM. (We do not want to get boring on the subject, but if management does not visibly support LCM, and mean it, then all of these efforts are complete wastes of time!) It is helpful for the credibility of the training if selected project leaders and brand directors also present their experiences of LCM.

When should the training sessions take place? Ideally, we see two time points, first, as a part of the basic training of staff joining project or brand teams, and of their colleagues in the functions who will be getting involved in LCM, and second, on a team-by-team basis as project teams approach development decision milestones or brand teams approach important strategic decisions which involve presenting their LCM Plans to senior management.

One very valuable training instrument is wargaming. In this exercise, a team will present its LCM Plan to another team who is asked to play the role of a key competitor (brand or generic), or another stakeholder like a payer, and try to counter the plan. This can be very instructive and very sobering, and is an effective way of squeezing wishful thinking out of LCM Plans before they are presented to senior management, thus preventing project leaders and brand directors looking naïve in front of their superiors.

Another form of on-the-job training is to add a member of the LCM CoE to key project or brand teams. It is unlikely that the CoE will comprise enough staff to make this the norm, but it can be a valuable move for very important projects or brands, as a temporary step when teams are approaching decision points or reviews at which their LCM Plans will be updated, or for key brands approaching patent expiry when all late-stage lifecycle management (LLCM) options need to be expertly evaluated by the team.

Borrowing the terminology we used to describe matrix project management structures earlier in the chapter, we would call an LCM CoE which is used only to raise awareness and to train a "weak" CoE.

Designing and Owning the LCM Planning Process. We will be considering the LCM planning process itself later, and going into considerable detail on how to create, write, and present an LCM Plan in the next chapter. A formal LCM planning process will certainly be required by mid- and large-sized drug companies with approximately 20 or more project and brand teams. This whole process can be entrusted to the LCM CoE. In that case, the CoE designs the LCM process, takes the lead on creating the tools and templates required by the process, and supports project and brand teams through the process. The CoE also acts as a repository for all LCM Plans and can disseminate best practices—and learnings of the more negative kind—throughout the organization.

A strongly empowered LCM CoE may be asked to help to identify skill gaps in the teams and functions, first, to adapt internal training programs to address company weaknesses, and second, to support line functions in recruiting external experts to boost their internal capabilities.

But even in the case of such a strong LCM CoE we would still very much recommend that the responsibility for the LCM Plan itself (as opposed to the process for creating it) remains very firmly in the hands of the project leader or brand director.

A strong LCM CoE will also be expected to benchmark other companies, and other relevant industries, to identify ways to upgrade the company's LCM knowledge, capabilities, and processes.

A final but very important point regarding the duties of the LCM team: in several companies who have major brands approaching patent expiry and a pipeline which is inadequate to replace them, the LCM CoE is really synonymous with the LLCM CoE. Virtually all of the capacity of the unit is consumed in simply trying to prevent or delay the entry of generics to the market, and occasionally also with designing strategies to retain more market share after the generics arrive, which in most cases they inevitably will despite the best efforts of the LLCM CoE. Even in companies which claim that this is not what they are doing, and who have an LCM CoE which is nominally responsible for advising teams over the entire life cycle, the available capacity is often fully occupied with the LLCM priorities and has little time for anything else. We believe that this is a short-sighted approach. Obviously, it is easy for us to say this as consultants rather than as the CEO of a company about to lose 70% or more of the sales on a multibillion dollar brand. But do bear in mind that many of the attempts to prolong the exclusivity of an aging brand are destined to fail, and even if the company believes it is their duty to do everything that they can for the brand even if the chances of success are low, there may be a better return on investing the available expertise and effort into enhancing the LCM of a younger brand.

30.4   COMPOSITION OF THE LCM CoE

Who actually works within the LCM CoE will be largely determined by the resources that the company is willing to invest in it, and the scope of the responsibilities and authority given to it. We will try here to cover the whole spectrum of possible alternatives, starting with the one that represents the smallest investment and moving upward from there.

In a small company, there may well be insufficient resources and knowledge to even nominate one person into the role of LCM expert. An alternative here is to identify staff members in the key functions involved in LCM (at least marketing, clinical, formulations, regulatory, and patents) and ask them to serve as ad hoc advisors to the project and brand leaders. As much of LCM is cross-functional, these experts should meet at least twice yearly to exchange their views and experiences on LCM, thus both increasing their ability to support the teams while also giving this virtual LCM team its own identity.

If the company decides that it has the will and the capacity to create a full-time, one-man LCM CoE, then the question comes as to who should be considered for the role. As mentioned earlier, the company's priorities when they take this decision are likely to be in the LLCM arena. In that case, we would propose that an ex-manager from a leading generics company may be the best choice. A one-man show can do little more than offer advice to the various project—and in this case mostly brand—teams, and the best return on this small investment is probably obtained when this person can play devil's advocate and, based on his generics experience, tell the teams where their LLCM efforts are likely to prove successful and where not. Such a person can usually not be found internally and must be recruited from outside. However, one must be aware of a potential problem. It may prove difficult to integrate him into the entirely different culture of a brand company, and there is then a real danger that he may soon decide to resign and return to a generics company with insider knowledge of the planned LLCM strategies!

One effective and relatively economical option is to combine the one-man LCM CoE and virtual team options. In this case, the person must have the organizational and personal skills to bring the virtual team together and optimize its performance. Clearly, this is still rather a weak structure, and often the virtual team members will not be able to free up enough time from their "day jobs" to optimize their input to the virtual team, and thus to the project leaders and brand directors. This problem can be corrected by freeing up the virtual team members from some of their functional work, and making their contribution to the virtual team part of their annual objectives; the more this is done, the more the virtual team with its full-time leader, the LCM expert in the CoE, looks like any other matrix team in the organization. The objectives of the virtual team would then be parameters like the number of project/brand teams with which LCM workshops have been conducted and the quality of the ensuing LCM Plans that these teams write.

The one-man show, with at least some secretarial support, may be sufficient to allow the CoE to perform at least some of the "Raising Awareness" tasks mentioned above, and providing training is also possible if the virtual team has the skills and capacity to prepare and conduct this. However, this structure will not be enough to enable the CoE to take on the role of designing and owning the LCM process. For this to be added to the duties of the LCM CoE, we would suggest a structure consisting of at least one full-time equivalent (FTE) each from development and marketing, and a full-time administrative assistant. Even then, a virtual team of functional experts will still be an essential component, as it is not possible for the expertise of these three persons to cover the whole gamut of LCM options.

CHAPTER 31

The LCM Process: Description, Timing, and Participants

In this chapter we will consider at what points in the brand life cycle the Life-cycle Management (LCM) Process should be conducted, and who should be involved in the process. Again, we will use as the basis for these discussions a typical brand company structure of a development-led matrix project team for molecules that have not yet been marketed followed by a marketing-led matrix brand team once the molecule has been introduced to the market for the first time. As mentioned in the previous chapter, this structure may become more complicated in the case of molecules that can be utilized in different therapeutic areas, even under different brand names, and we will refer to this special situation as and when appropriate. This is typically the case for biologics whose mechanism of action may be relevant to multiple disease states.

31.1 PURPOSE OF THE LCM PROCESS

The purpose of the LCM Process is to map out the future strategy for the brand, and to capture this in a document, the LCM Plan, which is approved by management. The process has the following underlying principles:

- It brings together all experts in the company who can contribute to the LCM strategy.
- It provides a framework for these experts, and possibly external consultants, to interact in forming the LCM strategy.
- It identifies and reviews all possible LCM options, combining them into different constellations and selecting the constellation that appears to offer the most potential to maximize the value of the brand asset to the company. We will call this best of all possible constellations the "LCM Strategy Proposal."

Pharmaceutical Lifecycle Management: Making the Most of Each and Every Brand, First Edition. Tony Ellery and Neal Hansen.
© 2012 John Wiley & Sons, Inc. Published 2012 by John Wiley & Sons, Inc.

- It estimates at a high, strategic level the resources that will be required to implement the LCM Strategy Proposal.
- It solicits senior management acceptance for the LCM Strategy Proposal to ensure their support, and to obtain allocation of the resources required to implement the strategy. Senior management may, of course, require changes to the LCM Strategy Proposal. Once any changes have been implemented and the strategy approved by senior management, the strategy can be finalized. We will call this the "Approved LCM Proposal."
- By involving all of the functions required to implement the strategy in its elaboration, the process ensures a high level of buy-in which will facilitate efficient implementation.

In the sense of the journey being the destination, going through this LCM Process is itself of immeasurable value for the brand and the project/brand team, but the tangible product of the process is the LCM Plan which we have repeatedly referred to already in this book, and which we will be describing in detail in the next chapter.

31.2 TIMING OF THE LCM PROCESS

Let us look at the LCM Process in more detail, and one question that immediately arises is when it should be employed. We should again like to emphasize that LCM is not just a process or a plan. Rather it is a mind-set that some companies seem to have fully bought into and accept while others still struggle with. Conceptually, LCM is something that should be being considered long before the formal process starts. Research management should be thinking about the applicability to different disease states when selecting the molecular targets for its programs. Researchers and patent attorneys should be evaluating lifecycle aspects when they formulate the first patents around a molecule or class of molecules. Researchers and early development functions should be aware of the importance of indication sequencing when selecting their patients for proof-of-concept (PoC) studies.

When we come to talk about the formal LCM Process, we believe that this should be initiated once the first positive PoC study or studies indicate that the molecule is a candidate for inclusion in the development portfolio. Particularly in the case of molecules that are being tested—or could be tested—in other indications there is no option but to start the process this early as indication sequencing will already be an issue, and this will in turn impact route of administration, formulation, dose, and other elements of LCM besides. Obviously, not all elements of an LCM Plan can be addressed at this early stage, first, because it makes no sense to consider aspects like over-the-counter (OTC) switching or repositioning at such an early stage, but also because not yet enough is known about the molecule anyway. The first version of the LCM Plan, elaborated immediately post-PoC, will then be modified and updated at intervals as the brand progresses through its life cycle. When should these revisions be made? There are three possible drivers of this:

- Development milestones
- Events
- Calendar

During development of the new brand, LCM Plan revisions should be made at the same time as major development milestones are reached, because this is the point at which the project team will be going to senior management anyway to request the next block of investments in the project. Typically, these milestones would be when the project is approved for entry into full development, that is, before expensive Phase IIb and Phase III trials get started, and at the point at which submission of a registration dossier is approved, upon the completion of Phase III trials.

Project teams may be extremely busy at these development milestones, especially just prior to submission of the registration dossier. Because the LCM Plan is less urgent than the short-term development and launch priorities, it may make sense to stagger the presentations to management of the development plans and the LCM Plan, although management needs to consider both in deciding whether to proceed with the project, and with what prioritization. Particularly now the value of a dedicated LCM subteam becomes evident. Moreover, if there is a long gap—say more than 2 years—between the entry into full clinical development and dossier submission, it is worth considering an additional intermediate LCM Plan revision.

We do not consider that approval/launch is a very sensible milestone for senior management to ask for an LCM Plan revision. Not only are the teams rushed off their feet at this time, but the team itself may be transitioning from being a project team to becoming a brand team, the leadership is transitioning from development to marketing, and team members are probably being replaced or added. Choosing a time point such as "first major launch + 6 months" for the LCM Plan revision makes more sense, by which time the new team should also have formed and be ready to perform as an established cross-functional unit.

Up until now, the LCM Plan revisions have been milestone-driven, but subsequently, this will usually switch to a calendar-driven mode, with the revisions coinciding with the annual brand-planning and budgeting process.

The driver of LCM Plans that companies sometimes forget are major external events. These are not tied to internal development plans, or to the calendar, but they can be the cause of huge changes in the LCM Plan. Let us take a couple of examples. Perhaps your company is developing a fast-follower me-too molecule which will hit market 2 years after the new class leader, and this class leader suddenly crashes because of major adverse events during

Phase III trials. This may mean the end of the road for your molecule too if it shares the mechanism that caused the adverse events, or it may mean that your molecule can become the new class leader if it lacks this mechanism. Alternatively, this new class leader may reach market a year before you had expected because of spectacularly good clinical results, and this could either make your project obsolete or increase the attractiveness of the new class as a whole. Either way, your LCM Plan is likely to require major revisions. Sometimes these external events can really blind-side companies. In the late 1990s, Isis developed and gained approval for an antiviral oligonucleotide called Vitravene® (fomivirsen), indicated for the treatment of cytomegalovirus retinitis in AIDS patients. Almost immediately after its introduction, Highly Active AntiRetroviral Treatment (HAART) therapy was introduced for AIDS patients and the retinitis problem went away.

31.3 DESCRIPTION OF THE LCM PROCESS

We have looked at the purpose of the LCM Process, and decided when it should be applied before and after approval. Now it is time to consider what actually happens in the process, how it is structured, and who gets involved.

Often the biggest mistake in creating LCM Plans is to start the process by thinking of clever ideas of what could be done with the molecule, and then unconsciously assuming that the marketplace will develop in a way that is favorable for these ideas. Inhaled insulin, discussed in Case History 12 in the Appendix, on Exubera®, is a fine example of how this can go very wrong. It is a lot more sensible to flip the order and first consider the marketplace before generating ideas for the molecule.

So what does that mean in practical terms at the first point of time that the LCM Process is required to generate the very first LCM Plan immediately post-PoC? The mechanism of action of the molecule is likely to be known, though this knowledge will probably be far from complete. Per definition, it is known that the molecule has proven its worth in the PoC trial, or we would not be looking to create an LCM Plan. The PoC trial may have involved confirming the mechanism of action, or showing that the molecule is efficacious measured against a biomarker, or a surrogate, or a real disease end point. Whichever is the case, there should now be an indication of which disease or diseases the molecule might be developed to treat. Some of these may look like safer bets than others.

So, we have a positive PoC and now it is time to initiate the formal process that will enable us to define our LCM Strategy for the molecule for the first time. This LCM Strategy will then serve as the basis for the LCM Plan itself. Companies differ, but the LCM Plan is likely to have a time horizon of something like launch + 5 years at this early stage in the life cycle. Other companies may try to project the plan right out to basic patent expiry.

There are many different approaches to writing the LCM Plan, and each company will have its own way of doing this. In the following we will describe just one variant which has proven its effectiveness in practice. Whether you, the reader, follow this process or a different one does not matter, just as long as the same principles are applied. The process as described here has the following six serial steps:

1. Situation Analysis Today
2. Situation Analysis Future
3. Key Assumptions
4. Option Generation and Selection
5. LCM Strategy
6. LCM Plan(s)

Let us look at each step in a little more detail:

1. *Situation Analysis Today*
As soon as a list of possible indications has been made, it is time to forget all about our molecule and to concentrate on the external world in which it would be expected to perform. Our starting point is the list of diseases.

We start by defining each potential target disease, according to the following criteria:

- Disease definition
- Epidemiology
- Signs and symptoms
- Cause(s)
- Pathophysiology
- Diagnosis
- Management
- Prognosis

The next job is to evaluate the current situation of each disease as it relates to all of the stakeholders who have an interest in it. This may vary a lot by market, in which case the evaluation has to be repeated for each of our key markets. The list of stakeholders may be a long one:

- Physicians (family, specialist, and hospital)
- Nursing staff
- Patients
- Potential patients (e.g., risk groups)
- Patient family (e.g., parent or children)

- Patient support (e.g., patient advocacy groups)
- Regulatory authorities
- Payers
- Pharmacists
- Competitors

Let us look at a couple of these more closely to better understand the kind of thing that requires evaluating.

Patient

- Segmentation
- Degree of satisfaction with current therapeutic options
- Unmet needs (e.g., more efficacy, easier compliance, better tolerance)
- First presenting symptoms, and type of physician first visited (family doctor, specialist, hospital); subsequent referral pathways
- Diagnostic methods and reliability thereof
- Degree to which patient influences choice of therapy
- Role of caregivers
- Options for disease prevention

Payers

- Who are the key decision makers and who influences them?
- Who pays for the treatment?
- How do payers measure the value of different treatments of the disease? What parameters do they use to determine cost-effectiveness?
- Which competitive offerings are reimbursed? Why? At what price? Which have not obtained reimbursement, or only at a poor price, and why?

We want to develop a comprehensive and clear view of how each disease is viewed today by the various audiences that impact or are impacted by it.

2. *Situation Analysis Future*
Next, we need to gaze into the future and forecast how the situation is going to change for each of the shareholders and each of the target diseases right up to the horizon of the LCM Plan. This is a major task for the team and will take a period of some weeks of full-time dedicated work by the team members and other experts in the company to be performed well. It will mean estimating how prices and reimbursement will evolve in the major markets, which competitors will come to market when, and what the profile of their products is most likely to be, how regulatory hurdles will evolve, and so on. Near-time forecasts are likely to be fairly accurate, but long-term forecasts over the whole plan horizon will of necessity be much more tentative. There may be

opportunities to mold the market to make it more receptive to the new molecule that is the subject of the LCM Plan, but at this stage, the forecasts should all be made without the team considering its own molecule. In the situation analysis, the team is trying to foresee the future environment in which the new molecule would be introduced and would have to operate. The position of your own molecule in this future environment and attempts to change the environment will be part of the next section of the LCM Plan, but for the time being, these should be ignored.

3. *Key Assumptions*

And now follows an extremely important step that some companies neglect. We must document the rationale for each of the differences between the situation today and the future situation, including key assumptions. Later, if any key assumption turns out to be wrong, this will almost automatically necessitate a revision of the LCM Plan. If the team has failed to document the key assumptions, it is very easy to forget what they were and to continue blindly following an LCM Plan which is no longer going to lead to commercial success. Key assumptions can relate to things like patent robustness, pricing and reimbursement policies, timelines and labeling of future competitors, and so on. The key assumptions may also provide the raw material for later market molding efforts. There is another pragmatic reason for ensuring that all the key assumptions are documented. If senior management accepts those key assumptions when it is presented with the LCM Plan for approval, then the team will not be unfairly criticized if one of those assumptions turns out to have been wrong.

4. *Option Generation and Selection*

The team now has all the raw material that it needs to start thinking about the future of the molecule. It knows the status of the disease today in the eyes of the different stakeholders, how it will evolve in the future, and why. It also knows and has documented where uncertainties may lie. It also obviously knows the current status, the "situation today," of the molecule itself. Now it can start considering the "situation future" of the molecule, which is, of course, the LCM Plan itself.

One additional loop can be useful at this stage of the process. In completely new indications, or in situations where there are disagreements in the team or in management with regard to the future environment, it can be a good idea for the project/brand team to present the situation analyses and key assumptions to senior management before moving on to the next stage of planning. After all, the LCM Strategy is going to be based upon the situation analyses, and there is nothing more frustrating for a team than writing a plan and then later discovering that management does not agree with an important aspect of the situation analyses which are the foundation of the LCM Strategy itself.

It would now be easy to dive straight into the detailed clinical planning for the lead indication, but we would suggest that it is valuable to spend some more time thinking before switching into this active mode. Even when a molecule only has the capacity to address one defined disease, there are likely to be different options as to how it should be developed. Let us take a really simple hypothetical case—the first of a new molecular class of antihypertensive. Even here there are so many options as to how to develop the molecule. Should we try for mass-market first-line therapy, or try to get a high price by only treating nonresponders to other drug classes? Which classes? Should we go for combination therapy? With which of the other classes should we go, and should we start parallel developing a fixed-dose combination (FDC) right from the start? Do we include Japan in the clinical program? How about China? Should we start clinical outcomes trials now to see if this new class prevents end-organ damage more effectively that existing classes? What about trying to expand the indication to cover cardiac failure? And so on.

We would argue that it is always better to go through a step of generating and evaluating different options before marching off in any one particular direction. The options will be based on what has been learned in the situation analyses plus what is known about the molecule itself. If there are important information gaps regarding any of the stakeholders, then these must first be filled. This could involve primary market research, discussions with patient, physician, and payer groups, and other measures.

The team should now be in a position to define what the opportunities and threats might be for the molecule in the marketplace, and from these to derive the strategic imperatives for the brand and the different ways in which these strategic imperatives might be achieved. These will constitute the options. It is often helpful to hold workshops to generate these options, using these workshops as an opportunity to bring in additional scientific, clinical, and regulatory experts from outside of the project team, plus representatives of the major markets.

At the end of these deliberations, the team will be able to select its preferred option, what we earlier called the "LCM Strategy Proposal." How might this look in practice? Again, let us take our simple hypothetical example. Perhaps we have decided that the best approach would be to develop the molecule as monotherapy for hypertension, immediately also starting a long-term outcomes study to get a readout on prevention of end-organ damage at least 5 years before patent expiry. We will also start short-term trials to see how our molecule performs in free combination with diuretics and calcium antagonists, and design the studies in such a way that we can switch at the end of Phase II to an FDC, which the formulations folk should have ready by then, for the Phase III trials, and so on.

The next step in our process is a presentation to senior management—better still, another workshop where the senior managers can contribute their concerns and ideas to the team effort rather than just sitting in judgment. At this workshop the team presents a summary of the situation analyses, the options they generated, and their "LCM Strategy Proposal." Very importantly, they explain why they selected the one option and why they rejected the others.

The purpose of the presentation/workshop is to get senior management to accept the "LCM Strategy Proposal," with or without modifications. More than one iteration may be necessary, with senior management sending the team back to clear up inconsistencies or answer open questions before the proposal is accepted at a second or even third presentation/workshop.

Once senior management has accepted the team's preferred option, and the team is in possession of an "Approved LCM Proposal," then it can proceed into the next stage of the planning process.

5. *LCM Strategy*

The LCM Strategy is essentially a more comprehensive version of the "Approved LCM Proposal." It will contain a summary of the situation analyses and list and outline all of the different activities required to achieve the deliverables of the strategy. There may be several different projects in this strategy. In the hypothetical example that we created, one project may be directed at developing the monotherapy while a second may target the FDC. In reality, two such related projects might well be handled by the same project team or even in the same project. But in other cases, different teams with different expertise will be needed, also because one team will not have the capacity to handle everything. A biological that is to be developed for psoriasis, rheumatoid arthritis, and ulcerative colitis, for example, will probably require three different project teams (or subteams), in three different therapeutic areas. We discussed how to handle such a situation in the previous chapter.

The resource requirements implied by the strategy will probably not be approved by senior management at this stage, as detailed planning of each project within the line functions is necessary before these resources can be estimated. There is obviously a potential problem when senior management approves an LCM Strategy before the costs are known, but equally, it is wasteful of planning resources to go through the detailed intra- and cross-functional project planning process for projects which senior management has not yet even directionally approved. Uncoupling the strategic decision making from the resource allocation decision making seems to us to be the lesser evil, and this is the trade-off accepted by most large companies.

6. *LCM Plan(s)*

These are simply the project plans of the individual projects within the overall LCM Strategy. They contain the activities, timing, and resource requirements of the overall project, and are supported by even more detailed plans within the involved line functions. We will not go into these in detail here, as this is just the normal project planning process and is not in any way specific to LCM.

INTEGRATING LCM WITH PORTFOLIO MANAGEMENT

CHAPTER 32

Principles of Portfolio Management

At the most general level, Project Portfolio Management (PPM) in the context of the drug development portfolio can be described as the science and practice of determining the optimal constellation of projects to support a drug company in achieving its strategic goals. It involves not only the initial selection of the best mix of projects, but also the sequencing of those projects, the level of resources they will receive, and their prioritization in case of resource constraints. It is a dynamic process. Any change in the value or resource requirements of one project may have an impact on other parts of the portfolio.

To understand how this works in practice, it is necessary to remember that every project has four dimensions:

1. *Specification.* (i.e., what the project is expected to deliver)
2. *Timeline.* (i.e., when that deliverable is required)
3. *Resources.* (i.e., what external—money—and internal—headcount—resources are required to achieve the deliverable at the required time)
4. *Risk.* (i.e., the likelihood that the deliverable will be achieved at the required time within the resource budget)

The project and portfolio organization can make conscious decisions to change the values of these parameters, or changes may be imposed from the environment, but whenever the value of one parameter changes, the value of at least one other parameter will also be affected. Let us take the simplest—and commonest—example of how this works in practice. The project timeline is slipping. If the company does nothing to compensate for this, then *either* the risk to timely completion of the project increases *or* the risk that the project specification will not be achieved within the timeline increases, or both. Often the company can decide to stop risk increasing, typically by throwing more resources at the project. In some cases, it may be able to keep the risk and the

Pharmaceutical Lifecycle Management: Making the Most of Each and Every Brand, First Edition. Tony Ellery and Neal Hansen.
© 2012 John Wiley & Sons, Inc. Published 2012 by John Wiley & Sons, Inc.

resources constant if the project specification is lowered. All of these trade-offs are limited by constraints. For example, however many resources are thrown at a preclinical lifetime cancerogenicity study in rodents, the time it will take has a lower limit which cannot be reduced further. And in practice, the maximum possible resource allocation is always limited by headcount and external budget.

Optimizing resource allocation is perhaps the single most important justification for portfolio management. In principle, any time that the portfolio must be reassessed as is the case, for example, when an important new project is in-licensed or an existing project fails, the resourcing of the other projects in the development portfolio can be adjusted in one of several ways:

- Increased (to reduce risk, improve the specification, and/or get to market earlier)
- Held constant
- Reduced (thus accepting higher risk, reducing the specification, and/or accepting delays)
- Frozen, to be activated again later when resources free up (accepting delays, and thus a risk that the specification becomes noncompetitive if the project falls too far behind)
- Withdrawn (this means discontinuing the project, selling or out-licensing it, or seeking a development partner)

We have stated that the portfolio management process should determine the optimal constellation of projects to support strategic goals. It follows that different companies would see different constellations as optimal, because they are following different strategies. Again, a simple example will suffice. A company which is eager to enter a new therapeutic area will rate a project in a therapeutic area of which they have no prior experience much higher than will a company which has decided to stick with what it knows best. The logical conclusion is that portfolio management can only function well if the company is clear in its own mind what its strategic goals are, and has communicated them to the portfolio management team in a transparent way. Perhaps surprisingly, this precondition is not always met.

The ability to manage the portfolio depends entirely on the quality of the information coming from the individual project teams and project plans. The attributes that must be analyzed to enable a project to be evaluated in the context of the overall portfolio include

- Specification (Target Product Profile [TPP], often in three versions—"base case," "optimal," and "worst acceptable"; annualized sales forecasts)
- Resource requirements (internal manpower and external costs, for the total project, for activities up to the next decision milestone, and for the current budget period)

- Timeline (total project; decision milestone schedule)
- Risk (likelihood of technical success; likelihood of commercial success; compilation of risks including potential impact and mitigation and contingency plans)

In addition to the TPP, some companies generate a separate document, the Value Proposition of the project. In these cases, the TPP restricts itself to a description of the draft label, with the Value Proposition describing the less tangible differentiated customer value proposition that the project is intended to deliver.

Based upon this input for all potential projects, the portfolio management team can generate a whole series of different possible project portfolios. This is typically done manually in small companies, but large companies will use sophisticated software to generate huge numbers of alternative portfolios with a wide range of values, costs, resource requirements, and risk profiles. It goes beyond the scope of this book to go into details of these methodologies. One much-used example is Monte Carlo simulations.

An additional layer of complexity and value can be added to these evaluations if project teams are asked to come up not just with one plan, but with alternative plans that emphasize different aspects of the four parameters mentioned at the start of this chapter. Thus, there may be a "best TPP" version and a "fastest to market" version, among others. The optimal portfolio will not just then consist of the optimal selection of projects, but also the optimal development strategy for each of those projects. Adding this degree of sophistication again vastly increases the number of possible portfolios. This should not be confused with the "base case," "optimal," and "worst acceptable" TPP versions mentioned above, which describe the possible range of outcomes of one defined project plan. Yet another level of complexity can be added if for each plan variant an optimistic and a pessimistic sales forecast is included. For companies that choose this very numerical approach to selecting the best project portfolio, computer software programs really are a must. Let us look at an example. A company decides to develop a new formulation of an existing drug. It decides to compare two alternative development strategies, a "fastest to market" strategy and a "lowest technical risk" strategy. For each of these, it creates a "base case," an "optimal," and a "worst acceptable" TPP. For each of these, it wants to see variants with optimistic and pessimistic sales forecasts. This approach would mean that there were $2 \times 3 \times 2 = 12$ different possible versions of the business case for the new formulation project. The work that must be invested by a project team in generating all of this information must be set against the value of the additional information in making a better portfolio decision. Undoubtedly, the law of diminishing returns will start to apply at some point, but companies differ in their opinions as to where that point is. Very frequently, the point at which a project team would like to stop generating alternative scenarios falls short of the point at which senior management considers that it has enough information to make informed decisions.

We have spoken loosely of the "optimal portfolio," but how is this determined? Well, that depends upon the company strategy. In the simplest case, of a company that is driven only by short-term profit maximization, the net present value (NPV) or expected net present value (eNPV) determines the best constellation of projects. The NPV is the difference between the present value of cash inflows and the present value of cash outflows of each project, and thus of each possible portfolio of projects. The eNPV is the same as the NPV, but with the value of each project discounted to reflect project risk. In principle, any project that has a positive eNPV can be expected to make the company money, and any project with a negative eNPV should generate a loss.

It is very important to remember that NPVs and eNPVs are numbers that look "hard," but they are in fact based upon very uncertain input and should not therefore be overvalued. Again, one example is enough to illustrate this. The eNPV is greatly influenced by the future sales forecasts ("cash inflows") five and more years in the future, and retrospective analyses of project plans have shown what one would expect to see—that these are often wildly at variance with reality. It is questionable whether eNPV is of any value at all in evaluating the early development pipeline. Not only are the sales forecasts very tentative as the TPP is not yet fully developed, but the chances of success are so low for every project that risk-discounting the NPV often turns the figures negative. More science-driven parameters are appropriate for the early pipeline. These may include things like the predictability of the animal models used, or whether the molecular target has been validated.

One should always remember that the primary use of eNPV is to provide comparability between projects, and that retrospectively, accurate values are not only impossible to obtain but are also unnecessary. Some companies waste a lot of time in refining their eNPV calculations when it is really not helpful to do so. It is like measuring clouds to the nearest centimeter; you can do it, but it does not benefit anybody, and 5 minutes later, it will be different anyway!

Most companies also use additional parameters to differentiate between possible late-development portfolios, first, because their strategies are more complex than just trying to make as much money as possible, second, because they need to differentiate between possible portfolios whose values are too close together considering the inaccuracy of eNPV calculations, and third, to reflect company strengths and weaknesses and resource constraints. The overall strategy, and therefore the selection of the optimal portfolio, will have to consider aspects like ensuring that each strategically important therapeutic area has a development pipeline, that new products come to market in a steady stream and not all at once, that there is a mix of lower- and higher-risk projects, a mix of new molecular entity (NME) and LCM projects, perhaps a mix of small molecules and biologics, and so on. Other more operational criteria for defining the optimal portfolio will include the availability of key resources. For example, there is little point—at least in the short term—in selecting a portfolio that requires twice as many clinical scientists as the company has access to but leaves half of the formulation chemists without work.

At this point, LCM deserves its first mention in the chapter. Portfolio analyses tend to evaluate only the importance to the company of the existing and imminent projects. But some molecules are going to be more suited for subsequent LCM projects than others, and therefore, a lower-value initial project may lead to higher lifetime brand value than a higher-value initial project. This is sometimes hard to quantify, but it is an essential consideration in LCM now that biologics are often first launched in quite minor indications and broader indications added only later. In companies with multiple health-care businesses, cross-sector LCM opportunities also need to be considered, including over-the-counter (OTC) switching, drug-device combinations, and animal health products.

CHAPTER 33

LCM Projects in the Development Portfolio

We could go into more detail regarding the fascinating field of portfolio management, but that would take us further away from lifecycle management (LCM) which is the subject of our book. Let us therefore now narrow the discussion down to consider the place of LCM projects in the development portfolio.

There is little doubt that the weak new molecular entity (NME) pipelines of most large companies will continue to encourage LCM projects. But how many R&D resources should be invested in NME projects and how many in LCM projects? This is one of the most important portfolio management decisions of them all, and it is therefore valuable to consider the main differences between NME and LCM projects.

LCM projects generally have lower net present values (NPVs) than NME projects, at least historically. An add-on indication, a new formulation, a new fixed-dose combination, or new dosage strength provided incremental sales, but was usually less valuable to the company than the initial approval of the NME. As we have seen, the advent of biologics has changed the picture somewhat, as biologics are often first approved in smaller indications, sometimes for orphan diseases. But even with small molecules, health authorities are now increasingly requiring that new drugs are first introduced into small, high-unmet need diseases or subpopulations before allowing their usage in broader patient populations.

The probability of success of an LCM project is usually higher than that of an NME project. The reasons for this are rather obvious. Many of the factors that can cause pipeline attrition have already been successfully negotiated if the drug is already on the market. These include preclinical safety and manufacturing scale-up of the active substance, efficacy against placebo (except in the case of new indications), and much else besides. The regulatory authorities know and accept the molecule, and the sales force has experience selling it.

Pharmaceutical Lifecycle Management: Making the Most of Each and Every Brand, First Edition.
Tony Ellery and Neal Hansen.
© 2012 John Wiley & Sons, Inc. Published 2012 by John Wiley & Sons, Inc.

The right experts are already on board in the company. The closer the LCM project stays to the original NME project, the truer this will all be. A new dosage strength for an existing disease is likely to have a very high probability of success, both technical and commercial. A new indication in a new patient population using a new route of administration, on the other hand, may not be able to leverage much of the work that has already been done on the molecule, will therefore be more expensive, and the risks of failure climb.

As in just about any area of investment, higher risks mean potentially higher returns. The expected net present value (eNPV) tends to balance out these two aspects. Thus, the new dosage strength with the low incremental sales benefit may have a similar eNPV to the new indication with the higher incremental sales benefit, or indeed the early-stage NME which could become a blockbuster but is highly likely not even to make it to market. Companies with a strong emphasis on short-term financials sometimes invest too much of their R&D budget into low-risk LCM projects for this reason, and fail to fill their early-stage pipeline. To counter this tendency in such companies, it can be good practice to ring-fence the early development budget so that these projects do not have to compete for resources against the lower-risk and shorter-term moneymakers. Ring-fencing all NME projects to prevent overinvestment in LCM instead of true innovation is also an option.

How much of the development budget should be spent on LCM projects compared to NME projects is to some extent determined not only by the company strategy, but also of course by which good project proposals are available. A balance does have to be set. Too much emphasis on early and high-risk NME projects can cause short-term financial problems, falling share price, and a reduction in R&D investment, but too much emphasis on LCM may endanger the long-term existence of the company.

CHAPTER 34

Managing Established Brand Portfolios

In the last two chapters we have considered the key principles of portfolio management as they sit for on-patent brands, and in particular when considering significant investments such as developmental lifecycle management (LCM) tactics. This final chapter focuses on an increasingly important area of portfolio management which requires a rather specific approach to LCM, namely the management of established brand businesses.

Historically, large portfolios of mature brands have been managed by small teams, unloved by the rest of the organization and generally ignored. Their job was to keep old products alive and basically cope with issues that might come up at a market level. It was not a strategically important place to be, and for some companies that will not be named, working in mature brands was the equivalent of being sent to a far-flung outpost in the military—you must have done something wrong somewhere along the line to end up there!

However, this paradigm has shifted with the advent of the patent cliff, and many companies have bolstered the capabilities of mature brand teams, now rechristened established brands or diversified brand teams, to support the need to manage patent expiry effectively and build/optimize portfolios of established brands tailored to profit maximization and global growth. Big Pharma has sought out the expertise of players from the generics industry to understand better how to manage broad portfolios and has tried to implement decision-making processes to make established brand optimization easier. Even with these developments, established brands team still face the same challenge—how can you possibly optimize the performance of a portfolio containing sometimes hundreds of brands, with a team of likely no more than four or five people?

As we consider established brand portfolio management, it is firstly important to understand what such a portfolio could include, which can be some or all of the following:

Pharmaceutical Lifecycle Management: Making the Most of Each and Every Brand, First Edition.
Tony Ellery and Neal Hansen.
© 2012 John Wiley & Sons, Inc. Published 2012 by John Wiley & Sons, Inc.

- Brands approaching basic patent expiry (e.g., 2 years before or shorter)
- Patent-expired brands
- Zero-growth brands
- Nonpromoted brands
- Strategically de-emphasized brands
- Local brands (e.g., old brands that have already been discontinued in most markets)

Given the diversity of brand types within the portfolio, it is not surprising that taking a broad-brush, one-size-fits-all approach to such a portfolio is not usually the best way forward. Instead, companies must segment and prioritize their portfolios to identify not only potential candidates where additional investment could generate an improved return, but also candidates where market exit might also be the best way forward. That being said, there are some tactics and approaches that should be actively considered for all brands in a systematic way to maximize profitability. Many of these have been discussed in detail earlier in this book, and include

- Supply chain optimization
- Stock keeping unit (SKU) harmonization and rationalization
- Price optimization
- Geographic optimization

One basic factor essential in making these decisions, which is still sadly lacking in many companies, is the brand-level profit and loss (P&L). For companies to truly make the right decisions for established brands, they ideally need to know the profit return on each brand, and optimally each SKU, and be able to breakdown the cost centers. Without this information, companies struggle to justify any decision that may involve reducing top-line sales to improve margin. This is an area that the drug industry must focus on improving if it is to truly improve established brand portfolio management.

In deciding which brands to prioritize for further investment, established brands teams should consider the following factors:

- *Current Growth Profile*: Is this a brand that is losing share rapidly, or does it have an attractive growth profile, at least in certain markets?
- *Therapeutic Relevance*: Is the brand still a relevant therapeutic option for patients, does it still have a valuable place in a treatment paradigm?
- *Geographic Profile*: Is the global footprint of the brand restricted to Western markets with high generic penetration, or does it have a viable growth profile in markets with a longer product life cycle?
- *Competitive Landscape*: How is the competitive landscape evolving? Are there opportunities to differentiate from competitors in local markets,

or is there a need to simply keep up with the competition to maintain brand share?

· *Brand Heritage*: Is this a strong brand that stakeholders recognize and see value in continuing to use, or is the brand exposure very limited?

34.1 WHAT DO YOU DO WITH A PRIORITY ESTABLISHED BRAND?

For priority established brands, the key question is how and where to invest to gain the maximum return on investment. Traditionally, this process has been managed at a local level, with many individual countries developing their own local portfolio expansion options, including new dosages, packaging, combinations, and so on, to meet their own needs. Now while this approach has been successful, it is obviously not optimal. After all, if a new development makes sense for one market, surely it could also make sense for other countries around the world with a similar market dynamic?

Given this, many companies are now seeking more effective portfolio management and selection processes for LCM investments targeted to established brands. The processes are fundamentally the same as those described earlier in the book, but have a much stronger focus on clustering together individual market needs to determine the likely geographic impact of each tactic. A potential decision-making process for a priority established brand would look something like the following:

· Develop baseline situation analysis, with focus on market dynamics in specific target growth markets for the drug
· Gain input and insight from target markets, both from local brand teams and ideally local stakeholders on unmet needs, competitive differentiation, and potential tactics
· Collate tactical options from multiple markets and host further brainstorming sessions linking tactics to market needs
· Score each potential tactical option from commercial (based or preagreed geographic clusters) and technical/regulatory/clinical angles, to enable effective prioritization
· Prepare baseline business cases for prioritized tactics for input and feedback by target markets
· Develop final business cases for management approval.

Successful execution of LCM for established brands can help to initiate what is sometimes coined the "second life" of brand, where the decline after patent expiry is halted, and a second, longer phase of growth is born. The description of the Voltaren® franchise in Case History 30 in the Appendix is a classic example of a brand that has been successfully moved into a second life and remains to this day one of the largest brands within the Novartis portfolio.

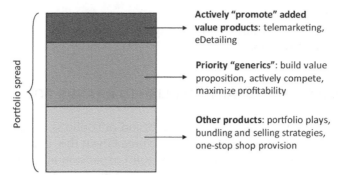

FIGURE 34.1. Generics company portfolio management. *Source*: Datamonitor.

34.2   WHAT ABOUT THE NONPRIORITY BRANDS?

So we have discussed what can be done with a priority brand, what about the brands where the return on investment of additional development work is just not strong enough? Should these drugs just be left on the shelf and ignored, or should they still be actively utilized but in a different way? Figure 34.1 illustrates a concept of how some generic companies look to manage their portfolios and is highly relevant for established brands team. Within a generic company portfolio, there could be three classes of product. The first group will be the value-added generics, where a company has invested in differentiating their drug from the competition, so the goal is to actively promote at a strong price and maximize returns. The second group will be the so-called priority generics, which will include those generics with barriers to entry (e.g., advanced formulations or 180-day exclusivities) and new generics for products facing very recent patent expiry. Again, these drugs will be prioritized for profit maximization, so the goal will be to compete aggressively, but to keep prices as high as possible. The third group contains everything else, including generics with lots of competition and no real differentiation. This group of products is used strategically by the generics company to drive the value of the first two groups. By selling portfolios of products containing all three classes of drug, the generic company is able to realize the higher prices desired for the first two clusters by offering attractive deals of the prices of the undifferentiated agents as part of the portfolio. By doing this, generic companies are able to generate a greater net profitability for their businesses. Moving forward, it may be in the interest of many established-brands businesses within the drug industry to consider such approaches with their broad portfolios to drive forward the overall profit returns for their businesses.

The alternative option for nonpriority brand is to consider exiting the market. Now much of this has already been discussed in Chapter 25, and so will not be repeated here, other than to say it makes sense that the ideal established brands portfolio will not always be what a company is left with after all its patent expiries. Actively managing products out of the portfolio should be just as important as prioritizing what to do within the portfolio to realize maximum returns.

34.3 BUILDING THE IDEAL ESTABLISHED BRANDS PORTFOLIO

As just highlighted, the ideal established brand portfolio is not always going to result from what falls out after patent expiry. Given this, it is important for established brands teams to consider portfolio expansion as well as contraction to build the most competitive portfolio moving forward. Again much of this has already been discussed in Chapter 24, given that the primary approach used for such portfolio expansion is through in-licensing or acquiring portfolios of generics drugs, or indeed full generic businesses in growth markets.

It is very much the authors' belief that while the impetus for new product development can never go away, the importance of the established brand teams and their portfolios can only increase over time, and it will be these teams and their portfolios that secure much of the platform for success in the key growth markets of the future. As such, those companies that can get their heads around optimizing established brand portfolio management earlier rather than later will be those that succeed in the coming years.

▰▰▰▰ CONCLUSIONS

So that is it, the authors' take on the why, what, where, when, who, and how of lifecycle management (LCM). This book has hopefully met its primary goal of bringing together the key information required for a reader to gain a full perspective on LCM. In addition, it is the authors' great desire that for at least some of the audience, this work has also provided inspiration to not just make LCM work in their companies, but to make it fly.

It is without doubt that LCM is increasing in importance within the pharmaceutical industry for the very reason described in our working definition of good LCM presented right at the start of the book. We described good LCM as "Optimizing lifetime performance of pharmaceutical prescription brands, every time, within the context of the company's overall business, product, and project portfolio," and this in essence describes what the branded drug industry needs today, even more than ever before—money from its existing assets! Great LCM is about optimizing return on investment of all brand spending, essentially focusing on de-risking the investment decision process, and as such is all about providing cash flow to the business. This cash flow is the lifeblood of the primary driver of the success of a branded drug company, new and innovative molecular entities. For those naysayers out there who constantly argue that they cannot invest in LCM because the business is focused on R&D, the critical argument back challenges the organization to say where the R&D cash is going to come from, if brand life cycles are not managed properly! Good LCM is not about taking money from R&D, it is about giving money back to R&D. As highlighted in the previous chapters, it is also not about spending more, it is about spending better. It is the process of knowing which decisions to make, at which point in time and of making them with the right intelligence, the right decision makers, and the right support, and of implementing them efficiently and effectively.

Pharmaceutical Lifecycle Management: Making the Most of Each and Every Brand, First Edition.
Tony Ellery and Neal Hansen.
© 2012 John Wiley & Sons, Inc. Published 2012 by John Wiley & Sons, Inc.

Now we have covered many different features of LCM in the book, from the drivers shaping the focus on LCM moving forward, to the tactical options available, to the internal processes needed to ensure LCM works. But to close out this piece, we would like to bring ourselves back to just three truly essential ingredients that can turn a good LCM program and process into a truly great one ... our three "P"s ... planning, people, and passion!

The first of the essential ingredients may sound a little boring, but it is absolutely the difference between success and failure of so many LCM plans that the authors have worked on and witnessed across the industry. Well-known quotes such as "Failing to plan is planning to fail" and "It's not the plan that is important, it's the planning" illustrate why it is critical, but it is the execution that is so central in LCM. Building a process that ensures the right level of planning at the right time, ensures decisions are not made too early, but also not too late, and enables updates and revisions to the plan that are responsive to market change is not easy. Indeed, telling a business that it should stop all work on a major new formulation because of a change in the market that would render the new version uncompetitive can be a real challenge. But what is the alternative? Not investing in the first place is not the right option, providing the intelligence base at the time the decision was first made was as strong as it could be. Similarly, keeping on with the launch plan in blind hope that reality will not kick in will just lead to more sunk costs without a viable return. LCM planning is not about making the right primary investment decision every time—we cannot expect to predict everything that will happen in a market sometimes 5 or 7 years out, but we can ensure we build in early indicators and fail-safes to ensure that all go/no-go decisions are constantly pressure-tested in an effective plan.

The second essential ingredient that truly enables the first is people. Throughout this book, we have highlighted the cross-functional nature of LCM, and it is this factor that is commonly a key roadblock to success. Trying to align so many different functions to a common plan is a key challenge that both authors have faced on many an occasion. But when it works, the results often speak for themselves, with faster decision making, aligned execution, and a better overall outcome. Indeed, in discussions with one of the authors at an LCM meeting, a key legal decision maker within a well-known branded drug company highlighted that it was great to be involved early in the planning process, because it meant he was much less likely to say "no" to tactics and plans he had witnessed from birth!

Trying to find a good analogy for how important people are for LCM is not always easy, but one of the authors was once asked to make LCM fit with the theme of an ongoing initiative within a brand team—ocean racing! Now initially, this was seen as something of a challenge. After all, how can you find similarities between such disparate activities, but after some head scratching, the analogy truly started to come to life. Ocean racing is one of the most technically challenging, strategic, and competitive sports. Teams compete to win with their boats (brands), with core boat design (R&D) essential, but success driven by excellence in route planning and strategy (global brand plans), sailing (local brand plans), and boat improvement and innovation (LCM), while coping with evolving race rules (regulations), weather conditions (payer attitudes), and local currents and waves (stakeholder behaviors). Even the concept of generic competition can be brought in, with a generic simply being a truly stripped-down version of your boat . . . with very big sails to ride the payer winds! The critical comparison here though is the role of the cross-functional team. The skipper of an ocean racing team plays a key role, but he is reliant on both his team of sailors to do their job, and also on many different land-based functions that shape his ability to succeed. From the boat designers who strive to make the boat withstand the elements, to the meteorologists who help predict the weather conditions and thus the best route and approach, an ocean racing team can only succeed if it has the right tools and intelligence on which to base strategy and tactics. Running a successful LCM team is no different—if your mast breaks halfway through a race, it is not just the responsibility of the sailors on board to come up with a solution, it means a reworking of the full plan. Similarly, when the meteorologists see a storm coming, not changing course or at the least the sailing trim would be disastrous. As the Noah principle highlights, "Predicting rain doesn't count. Building Arks does."

So our first two secret ingredients make sense, with planning and people essential to success. But what brings these together with real sparkle is passion. Many companies go through the motions on LCM—it is an afterthought, someone else's responsibility, something that interferes with the day job of making this month/quarter/year's numbers. Such companies, and individuals within the companies, need to step up and accept responsibility and "desire" to drive real optimization of brands to the benefits of both their organization and—even more importantly—their patients. There is a need for creativity and innovation and a burning drive to make the brand succeed irrespective of the internal and external barriers. We need new thinking, fresh ideas, all grounded in the reality of market needs. But principally, we need passion. Passion to make the plans work, passion to ensure any brand the individual is associated with is set on the best path for success. Passion to leave an imprint on a brand success that extends beyond that individual's involvement with the project itself.

The authors of the book have spent many years passionately driving LCM across a broad range of different organizations and would like to think that some of their passion has rubbed off on the current generation of lifecycle managers. We hope that the next phase of evolution in LCM will capture this essence for the benefits of patients and the industry alike. And with that, we wish you good luck!

Case Histories

A.1 MARKET AND PRODUCT-SHAPING DYNAMICS IN ACTION

Alzheimer's Disease Therapies: Aricept®, Exelon®, and Reminyl®/Razadyne®

Aricept is Eisai/Pfizer's donepezil, Exelon is Novartis's rivastigmine, and Reminyl/Razadyne is Shire/Janssen's galantamine. All three are cholinesterase inhibitors.

The market for the treatment of Alzheimer's disease (AD) essentially began with the launch in 1997 of Eisai and Pfizer's Aricept, the first-in-class cholinesterase inhibitor. Prior to Aricept, the AD market was very small with Warner-Lambert's Cognex® (approved in 1993) the only AD-specific treatment and rife with undesirable side effects. Aricept conferred significant advantages over Cognex, allowing it to rapidly become established and validated as the new gold standard for the treatment of AD.

The next task was to expand the potential use of the class, and Eisai/Pfizer's targeted promotional campaigns aimed at AD patients and their caregivers increased awareness of the disease and of Aricept as a viable treatment option. This resulted in treatment initiation in a previously untreated population, contributing to the growth of the new AD market and a sharp takeoff of Aricept's sales, which rose to over US$550 million within 2 years of launch. Continued focus on indication expansion saw Aricept become the first AD drug to gain approval for the full range of disease severities (mild, moderate, and severe), while studies of the drug in wide-ranging indications such as vascular dementia, attention-deficit disorder (ADD) and attention-deficit hyperactivity disorder (ADHD), mild cognitive impairment (MCI), dementia

Pharmaceutical Lifecycle Management: Making the Most of Each and Every Brand, First Edition. Tony Ellery and Neal Hansen.
© 2012 John Wiley & Sons, Inc. Published 2012 by John Wiley & Sons, Inc.

associated with Parkinson's disease (in Europe), migraine prevention (Europe and the United States) and Lewey body dementia (Japan) all expanded the experimental use of the drug, even without formal approvals for most of the non-AD indications. By 2009, Aricept was generating an estimated US\$3 billion in annual global sales, with the majority but not all of sales coming from use in AD patients.

The first competitor entered the U.S. market in June 2000. As the fast-follower second-in-class competitor, it was critical for Novartis's Exelon to differentiate from Aricept, and ideally to grow the market. Unfortunately for Novartis, although there was differentiation, this was not in the way that Novartis would have envisaged. The initial formulation of Exelon was dosed orally twice a day, compared to the well-established gold standard once a day for Aricept. Additionally, in the first head-to-head study of Aricept versus Exelon, released only 4 months after the launch of Exelon, it was reported that while both products showed a comparable improvement in the relevant measure of disease efficacy (AD Assessment Scale—cognitive subscale), twice as many patients discontinued treatment with Exelon due to side effects than with Aricept. Over the subsequent 2 years, Pfizer and Eisai continued to message further data from the study, demonstrating superiority over Exelon in safety, tolerability, and ease of use. Score one for Pfizer and Eisai on rear-guard defense!

Next up was Shire/Janssen's Reminyl/Razadyne, the third-in-class cholinesterase inhibitor, which claimed a dual mechanism of action as a differentiator (it also works on presynaptic nicotinic receptors), and which launched in early 2001. Once again, the new drug suffered an inferior dosing profile to Aricept, being also dosed twice a day as opposed to Aricept's once-daily dosing. Additionally, just as with Exelon, Pfizer and Eisai were quick with the comparative head-to-head data, releasing results from a study in early 2002 that showed more patients could tolerate the highest dose of Aricept than with Reminyl/Razadyne, that Reminyl/Razadyne was associated with a greater incidence of gastrointestinal (GI) side effects, and that significant improvements in cognition and activities of daily living were seen with Aricept compared with Reminyl/Razadyne. Score two for Pfizer and Eisai!

So what was left for Exelon and Reminyl/Razadyne? Was the game over? Were they limited to life as treatments for Aricept failures? Or was there an alternative approach to differentiation?

Let us start with Reminyl/Razadyne. So far, the drug was third in class, with an inferior dosing schedule, a different mechanism of action but with limited reason to believe this adds any value, and a poor head-to-head safety and efficacy profile. To address this, Shire and Janssen developed and launched a new once-daily formulation in 2005, while rebranding the entire franchise to Razadyne, now led by Razadyne ER®. While the rebranding was driven initially by the need to prevent confusion of the original brand name with a diabetes drug Amaryl®, it also provided an opportunity to relaunch the franchise with the now competitive once-daily formulation to go head-to-head with Aricept and to further damage Exelon. While this did indeed stabilize sales, sadly, the lack of any head-to-head advantage over Aricept prevented the drug from capturing first-line share, with global sales peaking at just over US$500 million, a good figure for a second-line drug, but less than one-sixth of the peak sales generated by Aricept.

So what about Exelon? Having been firmly put in its place by Aricept in the first 2 years after launch, and now fighting a seemingly losing battle with Reminyl/Razadyne on the daily dosing, Exelon needed to find a new avenue for differentiation. Two key approaches were taken to drive competitive value—first, new market penetration, and second, formulation innovation to target an untapped market need. In terms of new market penetration, Exelon was approved in 2006 for the treatment of mild to moderate dementia in Parkinson's disease, opening the potential use of the drug into a wider range of dementia patients. Even more significantly, Novartis launched the Exelon patch in 2007, the first patch formulation available for the treatment of AD. Novartis did not develop the patch in its own laboratories, the development being undertaken by a Japanese partner, Ono Pharmaceutical. Ono obtained the rights to comarket the product in Japan. While not offering an improvement in basic efficacy, what the patch did provide was a strong argument for improved compliance and a positive experience for the caregivers and the patient's family. The presence of the patch on the skin provided visual confirmation that the dose had not been missed, whether by patient, family member, or caregiver, and this was a real advantage in dementia patients. There was also an emotional aspect here relating to family members. In the case of institutionalized patients, the visiting family member could see the patch, and therefore knew that the patient was receiving his/her medication and, by inference, was being properly cared for. Moreover, dementia patients often resist swallowing capsules, and some Parkinson patients cannot even swallow tablets due to the loss of the swallow reflex. In addition to this, the patch provided continuous delivery of the drug to the bloodstream, avoiding the peak blood levels associated with oral delivery and allowing higher dosing. The patch therefore provided true differentiation for the Exelon franchise, enabling a unique positioning that could be owned by Novartis and built on for the long term. In 2009, the Exelon franchise grew to close to US$1 billion in annual sales, still some way from Aricept, but close to double Razadyne sales in the same year.

So was that the end of the story? Were Eisai and Pfizer happy to let the fast followers improve their competitive profiles and try to take share from Aricept? With patent expiry imminent, would Aricept make a late play to stay in the market? The answers to these questions are both yes and no—attempts have indeed been made to further improve the Aricept profile, but the later stages of lifecycle management (LCM), seemingly more under the control of Eisai than Pfizer, seem to have been significantly less successful. In July 2010, with less than 6 months until Aricept would take a swan dive off the patent cliff in the United States, Eisai and Pfizer received approval in the United States for a new high-dose 23-mg formulation of Aricept, based on a head-to-head study versus the 10-mg formulation. Meanwhile, the continued development of an Aricept patch looked to have hit a wall with a complete response letter from the Food and Drug Administration (FDA) in April 2011, 4 months after generics launched. Had these formulations been developed and launched earlier, the opportunities to capitalize on the brand equity of the US$3 billion Aricept franchise could have been enormous, particularly if a successful differentiation from the base product had been achieved. Instead, any success achieved by these line extensions should they ever launch will be against a background of generic competition, most likely relegating any developments in the Aricept-branded franchise to the same second-line positioning that the Exelon patch and Razadyne are currently fighting for.

Learnings

There are learnings here both for market leaders and for followers. Let us look at what happened from the LCM perspective, and from the perspective of the involved companies. Eisai/Pfizer got to market first and have retained clear market leadership until the present day. In a scientifically rather undifferentiated field of oral cholinesterase inhibitors, the advantage of once-daily dosing proved decisive, and the companies were aggressive and proactive in performing clinical comparisons with their new competitors. Did this success lead to some complacency later in the life cycle? Aricept could have been the first-to-market with a patch, but perhaps the companies were sitting on their laurels after so easily winning the battle for oral dominance.

Shire/Janssen took the conventional second-in-class route of playing catch-up with the market leader, but they were slow. They were 4 years behind Aricept in getting to market, and it was another 4 years before they were able to introduce a competitive once-daily formulation. Rebranding the franchise was a fortunate move to distance the new formulation from its unsuccessful twice-daily predecessor, but Razadyne remained a minor player in the AD game.

Novartis tried to change the game by moving the battle away from oral forms, where they were losing, and into the transdermal area where they were first to market and still have no competition. This strategy was rather effective, but it was implemented later in the life cycle than Novartis would no doubt have wanted. By the time Exelon patch was launched, Pfizer/Esai's lead was unassailable. It remains to be seen how the patch fares against oral generic donepezil. The withdrawal of Pfizer's heavy marketing support will help the Exelon patch somewhat, but it is hard to see how it can resist the onslaught of cheap oral generics, especially as all of the cholinesterase inhibitors demonstrate only a modest positive effect in dementia patients.

A.2 OPTIMIZING CLINICAL PROFILE VERSUS GOLD STANDARDS

Angiotensin II Receptor Blockers (ARBs): Cozaar®, Micardis®, and Benicar®

When Merck & Co. launched Cozaar (losartan), the first-in-class angiotensin-2 receptor blocker (ARB) for the treatment of hypertension, it was not all plain sailing from the start. A key challenge facing the new class was that, while the drug did show an improvement in side effects versus the previous gold standard, the ACE inhibitors, the improvement in efficacy was not significant. As such, establishing the new class relied on convincing physicians that the side effects were a big enough problem that the ARBs should be used as a priority. In reality, class growth only really took off once the market-leading ACE inhibitors lost patent protection. Once low-cost generic ACE inhibitors were moved to earlier lines of therapy, a greater market was created for patients whose blood pressure was not controlled using ACE inhibitors. To that extent, the LCM of Cozaar could be seen as a failure, as truly establishing "relevant" superiority to the earlier gold standard was never achieved.

This same challenge was faced by two key later players in the same class—Boehringer Ingelheim's Micardis (telmisartan) and Daiichi Sankyo's Benicar (olmesartan), which were approved as fifth and seventh within the ARB class. In terms of the base indication of hypertension, neither drug was able to significantly differentiate from the previous market entrants, and thus had to rely on alternative approaches to try to gain differentiation. Boehringer's approach with Micardis was to initiate a vast clinical program to prove effectiveness of Micardis in new patient populations and on critical outcomes, such as the prevention of cardiovascular events (stroke, myocardial infarction, etc.). The huge ONTARGET (>25,000 patients) and PROFESS (>20,000 patients) studies had the goal of establishing Micardis as the best ARB for the long-term prevention of adverse cardiovascular outcomes, much as the HOPE study had done for ramipril in the ACE inhibitor class almost 10 years earlier. However, the intended impact was not felt, both as a result of a failure to demonstrate significant superiority to alternative regimens in the trials themselves, and also because of a collective body of evidence from the other ARBs that suggested the class as a whole had similar protective effects. Indeed, even if the trials had been successful for telmisartan, there is no real evidence to suggest the results would not have been interpreted as a class effect, and thus equally relevant to the other six ARBs. The critical question that needs to be considered when evaluating whether this strategy was fundamentally good, but unlucky, or if it was indeed a poor choice, is whether Boehringer could have predicted the likely class effect that would have resulted from any positive outcome. If so, could they have designed studies better to demonstrate a difference between telmisartan and the other ARBs, so that there could have been a valid reason to believe that a positive result for Micardis could not be extrapolated to the other ARBs?

Interestingly, Daiichi Sankyo and Forest Labs took almost the complete opposite approach with Benicar, using the class effect to their advantage, and relying on a simple but strong marketing proposition (focused on "strength") and a good commercial proposition to drive uptake. Indeed, the indication expansion program supporting Benicar was one of the smallest in the ARB class, with only the bare bones of approval in place—usage in other indications or patient populations simply came with the class, and the developers could avoid the high costs of large trials. The success of this strategy—focusing on a clear single message and playing the class effect—is apparent with the Benicar franchise generating close to US$3 billion in annual sales in 2010 and still growing, ranking fourth globally despite launching seventh, and likely to rise to second after the impact of patent expiries in the coming years.

Learnings

Class effects can be good or bad news for a brand. Let us take the good news first. It is possible for a smaller brand with a limited marketing budget to benefit from a class effect when it is assumed that the brand will show the same safety and efficacy as its class competitors even if there is no extensive clinical evidence proving this assumption to be true. Working on the principle of "spend a little, earn a little," this strategy can be effective in a big-dollar drug class where even the crumbs from the feast can represent a substantial meal. But class effects can be bad news when vast sums of money are put behind a brand to differentiate it from other class members, and the results fail to convince the market that there are any real differences. One must also remember that the degree of differentiation required for success becomes enormously greater as soon as the first member of the drug class becomes available as a generic.

A.3 PARTNERING TO ENSURE REIMBURSEMENT AND COLLECTION OF COST-EFFECTIVENESS DATA

Aricept

Aricept (donepezil) is Eisai/Pfizer's once-daily oral cholinesterase inhibitor for treatment of AD. Other aspects of its LCM figure in AD treatments, described in Case History 1. The case history here describes one specific LCM strategy implemented in Germany. Aricept was approved in Germany in 1997, and its patent in Europe will expire in 2012.

Starting in mid-2005, Eisai, Pfizer, the German Federal association of the AOK (one of the largest statutory health insurances in Germany), and AOK Bavaria jointly sponsored the German IDA Study ("Initiative Demenzversorgung in der Allgemeinmedizin" = Dementia Care Initiative in Primary Practice), with the declared aim of optimizing the care of dementia patients living at home, and support for their informal caregivers, with respect to diagnostics, therapy, and support services. The study was designed to answer three questions:

1. Is it possible to change the care of patients with respect to diagnostics and drug therapy by means of training the general practitioners?
2. To what extent can the utilization of support services (caregiver counseling and support groups) be increased by recommendation of the general practitioner?
3. What effect does the utilization of family caregiver counseling have on the utilization of other available support services?

Patients and their informed caregivers were included in one of three groups, the first receiving usual care, and the second and third being given recommendations for additional support groups and caregiver counseling by the physicians. Included in the study were 390 patients and 129 general practitioners in the Central Franconian district of northern Bavaria. The results of the study were reported in 2010 (Donath et al. 2010. BMC Health Services Research 10:314). The study found that most physicians followed the relevant guidelines for treating AD patients, with about one-third of newly diagnosed patients being prescribed an antidementia drug. The level of usage of support groups and counseling was 4–5 times higher in the groups provided the additional support and counseling recommendations from their physicians compared to the "usual care" group. However, other support services not specifically addressed by the study, such as care groups and home nursing, were utilized at a low level by all three groups. The conclusion was that the specific recommendations for support services and counseling by the physician had been successful.

What had been the motivation of Pfizer/Eisai on the one hand and AOK on the other to sponsor this study? For the health insurer, the benefit was very clear. Any information regarding measures that might have the potential for keeping AD patients at home rather than institutionalized, at much higher costs for the insurer, is obviously of considerable interest. The drug companies were primarily interested in gaining data, including cost-effectiveness data, regarding the usage of Aricept, although no distinction was made between this and competitive drugs in the study design or publication of results. The very fact that Eisai/Pfizer sponsored the study could be read to indicate their confidence in their own drug, and certainly strengthened the link between the companies and AD in the eyes of physicians as patent expiry and the appearance of generics approached. The IDA project had its own website, http://www.projekt-ida.de—still active as this case history was written, but only in German—which is very clearly targeted at patients and informal caregivers. A short-term benefit for Eisai/Pfizer was that reimbursement of Aricept was pretty much guaranteed for the duration of the study, a not inconsiderable advantage considering the high levels of skepticism regarding the usage of cholinesterase-inhibitors in AD patients.

Learnings

This case demonstrates an alternative way of collaborating with health insurers in Germany which is a little more sophisticated than merely discounting prices. However, the amount of data regarding Aricept usage that emerged from the study was obviously rather modest, and one wonders if the companies could have constructed more of a win-win design with the health insurers that provided a greater volume of direct data regarding Aricept. One also wonders whether Eisai/Pfizer's main motivation for the study was simply to construct a creative deal structure to obtain listing and reimbursement by AOK without straight discounting. As Germany is a reference price market for many other European countries, drug firms are clearly reluctant to lower their prices as it would have a knock-on effect throughout the rest of Europe.

A.4   ACTIVE METABOLITES AND LATE-LISTED PATENTS

Buspar®

Buspar is Bristol-Myers Squibb (BMS)'s anxiolytic buspirone. It was launched in the United States in 1986 and lost exclusivity in 2001 despite an interesting and at that time unique late-stage lifecycle management (LLCM) strategy involving active metabolites and late-listed patents which at times reads like a Hollywood script.

The original composition-of-matter patent on buspirone was issued in 1973 and would have expired in 1990, but a second patent was issued with a 1997 expiry date. This date was extended to 2000 under the provisions of the Hatch–Waxman Act, and then by a further 6 months when BMS obtained pediatric exclusivity.

In anticipation of the final expiry of protection in 2000, three generic companies (Danbury, Watson, and Mylan) had obtained tentative approvals to market their generics on July 22, 2000, the day after the expiry of pediatric exclusivity.

Eleven hours(!) before expiry, BMS obtained a new patent on an active metabolite of buspirone and hand-delivered it to the FDA with the request that the new patent be listed in the Orange Book. However, the law does not allow a patent claiming only a metabolite to be listed in the Orange Book, so to overcome this hurdle, BMS claimed that its new patent covered a method of using Buspar itself, a claim the company had earlier abandoned in order to obtain the patent.

The FDA immediately informed the generic companies that they would have to update their Abbreviated New Drug Applications (ANDAs) to certify that their products would not infringe the new patent. Obviously, this was not possible, as there would have been infringement, and the generic companies responded by filing Paragraph IV certification against the new patent, whereupon BMS brought a patent infringement suit.

The essence of the new patent, the "365" patent, which would not expire until 2020, was that the 6-hydroxy metabolite of buspirone had an unexpected pharmacological activity. Any generic buspirone would also be converted to this metabolite, thus infringing the BMS patent.

The reaction of the generics industry and public opinion to this case was predictable. The Chairman of the Generic Pharmaceutical Association expressed the opinion that "This is probably the most outrageous manipulation of the system that I've ever seen," while Sidney Wolf, the outspoken director of Public Citizen, wrote "This is a whole new kind of patent extension that I find really objectionable. It's outrageous and the law needs to be changed immediately to stop this from happening."

The FDA requested clarification from BMS, asking whether the "365" patent actually affected Buspar at all in view of the fact that the patent covered the metabolite and not buspirone. BMS responded on December 6, 2000, stating that it interpreted the patent to cover buspirone as well as the metabolite since anyone taking Buspar would be producing the metabolite in their bodies.

But now BMS started to run into trouble. The judge disagreed with BMS's argumentation and ruled that they had misrepresented the scope and nature of the new patent to the FDA. He ordered that the patent be delisted from the Orange Book, and that Mylan be allowed to immediately start selling their generic. In his ruling, the judge said: "By creating new ways to extend its monopoly, BMS not only limits the public's access to low cost drugs but impedes the very innovation that Hatch–Waxman is designed to promote." Mylan and Watson began shipping generic buspirone in early April 2001 and had by June 2001 attained a 70% market share.

BMS' problems at this time involved more than just their LLCM of Buspar. In early March 2003, the Federal Trade Commission (FTC) announced that BMS had settled charges that it engaged in a series of anticompetitive acts over the past decade to obstruct the entry of low-price generic competition for three of its widely used pharmaceutical products: two anticancer drugs, Taxol® and Platinol®, and Buspar. According to the FTC's complaint, BMS's illegal conduct protected nearly US$2 billion in annual sales at a high cost to cancer patients and other consumers, who—being denied access to lower-cost alternatives—were forced to overpay by hundreds of millions of dollars for important and often life-saving medications.

In early April 2001, the Prescription Access Litigation (PAL) project filed six lawsuits against BMS, alleging that the company had employed illegal tactics to artificially maintain a monopoly on Buspar and lock generic competitors out of the Buspar market by filing a false secondary patent. In February 2002, Judge Koeltl issued an opinion denying the defendant's motion to dismiss the case and allowing the case to proceed. The Koeltl opinion included strong language indicating that pharmaceutical companies may not file invalid secondary patents to extend their patent monopoly on a drug without fear of legal attack.

In April 2003, PAL plaintiffs reached final settlement agreements with BMS including monetary damages, prohibitions on future bad conduct, and extensive reporting requirements.

Learnings

The FDA rules concerning "timely filing" of patents determines that patent information must be submitted with all new drug applications at the time of submission of the New Drug Application (NDA). For patents issued after approval of the NDA, the applicant holder has 30 days in which to file the patent to have it considered as a timely filed patent. Patents may still be submitted beyond the 30-day time frame but then the patent is not considered a timely filed patent. ANDA holders are not required to make a certification to an untimely filed patent if the generic application is submitted before the patent.

However, if a new patent really is granted late in the life cycle of a brand, then it can still be entered in the Orange Book and generic companies would be required to make a Paragraph IV certification to it. This was what occurred with Buspar, so the strategy would still have worked today. In the case of Buspar, however, the patent was delisted after it was determined that BMS had misrepresented the scope and nature of the new patent to the FDA.

A.5   A FIXED-DOSE COMBINATION (FDC) THAT COULD NOT FAIL, OR COULD IT?

Caduet®

Caduet is Pfizer's FDC of the calcium channel blocker Norvasc® (amlodipine) and the statin Lipitor® (atorvastatin). It was approved by the FDA in 2004, and is currently available in the United States as tablets in a wide range of 11 dose combinations, 2.5/10 mg, 2.5/20 mg, 2.5/40 mg, 5/10 mg, 5/20 mg, 5/40 mg, 5/80 mg, 10/10 mg, 10/20 mg, 10/40 mg, and 10/80 mg. It is indicated for use in patients who require both blood pressure reduction and blood cholesterol reduction, namely patients with either hypertension or coronary heart disease, and atherosclerotic vascular disease due to hypercholesterolemia.

At first glance, Caduet looked like it could not fail. Hypertension and hypercholesterolemia are two huge, mass-market indications. Pfizer pointed out that 35–50% of patients with one of the two conditions have the other as well, but that only 10% are treated for both. At the time of launch, Lipitor and Norvasc were the numbers one and six best-selling prescription drug brands in the world. Norvasc's basic patent was due to expire in 2007, which would give Pfizer plenty of time to switch eligible patients to the combination before amlodipine generics appeared on the market. The Lipitor patent extended until late 2011. Analysts were predicting multibillion peak annual sales for Caduet. Karen Katen, head of Pfizer's drug business, stated "We're very optimistic about Caduet's performance potential over the long term, not just because it works so well for patients but also because it's smart medicine. Treating two diseases with a single pill is the wave of the future. It simplifies complex treatment regimens and encourages patient compliance."

So what actually happened? Caduet had global sales of only US$527 million in 2010, having peaked 2 years earlier at less than US$600 million. This figure fell a long way short of forecasts at the time of its launch. Why did Caduet fail to fulfill expectations? Or were analyst expectations simply unrealistically high in the first place?

Well, very simply, Pfizer was unable to convince enough physicians of the benefits of their FDC in this patient population. The idea of using one pill to treat two separate diseases was rather new in 2004, and the marketing message was overcomplicated. As many physicians titrated the dose of each drug to find the optimal dosage for each individual patient, Pfizer had to make Caduet available in 11 different dosage combinations. Unfortunately, this did not help the physicians a great deal when titrating, but it did confuse them regarding which of the many dosage combinations to use. Moreover, the benefit of an FDC in this patient population was limited. Most patients were on more than one agent for reducing blood pressure, so combining just one of them with the statin did not really result in a significant reduction of the pill burden.

Finally, the specific FDC of atorvastatin and amlodipine simply made very little clinical sense. While many dyslipidemia patients were controlled on an atorvastatin monotherapy, very few hypertension patients would be prescribed amlodipine monotherapy. The role of amlodipine in therapy at the time was much more as a combination agent for other first-line ARBs or ACE inhibitors. Amlodipine was already available as an FDC with another antihypertensive, benazepril, in Novartis's widely used Lotrel®, and more such amlodipine FDCs would appear in the wake of the amlodipine patent expiry, including Exforge® also from Novartis. As such, it would be rare to have a patient fully controlled with Caduet, and if other agents would need to be added to the mix, then the value of the FDC would be questioned in the first place.

The most recent development in the Caduet story was the launch of an authorized generic FDC by Ranbaxy at the end of 2011, after Pfizer offered this pawn as part of their patent settlement with the generic company regarding Lipitor.

Learnings

The main learning is one that we will meet in several case histories in this book. It is very hard to change clinical practice patterns unless a new product offers such a big upside that the physicians are motivated to reject what they have been doing and move into a new paradigm. Caduet just did not provide a big enough motive for doing this. Perhaps Pfizer underestimated the marketing effort that would have had to be necessary to effect this change? Perhaps its attention was elsewhere, as another ill-fated Lipitor FDC—with an even higher expectation—was being developed at almost the same time.

A.6   INDICATION EXPANSION

Certican®/Zortress® and Afinitor®

Certican, Zortress, and Afinitor are brand names of Novartis's everolimus, which is a derivative of sirolimus (rapamycin) and acts similarly to this drug as an inhibitor of mammalian target of rapamycin (mTOR). The brand names are Certican (Europe) and Zortress (United States) where the drug is used for the prophylaxis of organ rejection after transplantation, and Afinitor where it is used for the treatment of cancer.

Certican was first approved in Sweden in 2003 for the prophylaxis, in combination with cyclosporine and corticosteroids, of organ rejection in adult patients at low-to-moderate immunological risk receiving an allogeneic renal or cardiac transplant. The drug subsequently gained approval in most European countries during 2004 via a Mutual Recognition Procedure (MRP). The road to approval in the United States was much rockier. The FDA issued an approvable letter in October 2003, requesting additional clinical data, and then a second approvable letter in August 2004, again requesting that Novartis provide additional information supporting a safe and effective dosing regimen for the combination with cyclosporine. Finally, following extensive additional clinical trials, the FDA granted an approval in April 2010 for the prevention of rejection of kidney transplants in adult patients at low-to-moderate immunologic risk, given in combination with reduced doses of cyclosporine, basiliximab, and corticosteroids. Zortress in the United States is not approved for heart transplant patients, whereas Certican in Europe is. Certican/Zortress is available in Europe and the United States as 0.25 mg, 0.5 mg, and 0.75 mg tablets, and the recommended initial dose is 0.75 mg twice daily.

During 2008, Novartis submitted regulatory filings in the United States and Europe for the usage of everolimus in a second indication, the treatment of renal carcinoma. The submission was based on the results of a Phase III trial in kidney-cancer patients whose disease was progressing despite antivascular endothelial growth factor (VEGF) therapy. This study showed that Afinitor, when compared with placebo, more than doubled the median time without tumor growth or death in patients with advanced kidney cancer, and that Afinitor reduced the risk of disease progression or death by 67% in these patients.

Accordingly, in March 2009, everolimus received its first approval in the United States for the treatment of patients with advanced renal carcinoma after failure of treatment with sunitinib (Sutent®) or sorafenib (Nexavar®), at a dose of 10 mg once daily. Afinitor is available in the United States as 5-mg and 10-mg tablets.

The approval of Afinitor in Europe followed in August 2009, for the treatment of patients with advanced renal carcinoma whose disease had progressed on or after treatment with VEGF-targeted therapy. The available dosage forms and recommended dosage are the same as in the United States.

The everolimus composition-of-matter patent is due to expire in September 2014. As the first approval in the United States was not until 2009, New Chemical Entity (NCE) Exclusivity also covers everolimus until March of the same year.

In July 2010, the United Kingdom's National Institute for Health and Clinical Excellence (NICE) decided not to recommend the use of Afinitor in renal cancer, concluding that it does not offer enough benefit to patients to justify the high cost. An 8-week cycle of treatment in the United Kingdom costs over £5264 per patient, and in a statement, Sir Andrew Dillon, Chief Executive at the NICE, stated that "A diagnosis of renal cancer is devastating for patients and those who care for them and we are disappointed not to be able to recommend everolimus as a second-line treatment option. However, we have to ensure that the money available to the National Health Service (NHS) is used to best effect, particularly when NHS funds, like the rest of the public sector, are under considerable financial pressure."

October 2010 saw the U.S. indications of Afinitor extended to cover subependymal giant cell astrocytoma, and in May 2011, Novartis gained FDA approval for advanced pancreatic neuroendocrine tumors (NET). European approval followed in September 2011.

Learnings

Everolimus provides a straightforward but good example of indication expansion where the second indication, cancer, provided access to a completely new physician and patient population. The gap of 7 years between the European Union (EU) and U.S. approvals of the transplantation indications, and the gap of 6 years between EU approval of the transplantation and cancer indications, were unfortunate, and heavily impacted the lifetime performance of the everolimus franchise. By the time the latest indication extension, pancreatic cancer, was obtained, there were only 4 years of patent life left.

The bottom line must be a thumbs-up to how well Novartis expanded the indications of everolimus, tempered by a thumbs-down for how long they took to do so.

A.7   KILLING A FRANCHISE THROUGH OVER-THE-COUNTER (OTC) SWITCHING

Claritin®

Claritin (loratadine) was Schering-Plough's tricyclic antihistamine which was first approved as a prescription drug for treating allergies in 1993. By 2001, it had grown to become Schering-Plough's biggest brand, selling for US$2.7 billion, or 28% of company sales. The composition-of matter-patent expired in 2002.

In 1998, the U.S. health plan company Wellpoint submitted a Citizen Petition to the FDA requesting that the allergy drugs Claritin, Allegra®, and Zyrtec® be switched to OTC status, a move opposed by Schering-Plough who stood to lose a lot of revenue if their premium-priced prescription drug were to move into the cheaper OTC arena. As patent expiry approached, at which time Schering-Plough would anyway lose most of its Claritin revenue, and following a positive recommendation from an FDA committee in 2001, Schering-Plough agreed to switch Claritin to OTC. Because Schering-Plough had decided early in the life cycle of Claritin not to seek regulatory approval for any additional dosages, it was forced to move the entire brand to OTC. Insurance companies promptly increased the self-pay for alternative prescription anti-allergics, effectively forcing patients to move to Claritin and pay for it themselves. In 2002, with the expiry of the loratadine patent, other OTC versions of loratadine entered the market and forced prices down.

Anticipating the patent expiry of loratadine, Schering-Plough had invested considerable efforts during the late 1990s to find a follow-on anti-allergic molecule. They were largely unsuccessful, and the only option they did find was to develop the active metabolite of loratadine, desloratadine, as the successor. Schering-Plough sought approval for this new brand, Clarinex®, in late 1999.

But Schering-Plough had been having quality issues which had soured the relationship with the FDA. After inspecting Schering-Plough's Puerto Rico manufacturing facilities, the FDA had concluded that the plant was not following proper procedures. The biggest deficiency—a very serious one—was that some asthma inhalers were being shipped which did not contain any drug. The FDA expressed the opinion that Schering-Plough had been less than diligent in correcting these shortcomings.

In January 2000, Schering-Plough announced that they had resolved all of the FDA's manufacturing issues, but this claim proved to be too optimistic and Clarinex was not finally approved by the FDA until early 2002, just a few months before the patent expiry of loratadine.

Schering-Plough invested massively in advertising campaigns to try to get physicians to move their prescription Claritin patients onto prescription Clarinex, but this was a pretty hopeless battle from the start. The time until patent expiry was short, the evidence that Clarinex was a better drug was, to say the least, weak, and during 2002, Claritin became available over the counter.

By 2003, Schering-Plough had lost its leadership position in the antihistamine market.

Learnings

As in the example of Nexium®, described in Case History 22, Schering-Plough attempted to save a strong company disease franchise—gastroesophageal reflux disease (GERD) in the case of Nexium and allergy in the case of Claritin—by introducing a minimally altered molecule before exclusivity expired on the original brand. But whereas AstraZeneca was spectacularly successful with Nexium, Schering-Plough fell short of this success with Claritin. There are several aspects which in retrospect Schering-Plough would probably wish to have handled differently:

- Clarinex just was not sufficiently better than Claritin. Whereas AstraZeneca had at least selected a slightly different indication for Nexium, Clarinex was less differentiated and had to compete directly with Claritin and its generics.
- Clarinex was developed too late in the Claritin life cycle, and then Schering-Plough's manufacturing issues delayed the launch still further, to a point where it was no longer possible to convert significant numbers of physicians and patients to the new brand.
- Schering-Plough's failure to invest in Claritin line extensions, such as a higher dose for more severely ill patients, looked like a mistake in retrospect and meant that the whole franchise had to be switched to OTC rather than just a low-dose formulation.

A.8 MOVING FDCS TO THE FORE IN DIABETES

Diabetes Therapies: Glucophage®, Avandia®, Actos®, and Januvia®

Glucophage is BMS/Merck KGaA's metformin, Avandia is GlaxoSmithKline (GSK)'s rosiglitazone, Actos is Takeda's pioglitazone, and Januvia is Merck's sitagliptin. All are oral drugs for the treatment of Type 2 diabetes mellitus.

The Type 2 diabetes market is a great example of how an FDC market can evolve, driven by the changing treatment paradigms of disease. In this case, the fundamental driver of FDC evolution was the success of metformin which was originally launched in 1958 in the United Kingdom, followed by the launch of the branded Glucophage by BMS in the United States in 1994. Metformin was so successful that no subsequent launch has been able to displace it from first-line therapy for the vast majority of Type 2 diabetics. Should a patient fail on metformin, the standard progression route is to add in an additional therapy as opposed to switching away from metformin. Indeed, it is only the small (less than 10%) proportion of patients that truly cannot tolerate metformin that are likely to be prescribed a different first-line therapy.

The success of metformin established the treatment paradigm for all new drugs, leaving them just two alternatives. Either the new drug will be restricted to the niche market of metformin-intolerant patients, or it must demonstrate use in combination with metformin. This led to the natural next step, FDCs of new drugs with metformin.

Indeed, Glucophage itself was the first brand to take this route, with the launch of Glucovance®, an FDC of metformin with the sulfonylurea glyburide shortly before the Glucophage patent expiry. While this product was moderately successful, it suffered a common problem of all FDCs, dosing flexibility. The common trend for physicians at the time was to carefully titrate patients to the correct dosage of sulfonylurea, resulting in real-world patients on a free combination being on a wide range of different dose combinations. This resulted in patients only moving onto the FDC if they had already been stabilized on the relevant free combination. As a result, the FDC would typically be restricted to third-line therapy.

Next up were the thiazolidinediones (TZDs), led by GSK's Avandia and Takeda's Actos. Following the high-profile withdrawal of the first-in-class TZD, Pfizer's Rezulin®, GSK, and Takeda established Avandia and Actos as a standard of care for second-line treatment of Type 2 diabetes. As expected, both drugs were most commonly prescribed in combination with metformin for patients who could not meet their treatment goals with metformin alone. Following the launch of the Avandia monotherapy in June 1999, GSK got to work on bringing an FDC to market as soon as possible and, in October 2002, launched Avandamet® in the United States. Takeda, by contrast, despite launching the Actos monotherapy only 3 months after Avandia, was not able to launch its FDC with metformin until 2005, a full 3 years after Avandamet hit the market.

So, were these FDCs successful? In its first year on the market, Avandamet captured 8% of the Avandia franchise sales, rising to own 10% of the entire TZD market, and close to 20% of Avandia sales in the United States by 2004. This launch helped GSK to take a slight upper hand in its battle with Actos, with the Avandia franchise taking the leadership share in the U.S. TZD market in 2004. When Actoplus Met® launched in 2005, the success was much more limited, with the product only taking 5% of the Actos franchise in the first year. In terms of market penetration, Actoplus Met took the majority of its patients from Avandamet, with the total share of FDCs in the TZD class remaining the same between 2005 and 2006, but with Avandamet's share dropping. For Takeda, the goal of the FDC seemed to be to drive intraclass competitive advantage (vs. Avandamet), and then simply to nullify it. There was not a sustained drive to change treatment practice and to position the FDC anywhere other than third line.

The latest page in the story of FDCs in diabetes comes with the DPP-IV class and its pioneering leader Januvia from Merck. When Januvia was in development, the clear role of metformin first line was well established, so Merck knew very well that Januvia would be competing head-to-head with the TZDs for second-line therapy in combination with metformin. This led to a different approach for Merck, with the launch of Janumet®, an FDC of Januvia with metformin within 6 months of Januvia's launch. The complementary marketing approach focused on "Start with the power of Janumet," with the goal of targeting patients that physicians believed would be unlikely to respond to metformin alone, and thus positioning the Janumet FDC for first-line patients, rather than the traditional third line for many FDCs. By contrast, the marketing for Januvia focused on "Add the power of Januvia," aiming for a second-line line positioning. This approach led to Janumet being positioned as the key element of the brand franchise as opposed to the base Januvia, with many of the marketing materials positioning Janumet ahead of Januvia. What was the end result? Within the first 12 months of launch, Janumet accounted for 14% of the franchise, rising to 29% of sales in 2010.

So what will happen next? Will the next-generation diabetes agents not even bother with monotherapy and just launch in combination with metformin? It is difficult to say whether the 29% share gained by Janumet is the upper limit in this market, but it will be interesting to watch how the market develops over the coming years.

Learnings

Changing medical practice is an uphill battle unless there is a real unmet need. When the gold-standard drug is satisfactory, and particularly once it has been genericized and is cheaply available, it is sometimes better to swim with the tide and accept that a new drug will not succeed in displacing it as first-line therapy. FDCs are one way of leveraging the success of the gold standard into building a franchise for the new drug. Merck was quicker to react to this reality than was Takeda, so Avandamet was more successful than Actoplus Met. By the time Merck brought Januvia to market, the recipe for success was so obvious that Merck decided to parallel-develop the metformin FDC with the monotherapy to ensure that they got to market as soon as possible after the launch of Januvia with Janumet.

Moving forward, companies will need to consider launching FDC programs much earlier in the life cycle. The historical ability to defend a franchise at patent expiry with FDCs is being nullified by payer policy and generic company success in overcoming secondary patents, so branded players should instead focus on using FDCs earlier in the life cycle to enable uptake. In the end, if the FDC cannot support driving uptake, it probably should not be used at all.

A.9 FDCS AND MULTIPLE DOSAGE STRENGTHS

Diovan® and Tekturna®/Rasilez®

Diovan is Novartis's angiotensin receptor blocker, valsartan. The Diovan family of products is currently Novartis's best-selling drug franchise, with the two main products Diovan and Co-Diovan® selling for US$6.1 billion in 2010.

Diovan was first approved for the treatment of essential hypertension in 1998. Four years later, in 2002, Novartis introduced Co-Diovan (an FDC of valsartan and the diuretic, hydrochlorothiazide). The name Co-Diovan was chosen to leverage the name Diovan, as the drug was selling well.

Five years later, in 2007, Exforge was approved. It is an FDC of valsartan and the calcium antagonist, amlodipine. Although Diovan/Co-Diovan were performing very well in the market in 2007, with well over US$5 billion sales, Novartis made the decision to use a completely different brand name rather than leveraging the Diovan name and reputation.

But Novartis needed a new, patent-protected molecule to sustain their cardiovascular franchise long term. In 2007, the FDA approved Novartis's novel renin inhibitor, Tekturna (aliskiren), for the treatment of essential hypertension. The basic patent on aliskiren is due to expire in 2015, 3 years later than valsartan. Tekturna is called Rasilez outside of the United States. In 2008, the FDC Tekturna HCT® (aliskiren + hydrochlorothiazide) gained approval, and, in late 2009, the FDC of Valturna® (valsartan + aliskiren) gained FDA approval, although the corresponding application in Europe, under the brand name Rasival®, was withdrawn by Novartis in September 2010, with the company explaining that it would not be able to meet the European Medicines Agency (EMA) requirements within the time frame required for a centralized procedure.

After using the Co-Diovan FDC to expand the Diovan franchise, Novartis is now using FDCs as part of its strategy to transfer the Diovan franchise into a Tekturna franchise. At the same time, the choice of the name Exforge for the late-entry valsartan + amlodipine FDC suggests that Novartis was trying to disassociate this brand from Diovan in anticipation of the launch of valsartan generics in 2012. However, in 2010, Exforge sales were less than US$1 billion and Tekturna sales a feeble US$400 million. Although Novartis pressed on with its FDC strategy, gaining FDA approval for Tekamlo® (the FDC of aliskiren and amlodipine) in August 2010, it appears that the Tekturna family will not be able to replace the Diovan family sales that will be lost following the expiry of the valsartan patent. With all the other classes of antihypertensives available as generics (diuretics, beta-blockers, calcium antagonists, ACE inhibitors, and ARBs), Tekturna would have to offer something rather special, and it just does not. Blood pressure reduction is not very impressive, and as yet there is no evidence that renin inhibitors are any more effective than the other classes in preventing end-organ damage in hypertensives. Indeed, just as we finish writing this book in December 2011, Novartis has announced that it has terminated the ALTITUDE study with Tekturna in high-risk patients with diabetes and renal impairment, after an independent data monitoring committee identified higher adverse events in patients receiving Tekturna. As a further consequence, Novartis announced that it would suspend promoting Tekturna-based products for use in combination with ACE-inhibitors or ARBs.

The LCM of Diovan is a good example of FDCs as a brand growth strategy. In addition, Diovan also shows the benefits of making multiple dosage forms available to the physician to maximize the potential of a brand. When the drug was initially approved by the FDA, in 1998, it was made available as 80-mg and 160-mg capsules. Within 3 years, Novartis changed the dosage form to tablets and added 40-mg and 320-mg dosages. Co-Diovan is available at dosages of 80 mg/12.5 mg, 160 mg/12.5 mg, 160 mg/25 mg, 320 mg/12.5 mg, and 320 mg/25 mg, and Exforge at dosages of 160 mg/5 mg, 160 mg/10 mg, 320 mg/5 mg, and 320 mg/10 mg. It is interesting to see how the lowest available dosage of valsartan has climbed from 40 mg with Diovan to 80 mg with Co-Diovan to 160 mg with Exforge. This reflects the physician's growing confidence over time in the low level of side effects caused by the drug.

Learnings

Novartis did a good job of maximizing the commercial potential of valsartan during its patent life by a combination of LCM strategies, including indication expansion into heart failure, new dosages, and FDCs. However, it appears that the company has been unable to find a credible successor to Diovan. Indeed, the Diovan/Tekturna FDC looks more like one of the last steps in the LCM of Diovan rather than a first step in the LCM of Tekturna. It can be anticipated that Novartis will therefore leave no LLCM stone unturned in trying to extend the exclusivity of Diovan, and in fighting for as high a market share as possible in the postpatent generic valsartan market from 2012 onward. It will also be interesting to observe how much the Diovan franchise has suffered during 2011 even before patent expiry. The patent on the first ARB, Merck's Cozaar (losartan) expired in the United States in April 2010, but Teva had 180-day exclusivity so the price did not come under pressure until late 2010. Although there are differences in the Cozaar and Diovan labels, both are primarily used as hypertensives, and it is to be expected that some patients will be switched from Diovan to cheap generic losartan.

At the end of 2010, Novartis completed its acquisition of Alcon, the eyecare company, from Nestle for US$52 billion. Alcon's sales in 2009 had been US$6.5 billion, almost exactly the same as those of the Diovan franchise. Many analysts saw the US$52 billion as the price tag for Novartis failing to develop a credible successor to Diovan.

A.10 BUILDING A COMPLIANCE SUPPORT PROGRAM

Enbrel®

Enbrel (etanercept) is a TNF-inhibitor developed initially by Immunex and marketed by Amgen and Pfizer in North America and by Wyeth in the rest of the world. It is indicated for the treatment of autoimmune diseases, including psoriasis and rheumatoid arthritis (RA). This case history looks at an example of commercial LCM of the brand implemented in Germany.

Enbrel was the second tumor necrosis factor (TNF) inhibitor to reach market, in 2000, following approval of Schering-Plough's Remicade® (infliximab) in 1999. The marketing authorization of Abbot's Humira® (adalimumab) was granted in 2003.

From 2003 onward, Wyeth found itself facing an increasingly tough battle for market share, particularly against Humira. New marketing ideas were urgently needed to boost sales, and these would have to be country-specific because of the disparity of national regulations regarding aspects like rebates and direct-to-consumer advertising.

In mid-2008, Wyeth signed a deal with one of the largest German sick funds, Taunus BKK. Under the terms of this so-called "Mehrwertvertrag" ("added-value contract"), Wyeth would finance individual service programs aimed at improving compliance in RA and psoriasis patients. The two programs were called RUDI ("Rheuma Unterstützungs-Dienst" = RA support service) and PIT (Psoriasis Information Team), and were developed in collaboration with BSMO, a specialty multimedia communication company which was part of the Springer publishing house, and Santis Patientenberatung (Santis Patient Advice).

The programs comprised two components aimed at increasing patient compliance: first, home care visits to psoriasis and RA patients by licensed nurses and doctor's assistants and second, a telephone-line support service with specially trained operators. Both of these approaches were permitted by German law. The home visits were particularly aimed at giving patients practical tips on how to inject themselves. Compliance is notoriously bad in RA, as patients who have joint pain and mechanical difficulties with their hands often give up on injecting themselves. And the injections may cause rashes that can persist for days. Both of these factors can heavily impact compliance. It is therefore important to underline the importance of persisting with the injections, and not giving up or switching to an alternative oral therapy. The telephone-line support service provided answers to questions regarding the dieases themselves and their treatment, and again underlined the importance of compliance. As Udo Sennlaub, a director of Taunus put it, "The two compliance programmes are aimed at providing patients an individual and holistic support which will contribute greatly to the success of treatment."

"In Vivo," Elsevier's Business and Medicine Report, analyzed the case in depth in their July/August 2009 issue. "In Vivo" assumed that Wyeth provided Enbrel at a discounted price within the scope of these programs, as by German law the basis of any deal between a sick fund and a drug manufacturer is classified as a rebate contract. Wyeth Germany had declined to confirm the actual discount. "In Vivo" stated that Wyeth also benefited from Taunus's significant publicity around the program, and that another benefit of the program for Wyeth was less parallel trade as pharmacists were encouraged by computer software to dispense the original product rather than an imported version—and according to Wyeth and Taunus, the deal was designed in such a way that it was more economical for them to do so. Wyeth has since expanded the deal to over 100 German payers, some of whom eliminated patient co-pays for Enbrel to further encourage drug uptake. Cited in "In Vivo," Booz estimated that the program cost Wyeth about €500 per patient. A significant improvement in Enbrel compliance would quickly justify such an investment.

Learnings

Local LCM marketing tactics must respect the local conditions of that particular market. Wyeth Germany partnered with a national sick fund to improve compliance and sell more Enbrel, and this appears to have been successful.

A.11 TARGETING RESPONDERS WITH HIGH-PRICE CANCER AGENTS

Erbitux®

Erbitux is Merck KgaA/BMS's monoclonal antibody cetuximab, an epidermal growth factor receptor (EGFR) inhibitor administered by intravenous infusion to patients with metastatic colorectal cancer or head and neck cancer. It was discovered by ImClone, which has been a subsidiary of Lilly since 2008, and licensed to BMS for North America and Merck KGaA for the rest of the world. Approval was gained in the United States in 2004 for the treatment of colorectal cancer in patients who are refractory or intolerant to treatment with Pfizer's Camptosar® (irinotecan). In 2006, the additional indication of treatment of advanced squamous cell carcinoma of the head and neck, in combination with radiotherapy, was approved by the FDA. European approval for colorectal cancer was obtained in 2004, but again only as second-line therapy after failure of Camptosar treatment. In 2006, European approval was obtained for the head and neck cancer indication, after failure of standard chemotherapy.

Several papers at the 2008 American Society of Clinical Oncology (ASCO) meeting reported data that treatment with EGFR inhibitors such as Erbitux is only effective among colorectal cancer patients with the normal, "wild-type" KRAS gene, while those with a mutated KRAS gene demonstrate virtually no response to these agents. It is estimated that up to 40% of all patients with colorectal cancers have a KRAS mutation that would therefore render them ineligible for EGFR-targeted therapy. Consensus was quickly reached in the oncologist community that all patients eligible for EGFR-targeted therapies should first undergo KRAS testing prior to initiation of therapy, and this became common practice among oncologists.

Merck KGaA had reacted immediately to the findings that while Erbitux would be ineffective in 40% of its target population, it would show enhanced efficacy in the remaining 60% of patients which lack the KRAS mutation. In

July 2008, European approval was duly granted for the first-line usage of Erbitux in combination with chemotherapy in colorectal cancer patients with the "wild-type" KRAS gene.

Since then, between 2008 and 2010, Merck KGaA has seen its sales of Erbitux increase by around 45%, despite losing 40% of its target population, primarily due to its winning first-line status in colrectal cancer patients in Europe.

In the United States, BMS failed to act decisively on the KRAS data and did not file for first-line status. With only second-line status, BMS has seen its sales of Erbitux drop by around 18% between 2008 and 2010. In mid-2009, the FDA added wording to BMS's Erbitux label stating that trials had not shown a treatment benefit for patients whose tumors had KRAS mutations, and that the use of the drug was not recommended for the treatment of colorectal cancer in such patients. However, BMS was still unable to obtain first-line labeling for colorectal cancer patients with the "wild-type" KRAS gene.

Learnings

The arrival of a diagnostic test which can differentiate between potential responders and nonresponders to a drug can be looked upon in different ways. In the event of a diagnostic test that stratifies the market appearing in the mid-life cycle of a brand, sales will inevitably contract as nonresponders are removed from the treatable pool unless the company takes measures to compensate for this. But it also means a higher success rate in the patients that are predicted to be responders. In the case of Erbitux, where 60% of patients could be expected to respond, the introduction of the KRAS test was clearly of benefit to the brand, and Merck KGaA reaped the rewards while BMS was unable to benefit in the same way. Merck KGaA in the EU turned the situation to its advantage by actively pursuing with regulators evidence that the drug shows enhanced efficacy in the responder subpopulation. The test offered the potential of promotion to earlier stages in the treatment regime, and consequently, a boost in sales that could more than offset the nonresponder-driven decline. The story might had been different had the responder rate been, say, only 10%. Increasingly, however, high-priced drugs are much more likely to get used if they can promise a high response rate. In the United States, Erbitux costs US$3000 or more per week, and a course of treatment lasts for 8 weeks. This lesson extends beyond oncology and applies to any disease area facing the introduction of a new diagnostic test that stratifies patient populations.

A.12   FAILURE OF A "NO-BRAINER" LCM STRATEGY

Exubera®

Exubera was Pfizer's brand of inhalable insulin, and represented the first ever noninjected insulin when it was approved in both the United States and

Europe in January 2006. Before its launch, it was already being welcomed as one of the most significant medical breakthroughs of recent years. Never again would diabetics have to insert a needle into the skin of their belly or buttocks from one to four times a day. This would mean no more pain, and no more buildup of unsightly scar tissue. Predictably, patient satisfaction trials had shown that a clear majority of diabetics would prefer to be prescribed inhaled insulin rather than the traditional subcutaneous injections.

What a fantastic example of cutting-edge LCM this would be! To take a nearly century-old active substance, and a biologic at that, and create a new, infinitely more patient-friendly route of administration. What a superb example of patient-oriented LCM to set alongside the rather more cynically perceived examples of LLCM such as Nexium. And what a huge commercial opportunity for Pfizer!

But in October 2007, less than 2 years after FDA approval, Pfizer voluntarily withdrew Exubera from the U.S. market, citing poor sales as the reason. A year later, in September 2008, the European Commission issued a decision to withdraw the marketing authorization for Exubera. What had gone wrong? Why did the fairy tale have such a miserable ending, both for diabetic patients and for Pfizer's shareholders?

Within 3 years of the discovery of insulin in 1921, German scientists were already experimenting with the possibility of delivering it to the patient by inhalation. Decades of failure followed, because the required insulin dose was always too high and the resultant blood levels too low. It was not until the 1990s that the problem seemed, at last, to have been solved.

Nektar Therapeutics (formerly Inhale Therapeutic Systems) finally developed a delivery system that ensured that insulin powder could be delivered deep into the lungs where it is easily absorbed into the bloodstream, using a handheld inhalation device. The basis of Nektar's success was its use of an advanced PEGylation technology to develop a dry powder-inhaled polyethylene glycol (PEG) formulation for delivering peptides efficiently across the lungs, and to promote prolonged serum concentration of the peptide. The delivery device converted the insulin powder into an aerosol, and did not require the use of propellants. Nektar licensed the system to Pfizer, who themselves already had an agreement with Hoechst Marion Roussel (today Aventis) for the supply of recombinant insulin. The Nektar/Pfizer agreement stipulated that Pfizer would lead the clinical development of inhaled insulin, while working with Nektar Therapeutics to develop the technology required for packaging the product. Nektar Therapeutics would receive royalties on sales of inhaled insulin developed and marketed by Pfizer and Aventis, as well as milestone payments and research support from Pfizer.

Initially, the development of Exubera progressed well, with Phase III trials being completed in 2001 and Pfizer holding a considerable time lead over competitor efforts to develop an inhaled insulin, namely those of Lilly (collaborating with Alkermes) and Novo Nordisk (collaborating with Aradigm).

But then Pfizer announced that it expected to have to delay filing until 2002 after discussions with the FDA. Pfizer stated that the FDA was requesting additional data because of the novelty of the therapy, and also because of questions raised about the drug's long-term effectiveness. New clinical data had revealed that patients on Exubera were four times more likely to develop antibodies against their insulin than those taking injectable insulin. Then, in May 2002, a further delay occurred as treatment with Exubera was shown to be associated with a small reduction in lung function, as well as with cases of mild-to-moderate cough. It was estimated that the filing could still be made before the beginning of 2003. But further delays followed, and it was not until March 2004 that Pfizer and Aventis were finally able to announce that the EMA had accepted their regulatory submission of Exubera in Europe, stating at the same time that discussions with the FDA were ongoing to determine when the U.S. submission could be made. Almost exactly 1 year later, in March 2005, the companies were finally able to announce that the FDA had accepted their filing in the United States.

In early January 2006, a bullish Pfizer agreed to pay US$1.3 billion to Aventis to buy out their interest in Exubera. The deal included full ownership of the insulin production plant that they jointly owned in Frankfurt, Germany. At this time, analysts were predicting peak annual sales of Exubera of US$1–2 billion, and in one case, US$4.8 billion. And analysts were particularly impressed by Pfizer's bold move in acquiring the full rights to Exubera at a time when the company was struggling to find new blockbusters to replace drugs facing generic competition.

Finally, in January 2006, Exubera was approved in both Europe and the United States. Pfizer CEO McKinnell proudly announced "Exubera® is a major, first-of-its kind, medical breakthrough that marks another critical step forward in the treatment of diabetes, a disease that has taken an enormous human and economic toll worldwide." The sales bonanza was about to start. Or was it?

Take away all of the ballyhoo and Exubera was really just a cheap old generic drug in an expensive new device, a constellation not predestined to gain the instant and uncritical support of third-party payers.

Within just a couple of weeks of approval, skeptical voices were already making themselves heard. Writing in *Business Week* in February, 2006, Michael J. Russo and David Balekdjian pointed out that, under a rigorous outcomes-based access (OBA) analysis, Exubera did not offer an acceptable value proposition. No data has been generated to support Exubera's price, which was expected to be up to four times more than injected insulin. The authors reported that Pfizer might try to compare the cost of Exubera not with other insulins but with oral diabetes medications that carry similar price tags but are vastly different therapies, often used in combination with insulin. They expected that this "apples-to-oranges" comparison would be destined to fail, with payers either drastically limiting availability, imposing very high co-payments or rejecting coverage outright. To many observers, it seemed that Pfizer was neglecting to provide the clear proof that inhaled insulin would improve compliance and disease outcomes.

Although Exubera was now approved in the United States, the launch date kept getting put back. On July 11, 2006, the Pfizer website was still listing a mid-July launch, but on July 20, Pfizer Vice Chairman Karen Katen announced that "education programmes and manufacturing preparations are time-consuming," and that the company was "taking the time necessary to do the job right." In blogs, persons claiming to be Pfizer sales representatives stated that Pfizer was having technical problems with quality control failure in the inhaler and issues with blisters.

At last, on September 1, 2006, 5 years after completion of the original Phase III clinical program, Exubera was launched in the United States. In late September, at a UBS Global Life Sciences Conference, Pfizer told analysts and conference attendees that it was counting on Exubera to be an "important source of revenue growth" for the company. But just weeks later, the company announced that it was delaying the full-scale rollout of Exubera to general practitioners until early 2007.

By April 2007 *The New York Times* was reporting that Exubera looked like becoming an expensive flop. After 6 months of marketing to doctors, Exubera was receiving only about one of every 500 prescriptions for insulin written in the United States. Analysts were drastically cutting their peak sales forecasts for the product.

Pfizer's biggest selling argument for Exubera had been that inhaled insulin was more convenient than injections and avoided needle pricks. In the real world, this apparently "no-brainer" argument was just not working. The Exubera inhaler was cumbersome and unwieldy, about the size of a can of tennis balls, and doctors and patients alike were unhappy with it. Furthermore, it now seemed that most diabetics were not that dissatisfied with injections. The needles used today are smaller and less painful than they used to be. To add to these problems, Exubera dosages were not the same as injected dosages, and converting doses could be tricky.

Competition was getting stronger, with four new treatments approved since Pfizer had completed the development of Exubera (Januvia, Byetta®, Levemir®, and Symlin®).

And the safety problems first identified back in 2000 were not going away. In fact, concerns were growing that long-term insulin inhalation could reduce pulmonary function and damage the lungs. As a result, potential Exubera patients had to be screened using lung function tests before they could be prescribed the product, and this was discouraging both physicians and patients.

The unfavorable constellation of high cost, lack of convenience, and safety concerns were weighing heavily on Exubera's chances of success. And to add to the brand's woes, it was being marketed by Pfizer's cardiovascular division where sales representatives had a much easier job pushing high-margin products like Lipitor instead of trying to overcome physician resistance to lower-margin Exubera.

On October 19, 2007, just a year after launch, Pfizer announced that it was withdrawing Exubera from the market and taking a US$2.8 billion pretax charge in the third quarter. The product had sold only US$12 million in the first 9 months of the year. Nektar shares promptly lost 20% of their value.

In January 2008, Novo Nordisk discontinued its AERx® inhaled insulin development program, and Lilly followed suit with its AIR® insulin system in March. In April, Nektar announced that it was terminating all negotiations with potential partners to succeed Pfizer following the release of new data by Pfizer indicating an increased lung cancer risk in patients taking inhaled insulin.

Only Mannkind persisted with inhaled insulin. Their Afrezza® device was submitted to the FDA in May 2009 and received a complete response letter in May 2010. In early 2011, Mannkind announced that they were delaying the FDA submission until late 2012 at the earliest because of the need to conduct additional clinical trials. Mannkind lost 60% of its share value within a few days of the announcement.

Learnings

Rear vision is always 20/20, and it is easy to be wise after the event. It would seem at first sight that diabetics should have been very happy to accept even a clumsy inhaler if it would stop them having to inject themselves. But they were not, and it does seem that in this case, mighty Pfizer's market research apparatus rather let it down. For most patients, injecting themselves was just not so big a deal. The safety concerns compounded the problem, and also Pfizer clearly did not do enough to convince third-party payers that Exubera was a value proposition. Mannkind has developed a lightweight inhaler that fits easily in the palm of the patient's hand for its inhaled insulin development, and also utilizes single-use, disposable, plastic cartridges which they hope will facilitate patient compliance. And their patented, dry-powder formulation of rapid-acting insulin is claimed to penetrate deeper into the lung when inhaled, therefore offering significant pharmacokinetic advances over Exubera. But concerns about long-term safety of inhaled insulin persist, and Mannkind has so far been unable to find a marketing partner.

One of the most important learnings from the Exubera fiasco is that it is getting more difficult to earn money with reformulations late in a brand (or molecule) life cycle. The degree of advantage that the new formulation must show over the old formulation to get listing and a premium price over generics is very hard to achieve. Exubera demonstrates that even moving to a more preferable route of administration may not be a sufficient motivation for third-party payers to join the party.

A.13 AT-RISK LAUNCHES AND PRODRUG PATENTS

Famvir®

In 2000, SmithKline Beecham divested its antiviral, Famvir (famciclovir), to Novartis. The divestiture was undertaken to secure regulatory approval for SmithKline Beecham's merger with Glaxo Wellcome, which already marketed the direct competitor product, Valtrex®. The Famvir composition-of-matter patent was due to expire in 2010.

Teva submitted an ANDA for famciclovir in 2005, with Paragraph IV certification. Novartis filed a patent infringement lawsuit, and the FDA imposed a 30-month stay on the approval of the ANDA. Novartis and Teva remained in litigation without resolution until the 30-month stay expired in August, 2007, at which time Teva prepared to launch its generic "at risk." To prevent the launch, Novartis filed a preliminary injunction, claiming that Teva infringed the famciclovir composition-of-matter patent.

To understand how the litigation moved backward and forward subsequently, it is important to review the chemistry. Penciclovir is the active substance of a topical preparation for the treatment of herpes infections. It is available as a cream, and the composition-of-matter patent expired in different countries between 2009 and 2010. But penciclovir has poor oral bioavailability, and this was the rationale behind taking a prodrug with good oral availability, famciclovir, as the active substance for the oral antiviral Famvir. Famciclovir undergoes rapid biotransformation in the body to form the biologically active penciclovir.

Teva's rationale behind their Paragraph IV certification was that it was obvious to take famciclovir as a prodrug, and that therefore the patent on famciclovir should never have been granted.

The district court denied Novartis's motion, stating that it had concluded that Novartis was unlikely to succeed on the merits of its case, and that Novartis would not suffer irreparable harm from denial of the injunction. Specifically, the court ruled that Novartis failed to show that Teva's obviousness defense lacked substantial merit. The court determined that it had indeed been obvious to select penciclovir as a lead compound from which to design famciclovir because it was "one of only five known acyclic nucleosides to have strong activity and low toxicity." It specifically referred to the KSR versus Teleflex judgment in making this call, stating that "selecting penciclovir was a matter of ordinary skill and common sense." The court further ruled that any economic harm to Novartis would not be irreparable, since Teva would be able to pay any damages that might be suffered by Novartis should Novartis win the litigation, and that Novartis's research activities would not be disrupted by a temporary reduction in Famvir sales revenue.

Novartis immediately filed an Emergency Motion for an Injunction Pending Appeal with the Federal Circuit, but 1 day later, Teva announced that it had "commenced shipment of famciclovir Tablets" and that it was the 180-day exclusivity holder. Later on the same day, the Federal Circuit ordered that

Teva be "temporarily enjoined from selling its generic famciclovir product, pending the court's receipt of Teva's response and the court's consideration of the papers submitted." Teva filed its opposition brief the week after, Novartis then filed its reply brief.

The Court of Appeals rejected Novartis's Emergency Motion, clearing the way for Teva to resume selling of generic famciclovir.

The patent infringement lawsuit between Novartis and Teva dragged on. In November 2009, a jury in the New Jersey District Court returned a verdict in favor of Novartis, and at this stage, it seemed likely that Novartis could ultimately prevail, leaving Teva open to damages.

Then, in February 2010, Teva and Novartis announced that they had signed an agreement to settle the famciclovir litigation, including all claims for patent infringement and damages. This agreement released Teva for all past and future activities in connection with the U.S. marketing and sale of generic famciclovir. Under the terms of the agreement, Teva would make a one-time payment to Novartis, stated to be US$42 million in the Novartis annual report for 2010, in addition to an ongoing royalty on U.S. sales of the generic.

In some ways, this is a typical case of a generic launch at risk, but there are a couple of especially interesting points.

- In allowing Teva to resume sales in 2007, the Court of Appeals was in effect saying that it believed it unlikely that Novartis would be able to defend a composition-of-matter patent, citing KSR versus Teleflex as the reason for coming to this conclusion.
- In its Annual Report 2007, Novartis stated that it had "recorded impairment charges of US$482 million principally relating to an impairment of US$320 million for Famvir® product rights due to an earlier than anticipated challenge to its patent and subsequent loss of sales in the Pharmaceuticals Division." In other words, it had not only lost sales and profits because of Teva's "at-risk" launch but had also suffered a hit on its balance sheet for the value of the Famvir asset which it had acquired from SmithKline Beecham. Had the litigation not been cut short by the February 2010 settlement, and had Novartis prevailed in defending its patent, then Teva would have been liable for the sales and profits that Novartis had lost but not for the reduction in book value of the asset. One could therefore argue that Novartis had indeed been liable to suffer "irreparable damage." As a result of the settlement, Novartis was able to reverse US$100 million of the impairment on its balance sheet.

Learnings

Following the KSR versus Teleflex ruling, we must look more critically even at our composition-of-matter patents. In particular, prodrug and active metabolite patents are under threat of being dismissed for reasons of obviousness. Although there have been no precedents as yet, some experts even speculate that the whole strategy of creating "me-too" drugs could be thrown into question. Me-too drugs are often created by companies which simply synthesize variants of a competitor's molecule in the hope of finding one which is at least as effective and as safe, but which lies just outside of the competitor's patents. Now doesn't that seem to be rather an "obvious" thing to try?

A.14   NEW DOSAGES, FDC, AND PATENT LITIGATION

Fosamax®

Fosamax is Merck's alendronate sodium, a bisphosphonate marketed for osteoporosis and several other related bone diseases. It is also available as an FDC with Vitamin D, under the brand name Fosamax Plus D®. The sales of the Fosamax family peaked in 2007 at US$3 billion but halved in the following year and dropped to one-third in 2009 after the entry of generics into the U.S. market in February 2008.

Fosamax was first approved by the FDA in 1995 for the treatment of osteoporosis in postmenopausal women and for Paget's disease. By 1997, the labeling was expanded to include the prevention of osteoporosis and the prevention of bone fractures in the postmenopausal population. The year 1999 saw another indication added to the label, the treatment of osteoporosis in men and women receiving cortisone resulting in low bone mineral density. One year later, male osteoporosis was added to the label. Up until 2000, Fosamax was available as 5-mg, 10-mg, and 40-mg tablets with the recommended dose ranging from 5 mg once daily for the prevention of osteoporosis, through 10 mg once daily for its treatment and 40 mg once daily for treating Paget's disease.

At the end of 2000, Merck changed the game within the bisphosphonate drug class for preventing and treating osteoporosis by introducing two additional new dosage strengths, 35 mg and 70 mg, the lower dose to be given just once weekly for prevention and the higher dose once weekly for treatment of the disease. Merck had been able to demonstrate that once-weekly Fosamax was therapeutically equivalent to daily dosing (e.g., one 70 mg weekly dose was equivalent to 10 mg daily doses). A 70-mg once-weekly oral solution was added in 2003. And then, in 2005, Merck gained pediatric exclusivity for Fosamax.

On April 7, 2005, Merck gained FDA approval for an FDC of alendronate sodium plus cholecalciferol (vitamin D3) tablets, under the brand name Fosamax Plus D, for the treatment of osteoporosis in postmenopausal women and to increase bone mass in men with osteoporosis. Approval was based firstly on the fact that it was already recommended that patients on Fosamax take concomitant Vitamin D, and secondly on bioequivalence studies confirming that there were no pharmacokinetic interactions between the two components. The initial approval was for once-weekly dosing of 70 mg of alendronate combined with 2800 i.U. of Vitamin D3, and then an additional approval was obtained for a 70 mg plus 5600 i.U. combination.

Another interesting aspect of Fosamax LCM is the long-standing and complicated story of Merck's efforts to maintain exclusivity of Fosamax and the efforts of generic companies to challenge it. The complexity is mirrored in the fact that when Teva filed its ANDA for a generic version of Fosamax, it had to certify against 10 separate patents which were listed in the Orange Book. Several generic companies were involved in the battle with Merck in the United States, but for the sake of clarity we will concentrate only on Teva.

The first of the 10 patents that should concern us here, the "077" patent, is a 1982 patent from the Italian company Instituto Gentili claiming the use of alendronate or its salt as the active ingredient in a pharmaceutical compound. The patent stated that alendronate had characteristics that made it suitable as an inhibitor of bone resorption *in vivo*, while other compounds which worked *in vitro* were incapable of therapeutic application due to rapid hydrolysis. The "077" patent was due to expire in August 2007, but Merck obtained pediatric exclusivity to extend protection until February 2008. The second patent of particular interest is a 1997 patent owned by Merck ("329" patent) claiming a particular dosing regime for the treatment of excessive bone desorption in humans, comprising the administration of a single dose of about 70 mg of active ingredient. The "329" patent was due to expire in 2018. Summarizing, the first patent thus covered the use of alendronate in osteoporosis, and the second patent the once-weekly dosage regimen.

After Teva filed in 1999, stating that each of the 10 patents in the Orange Book was invalid, unenforceable, or would not be infringed by the generic product, Merck filed for infringement on 9 of the 10 within the allowed 45-day period. These nine patents included the "077" and "329" patents and others related to formulations and methods of use.

In November 2002, the Delaware District Court found that Teva's ANDA filing infringed the "077" and "329" patents, and Teva immediately appealed the court's claim construction and nonobviousness findings. In October 2003, the Federal Circuit affirmed the judgment of the District Court. However, in January 2005, the Federal Circuit reversed the District Court judgment, holding the claims of the "329" patent to be not invalid but also not infringed by Teva's generic. This left the way free for Teva to launch the full range of aledronate generics once the "077" patent expired. Accordingly, in February 2008, Teva launched generic aledronate at the doses of 5 mg, 10 mg, and 40 mg (daily) and 35 mg and 70 mg (weekly).

The situation in Europe was rather more involved, to say the least. The equivalent of the "077" Gentili patent was a series of national patents throughout Europe, while the equivalent of the "329" patent was a Patent Cooperation Treaty (PCT) application, the "292" patent. Let us look in detail at what happened in just one European country as an example. The British High Court decided in early 2003 to support Teva as plaintiff in invalidating both of the key European patents for reasons of obviousness. The court found the patent covering use of the drug in osteoporosis to be an obvious extension of work performed in Switzerland by Professor Fleisch in the 1960s, and weekly alendronate to be an obvious development. The court did express regret for its decision, in the following statement: "Merck have only had a few years' exclusive exploitation of alendronate. They must surely have had to make a very considerable investment and incurred considerable risk in bringing it to market. And mankind is better off as a result. But the patent system does not confer monopolies on those who develop obvious or old products, even if they have never been exploited." The Court of Appeal upheld the decision in November 2003, and in a separate case brought by Merck against another generic company, the High Court dismissed Merck's claim that one of its process patents was being infringed.

Outside the United Kingdom, a preliminary injunction was granted in Belgium to prevent sales of the generic, in Italy an appeals court reversed a district court decision to deny a preliminary injunction, in Holland a preliminary injunction was granted which was then reversed on appeal, in Denmark a lower court denied a preliminary injunction, the appeals court overturned the decision, and then the lower court again ruled against the preliminary injunction. All in all, Teva had to litigate patent infringements in eight countries, Holland, Italy, the United Kingdom, Germany, France, Belgium, Sweden, and Spain. In all of the cases that reached a judgment on the merits of a patent, Teva was able to get the challenged patent revoked. In six of the eight countries (not the United Kingdom and Spain), Merck sought a preliminary injunction, and it was granted in four cases though later revoked in two of these.

Merck also took Teva to court, alleging that the Teva generic was not bioequivalent, but here, too, Teva finally always prevailed. In Holland, Teva had to take Merck to court after Merck sent letters to 12,000 doctors alleging that the Teva generic was of inferior quality. These letters subsequently had to be retracted. In Germany, Merck sued Teva for unfair competition, claiming that Teva illegally compared its product to that of Merck in advertisements. Merck initially obtained a preliminary injunction in Germany, which was later revoked.

Learnings

Merck did a fine job of maintaining its dominance within the bisphosphonate class by creating new formulations with novel dosage regimens. Regarding its struggles with generic companies, and especially Teva, at the end of the Fosamax patent life, the main learning is probably that the huge complexity and uncertainty around the final outcome of patent litigation is a massive incentive for brand and generic companies to seek settlements. This aspect of LLCM is often criticized, as settlements certainly do not benefit the consumer, but one must also have sympathy with the involved companies who seek a quick and clean end to the litigation. The inconsistent decisions in the different U.S. courts are problem enough, but even worse are the continuous inconsistencies and reversals within the many, independent EU jurisdictions. The dream would be a centralized European-level patent court which would be responsible for European patents instead of allowing them to cascade down into a plethora of national patents which may be handled differently in each jurisdiction. But as recently as March 2011, the Court of Justice of the European Union (CJEU) has stated that such a European patent would not be compatible with EU law, as it would require a new court to deal with disputes relating to the European patent, and in its present form, it does not include an appropriate mechanism by which that court could be challenged if it breached EU law. And so the unsatisfactory situation drags on.

(The LCM of Fosamax regarding formulations and dosage regimens within the context of the whole bisphosphonate class is examined in Case History 24.)

A.15   HIGH REGULATORY HURDLES FOR LIFESTYLE DRUGS

Girosa®

Girosa (flibanserin) is Boehringer Ingelheim's 5-HT1A receptor agonist and 5-HT2A receptor antagonist. Originally, based on preclinical data, Boehringer had hoped that flibanserin could be developed as a fast-acting antidepressant, which patients would respond to in just a few days rather than the weeks it takes for tricyclic antidepressants to exert their effect. They initiated an appropriate Phase II program comprising 11 clinical trials. During these trials, Boehringer monitored patient libido, as antidepressants can often cause a reduction in sexual desire due to an increase in serotonin levels. The results of the trials were totally unexpected. While flibanserin failed to exert a positive effect on depression, and had no effect on the libido of males in the trial, many female patients reported an increase in sexual desire and arousal.

Accordingly, Boehringer shifted its focus away from depression and conducted two proof-of-concept (PoC) trials of flibanserin in Hypoactive Sexual Desire Disorder (HSDD) in premenopausal women. These trials were followed, starting in 2007, by an 8000 patient, seven-trial Phase III clinical program in HSDD. Inevitably, the popular press was now full of references to the upcoming "female viagra" or "pink Viagra." Indeed, the parallels were there for all to see. Viagra® had also been under development for a completely different indication when its not unwelcome side effects on male libido were observed in clinical trials.

However, flibanserin was in for a rough ride. The first problem it had to face was the ongoing controversy about whether a true female analog to male erectile dysfunction even exists. Following the success of Viagra in men, there was a widespread perception that the pharmaceutical industry was trying to "invent" female sexual dysfunction as a defined—and common—disease. A

JAMA article in February 1999 titled "Sexual Dysfunction in the United States: Prevalence and Predictors" stated that, for women aged 18–59, the "total prevalence of sexual dysfunction" was a remarkably high 43%, a figure which was subsequently widely cited in both scientific literature and the popular press. Belatedly, two of the authors of this article admitted that they had close contacts with Pfizer, who at that time were also investigating the possible usage of Viagra for HSDD. But while penile erection is a quantifiable physical event, female sexual response is much more qualitative, involving a complicated sequence of desire, arousal, orgasm, and subsequent satisfaction which is extremely difficult to measure objectively, and where there are no established and recognized clinical end points. Indeed, no drugs had ever been approved for HSDD as Boehringer initiated their Phase III program.

The five U.S. Phase III trials were carried out under a Special Protocol Assessment (SPA), using end points, measures, and data collection methodologies which were broadly pre-agreed and in line with the FDA's "Guidance for Industry" regarding female sexual dysfunction. The results were reported in 2009. Patients in the flibanserin groups exhibited a statistically significant increase in the number of "satisfactory sexual events" compared to placebo in each of the U.S. studies, but no significant improvement in the coprimary end point of change in desire as measured by electronic diaries. During the trials Boehringer had requested use of an alternative desire measure instead of the eDiary, namely the female sexual function index, but the FDA had considered this to be unjustified statistically and unsupported by exploratory data. Boehringer claimed that a series of secondary end points supported the efficacy of flibanserin, but the FDA countered in its briefing document to Advisory Committee members that, since flibanserin failed to demonstrate statistically significant improvements in both coprimary efficacy end points, according to the protocols and statistical analysis plans analysis of the secondary end points should not have been conducted. While the evidence for efficacy was not compelling, there was clear evidence that flibanserin caused more adverse events than placebo, though none of them were serious. The adverse events included dizziness, nausea, anxiety, insomnia, and fatigue, and there were also depression-related adverse events that caused the FDA to speculate that this could be a predictor of an increased risk of suicidality were the drug to be used in a larger patient population. Some adverse events were worsened by concomitant contraceptive usage.

The FDA Advisory Committee met in June 2010 and voted 10 to 1 that flibanserin was not significantly better than placebo for HSDD, and 11 to 0 against flibanserin having an acceptable risk–benefit profile. The FDA issued a Complete Response Letter in August 2010, and Boehringer announced in October that it had discontinued the development of flibanserin. Professor Andreas Barner, Chairman of the Board of Boehringer, stated that "the decision was not made lightly, considering the advanced stage of development. We remain convinced of the positive benefit-risk ratio of flibanserin for women suffering with HSDD."

Learnings

The reason for including this interesting case history in a book on LCM is that flibanserin had originally been designed for treatment of a severe disease, depression, where its adverse event profile might well have been acceptable. But the hurdle is much higher for a lifestyle drug, especially for one where there is controversy as to what extent the disease actually exists and how to measure whether or not a treatment is exerting a benefit. Flibanserin was not the first HSDD drug to fall foul of the FDA, with Procter & Gamble (P&G)'s testosterone patch (Intrinsa®) already having failed to clear the risk–benefit hurdle in 2004.

Moreover, selection of "perception-based" end points, particularly for a disorder that may not be widely accepted, is a risky clinical strategy. Boehringer made this approach even riskier by attempting to change end points halfway through the trial, and this without doubt contributed to the negative vote of the Advisory Committee.

A.16   BIG MONEY FROM ORPHAN INDICATIONS

Gleevec®

Gleevec is Novartis's imatinib mesylate, used to treat a variety of rare types of cancer. At the time of its initial U.S. approval in 2001, Gleevec was the first representative of a new class of agents that act by specifically inhibiting an individual enzyme that is characteristic of a particular cancer cell, rather than by nonspecifically inhibiting and killing all rapidly dividing cells. In the case of Gleevec, the target is tyrosine kinase.

From the very start, Gleevec was welcomed as the vanguard of a revolution of new medicines. In the same month as the FDA approved it, in May 2001, it was the cover story in *Time* magazine, the story being titled "New Hope for Cancer." The first approval was for the treatment of patients with chronic myeloid leukemia (CML) in blast crisis, accelerated phase, or in chronic phase after failure of interferon-alpha therapy. In February 2002, the FDA narrowed the initial indication to Philadelphia-chromosome-positive CML patients, but at the same time approved the additional indication of Kit-positive unresectable and/or malignant gastrointestinal stromal tumors (GIST). In May 2003, Gleevec was granted the indication for pediatric CML. In April 2003, Novartis introduced Gleevec tablets to succeed the capsules that they had marketed since 2001.

In October 2006, a whole series of new indications was approved, namely dermafibrosarcoma protuberans, myelodysplastic syndrome/myeloproliferative diseases, Philadelphia-positive acute lymphoblastic leukemia, aggressive systemic mastocytosis, and hypereosinophilic syndrome/chronic eosinophilic leukemia.

There can be no doubt that Gleevec represented a major medical breakthrough, and completely changed the quality of life and survival prospects of

CML patients. Prior to Gleevec, CML patients were treated with high doses of interferon, and the survival rate after 10 years was a meager 10–20%. With the introduction of Gleevec this figure rose dramatically to over 90%, a level of success achieved by very few drugs in the modern age.

However, the success of Gleevec was not without its critics. CML patients in the United States taking one 400-mg Gleevec tablet per day faced annual treatment costs of about US$40,000, and many patients were taking daily doses as high as 800 mg. In 2010, Novartis reported that Gleevec's annual global sales had reached a remarkable US$4.3 billion, making it Novartis's second best-selling drug behind Diovan. And all of the diseases for which Gleevec was approved were orphan indications. Quoting from the Orphan Drug Act that the FDA uses as the basis for designating orphan drugs, ". . . so few individuals are affected by any one rare disease or condition, a pharmaceutical company which develops an orphan drug may reasonably expect the drug to generate relatively small sales in comparison to the cost of developing the drug and consequently to incur a financial loss." Looked at from this perspective, it certainly does appear that Novartis has been very astute in its LCM of Gleevec, fully utilizing the relevant legislation to build a powerful brand franchise.

The success and clinical importance of Gleevec led to it facing criticism in India too, where changes in the national patent legislation resulted in it being denied a patent by the Indian Patent Office (IPO) in 2006. Novartis appealed this ruling, but in July 2009, India's Intellectual Property Appellate Board (IPAB) upheld the decision of the IPO. Even though the beta-crystalline patent on imatinib had been approved in all developed countries, as well as in China, Russia, and Taiwan, IPAB agreed with IPO that it did not meet the specific requirements of the Indian legislation. How could this be? In 1993, Novartis had been granted a patent for the synthesis of the imatinib molecule, but this was only the initial step in creating a commercial product as Novartis first had to develop the mesylate salt and then the beta-crystalline form of this salt before the Gleevec pill could be introduced to the market in 2001. In other words, this was a case where a "new" salt was required before the drug could be used in the first place, a far cry from the LLCM strategy of tweaking crystalline forms to prolong the exclusivity period of existing brands. Nevertheless, in rejecting the patent, the IPO cited paragraph 3(d) of the new legislation which states that "a patent is granted only if a product proves to be more efficacious than an existing drug molecule."

In its 2009 ruling, the IPAB not only called on this paragraph 3(d) but also stated that "any patent granted to support such a high monopoly price would be against 'public order.'" The board pointed out that Gleevec's price tag of US$2500 per month was too expensive for Indian cancer patients to afford. This statement needs to be closely scrutinized for two reasons:

1. According to the Institute of International Trade, this is the very first time that a patent has been denied because of an "unaffordable price."

The idea that cost containment is now influencing an innovator's ability to protect health-care inventions is scary indeed.

2. Generic imatinib is available in India at US$250 per month, one-tenth of the price of Gleevec. But even this price is a multiple of the average salary in India, putting even generic imatinib treatment far out of reach of the majority of the population. And Novartis was already in 2006 giving away free Gleevec to 99% of all Indian patients that were pre-scribed imatinib under its Gleevec International Patient Assistance Programme (GIPAP).

It was announced in September 2011 that Novartis has once again challenged the relevant passage of Indian patent law and that the case has been elevated to the Indian Supreme Court.

A further interesting aspect of the Gleevec story is that Novartis appears to have succeeded where many other companies have failed in developing a slightly modified successor molecule which represents a real advance in treat-ment and not merely an attempt to limit generic erosion of the franchise when the existing product becomes generic.

Tasigna® (nilotinib) was approved by the FDA in 2007 for the treatment in CML in patients who were unresponsive to Gleevec therapy. Tasigna was specifically designed to target the Bcr-Abl protein more preferentially than Gleevec® without adding any new mechanisms of action. And then, in June 2010, Tasigna gained approval as first-line therapy after clinical trial results showed that 44% of patients taking Tasigna had a "major molecular response" compared with only 22% for Gleevec at 12 months. A major molecular response is defined by a reduction of disease by 99.9%, and has been associ-ated with higher rates of long-term survival. But Tasigna will not have it all its own way, as BMS's similar CML drug Sprycel® also beat Gleevec in a head-to-head trial.

CML is an uncommon disease, and the cost burden to health insurances is therefore low despite the high price of the drugs used to treat it. Both com-panies are no doubt hoping that this will ensure that the newer drug are used as first-line treatment rather than only in patients unresponsive to Gleevec once the Gleevec patent expires in 2015 and generic imatinib appears on the market. The Sprycel patent expires in 2020 and the Tasigna patent not until 2023.

Learnings

Orphan indications can be big business! Not only are they valuable in getting new molecules onto the market in small, high unmet need and high price patient populations, but in some situations, they can be financially very reward-ing in their own right.

The Gleevec patent dispute in India is not really about Gleevec at all. The Indian government is trying to make patenting more difficult in support of its own generics industry, while Novartis is trying to ensure that patents—and therefore prices—are maintained in this important emerging market. Who will win? Novartis is unlikely to surrender, but other governments—especially in emerging markets—will no doubt be observing the Indian situation with great interest.

It is hard to look like the good guy these days if you are a Big Pharma company. Gleevec is a wonderful drug, and Novartis is giving it away to the vast majority of Indian CML patients, but much of the popular press still sees Gleevec in India as an example of how Big Pharma exploits economically disadvantaged patients to line their own pockets. A wrong conclusion in this case, but one that has been reached based on earlier "new salt" LCM strategies with other brands and at other companies that were indeed designed to keep generics off the market, to the detriment of patients. In a recent step, a group of NGOs wrote to Novartis in February 2011 urging the company to stop challenging Indian patent law and claiming that the GIPAP was only covering one-third of the Indian patients who were in need of Gleevec therapy.

Creating successor molecules to drugs nearing patent expiry is often viewed as a rather suspect way of preventing generic success, as described elsewhere in this book, based on the many cases where companies have exploited the potential of isomerism, polymorphism, prodrugs, active metabolites, novel salts, and so on. Tasigna appears to be good example of a successor molecule where any such criticism is inappropriate; Tasigna represents a significant incremental improvement over a breakthrough in medicine and should be applauded as such.

A.17 NOT GIVING UP ON A CONTROVERSIAL BRAND

Iressa®

Iressa is AstraZeneca's gefitinib, and it was the first selective inhibitor of EGFR's tyrosine kinase domain. It was first approved in Japan in 2002 for the treatment of non-small cell lung cancer (NSCLC). Interestingly, it was the first globally developed drug from a major pharmaceutical company to gain approval in Japan before either the United States or Europe. Japanese approval was granted on the basis of two large Phase II trials in patients with locally advanced or metastatic NSCLC who had received platinum-based chemotherapy. In these trials, tumor size was shown to reduce under Iressa therapy, and this surrogate end point was accepted as the basis for approval by the Japanese health authority.

The FDA subsequently approved Iressa based on the same clinical evidence in May 2003, under its accelerated approval program, for the treatment of patients with NSCLC who had previously failed two or more courses of chemotherapy. AstraZeneca CEO Tom McKillop predicted the pill would become a "megabrand" with sales of more than US$1 billion. However, the FDA asked AstraZeneca to study the drug further to verify the clinical benefit. Required was a clinical trial in 1700 patients to determine whether the drug would in fact prolong survival in comparison to patients taking placebo. The results of this trial program were released by AstraZeneca in December 2004, and they demonstrated no survival benefit of patients taking Iressa compared with those receiving placebo. The FDA decided not to withdraw the drug from the market completely, but immediately restricted its use to patients who were already receiving or had received Iressa and who responded positively to the therapy. The life expectancy of these patients was short, and Iressa has now disappeared from the United States market.

In January 2005, AstraZeneca announced that it was withdrawing its European submission as the survival rates in the Phase III program did not support European approval. Also in January 2005, the Japanese Ministry of Health and Welfare stated that it was considering banning Iressa after accepting a report that linked the medicine to 588 deaths in the country. These were mainly caused by acute interstitial pneumonia, and the Ministry created a study team to evaluate Iressa. At this point, it really did appear as if the days of Iressa might be numbered. But AstraZeneca refused to give up on the drug.

Instead of banning Iressa, the Japanese study group drew up guidelines for its usage, and in March 2005, the Ministry accepted the recommendation and authorized the continued usage of Iressa in Japan under this guideline. (It subsequently emerged in a court of law that 3 of the 10 doctors involved in drawing up the guideline had received donations from AstraZeneca, but that is another story).

AstraZeneca continued to conduct clinical trials to prove the value of Iressa. In July 2005, it was reported that subgroup analysis of the Phase III trials indicated that a survival benefit could be demonstrated in patients with Asian ethnicity and in patients who had never smoked. These findings appeared in various published forms, and a rationale was found for the phenomenon. Only patients with EGFR mutations would respond positively to Iressa therapy, and such mutations were shown to be more common in females, in patients with a history of adenocarcinoma, in Asians, and in patients who had never smoked. Approximately 30–40% of Asian NSCLC patients have EGFR mutation positive tumors compared with only 10–15% of Caucasians. These findings spawned a 22-month study in six Asian countries involving more than 1200 nonsmoking lung cancer patients who had never received chemotherapy. The results of this trial, which were released in 2008, showed that, in the patient population tested, Iressa was better tolerated and resulted in a greater likelihood of response than a conventional chemotherapy regimen of carboplatin and paclitaxel. Based on the results of these and other clinical studies, AstraZeneca resubmitted in Europe.

Iressa had survived in Japan, and approvals and sales were also satisfactory in other Asian countries. The extremely restrictive labeling in the United States persisted, but in July 2009, AstraZeneca was finally able to announce that the European Commission had approved Iressa for the treatment of adults with locally advanced or metastatic NSCLC with activating EGFR mutations. In January 2010, the influential British NICE stated that it needed more data before deciding whether Iressa could be offered to patients via the NHS, and in June 2010 decided to back the drug after AstraZeneca agreed to offer it for a fixed price whatever the length of treatment, and free to patients who remain on the drug for less than 3 months.

In January 2011, the Japanese government rejected a court settlement plan for damages suits over side effects caused by Iressa.

In 2010, Iressa sold for US$400 million worldwide, the majority of this turnover coming from Asia.

Learnings

Iressa overcame the challenges of a failed Phase III clinical program, serious efficacy concerns, and a submission withdrawal in Europe to finally establish itself as an accepted item in the oncologist toolbox. This was achieved by a combination of strategies including postapproval trials, segmentation of the patient population, and the development of a biomarker. In addition, a bespoke pricing system was offered in the United Kingdom to get the support of NICE. Iressa is not a major product for AstraZeneca, but without their persistence, it would probably not exist at all. As discussed in Case Histories 22 and 23, on Nexium, AstraZeneca was faced with a series of high-profile Phase III development failures in the early to mid-2000s and just could not afford to let Iressa go without a fight. The best LCM is often performed by companies with a pipeline crisis which heightens the importance of the existing brand portfolio and the willingness of top management to continue to invest in them.

A.18 EXPANDING A MEDICAL AESTHETICS FRANCHISE WITH AN OPHTHALMIC DRUG

Latisse®

Latisse is Allergan's prostaglandin analog/prodrug bimatoprost for the treatment of hypotrichosis of the eyelashes by increasing their growth including length, thickness, and darkness. It was approved by the FDA on Christmas Eve, 2008, as a 0.03% ophthalmic solution.

Allergan had already obtained FDA approval for bimatoprost in 2001 under the tradename Lumigan® for the treatment of elevated intraocular pressure in patients with glaucoma or ocular hypertension, initially as second-line therapy and from 2006 as first line. The first prostaglandin analog to be approved for this serious indication had been Pfizer's Xalatan® (latanoprost), back in the mid-1990s, and Alcon had launched their me-too, Travatan® (travoprost) a few months earlier than Allergan.

The prostaglandin analogs were very effective in treating elevated intraocular pressures, which gave them a decisive advantage over earlier drug classes. The carbonic anhydrase inhibitors were less effective, and beta-blockers, even when given as eye drops, could have serious side effects. But the prostaglandin analogs were also not without their problems. They were less well tolerated locally, and they caused two very strange side effects—darkening of the iris of the treated eye, and lengthening and thickening of the eyelashes. Indeed, it was primarily these side effects that limited their initial approval to second-line therapy, especially behind Merck's beta-blocker, Timoptic® (timolol). However, even after Merck had launched an FDC, Cosopt®, containing timolol and a carbonic anhydrase inhibitor (dorzolamide), the perception among opthalmologists that the prostaglandin analogs were still more effective led to high levels of off-label first-line use even before the FDA granted first-line approval. Xalatan, the first prostaglandin analog to be launched, propelled by the marketing muscle of Pfizer, became the biggest-selling drug in the history of ophthalmic pharmaceuticals.

Allergan launched a lower dose 0.01% ophthalmic solution of Lumigan in 2009 (EU) resp. 2010 (United States), claiming a reduction in reddening of the eye and similar efficacy. All three companies developed FDCs of their own prostaglandin analog with timolol, namely Xalacom® (Pfizer), DuoTrav® (Alcon), and Ganfort® (Allergan). They were all approved in Europe, but none gained FDA approval owing to regulatory challenges following changes in the FDA guidance for combination products.

The prostaglandin analogs used for treating elevated intraocular pressure are nearing the end of their patent lives. The patent of the market leader, Xalatan, expired in the United States in March, 2011, and although the patents of the other two products expire later, in 2012–2014, generic latanoprost is certain to hit their sales.

Apart from FDCs, there seemed to be few options for LCM of the prostaglandin analogs. The eye drops were already once daily, the active substances could not be given systemically, and no other local indications appeared feasible.

But Allergan had one in-house success story that had initially astounded the pharmaceutical industry and the medical community, and which had generated huge sales and profits. Botox®! Who would have thought of taking one of the most potent neurotoxins known to man, botulinum toxin, and turning it into a cosmetic drug? Suffice it say here that the unwanted side effect of latanoprost, lengthening and darkening of eyelashes, rang some bells in Allergan's "medical aesthetics" department.

Allergan saw the opportunity of turning this unwanted side effect into a line extension that offered significant commercial potential. Women spend millions of dollars every year on mascara to accentuate their eyelashes, and Lumigan was doing exactly that.

Developing the new indication was not difficult. Allergan took exactly the same formulation as 0.03% Lumigan for glaucoma but added a disposable sterile applicator to the packaging to enable patients to apply the solution along the skin of the upper eyelid margin at the base of the eyelashes instead of dropping it into the eye, to minimize the risk of darkening of the iris. Thus, a new route of administration was added without any need to reformulate, a clever move that saved both time and development costs. A clinical trial was conducted against vehicle at 16 sites across the United States and included 278 patients. After 4 months of treatment, Latisse proved effective for 78% of patients compared with 18% for the vehicle group in improving eyelash quality (length, thickness, and darkness) in a Global Eyelash Assessment (GEA). The FDA approval duly followed, and Allergan leveraged the power of its Botox sales force and experience to make the launch a success. They used the same model they had deployed for Botox, setting up partnerships with local doctors. They started a national campaign to drive in patients. Their advertising featured actresses like Brooke Shields and Claire Danes, whose eyes had hitherto apparently suffered from the ravages of hypotrichosis.

Latisse did have to carry the existing baggage of Lumigan side effects on its label—including iris and lid pigmentation, hair growth away from the treatment area, ocular inflammation, and macular edema—but this did not prevent Latisse providing a significant boost to bimatoprost sales. Like Botox, Latisse has been positioned as a luxury product which has enabled it to command more or less the same high pricing as Lumigan. Latisse sold US$75 million in 2010, and predictions were for this to increase by a third to US$100 million in 2011. This would represent a nearly 20% increment over the predicted Lumigan sales of US$550 million. One leading analyst has estimated that Latisse sales could top US$250 million by 2013. Latisse is currently being investigated in clinical trials in Europe, where it has not yet been submitted for approval.

Allergan is now also developing Latisse for male-pattern baldness, increasing prospects for the bimatoprost franchise further.

Learnings

Like Viagra, Latisse is another fine example of a drug being developed opportunistically to exploit a side effect seen in patients being treated for a different condition. By leveraging the considerable preclinical safety data already generated for Lumigan, sticking with the same formulation, and meeting FDA demands with a modestly sized clinical trial, Allergan was able to gain a lucrative indication extension for bimatoprost quickly and cheaply. The excellent fit with the rest of their medical aesthetics business meant Allergan was able to cross-sell using its existing sales force and apply its considerable direct-to-consumer advertising experience and muscle. The credibility that Allergan had already won with Botox in the same target population and with the same physicians facilitated the speedy acceptance of Latisse.

Did Pfizer and Alcon miss opportunities of doing the same with their prostaglandin analogs? Probably not, as they lack the business synergies, experience, infrastructure, and reputation enjoyed by Allergan in the medical aesthetics field and could not have expected to take a significant share of the eyelash market.

A.19   PATENT EXPIRY OF THE BIGGEST DRUG BRAND EVER

Lipitor®

Lipitor is Pfizer's atorvastatin, a statin indicated for the treatment of dyslipidemia and the prevention of cardiovascular disease. It was first approved in the United States in December 1996, at which time it was owned by Warner-Lambert which was subsequently acquired by Pfizer in 2000. Lipitor grew to be the world's best-selling drug ever, with cumulative sales to date of over US$130 billion. Its primary composition-of-matter patent expired on November 30, 2011, and Ranbaxy, the holder of 180-day exclusivity, launched its generic on the same day, just 3 weeks ago as we finalize our book. The Ranbaxy generic is manufactured at their Ohm Laboratories plant in the United States, thus avoiding problems that the company had experienced with the FDA regarding some of their Indian production sites. Other generics will follow in 6 months, once Ranbaxy's 180-day exclusivity expires, and this is bound to cause major revisions in Pfizer's postpatent strategy.

The first elements of the early postpatent strategy for preserving as many Lipitor sales as possible in the United States are starting to become clear, but the reader is encouraged to study the latest developments as what we have written will already have been overtaken by events by the time the book is published.

Pfizer is switching the emphasis of its marketing to pharmacists, payers, and patients. First, patients on Lipitor can obtain a US$4 co-pay card which they present to pharmacists when filling their prescription, and this means they will only have to pay US$4 per prescription out of their own pockets. This so-called "Lipitor for You" program is described in detail on the following website: http://www.lipitor.com/patients/lipitorforyoufaq.aspx.

Second, Pfizer is dropping the price of Lipitor to the level of the first-entry generic for health plans and for pharmacies and pharmaceutical distributors who agree to fill prescriptions with Lipitor instead of with the generic. Investigations are currently underway to decide whether patients will be forced by these agreements to take Lipitor instead of either of the two generics (first filer and authorized).

Third, Pfizer has created an authorized generic which is being marketed by Watson Laboratories.

Estimates in mid-December indicate that branded Lipitor has already lost around half of its U.S. sales volume.

Learnings

Clearly it is too early to talk authoritatively about learnings in this case. One learning, however, is that even mighty Pfizer with its biggest brand has had to accept the reality of basic patent expiry. A second learning is that there is no magic remedy once that event has occurred. Pfizer is falling back on exactly those tactics which are mentioned in our book, and have still lost 50% of their brand sales even before the floodgates open at the end of Ranbaxy's period of exclusivity. And despite this, industry critics are still leaving no stone unturned in their attempts to discover whether Pfizer has contravened any laws in its attempts to get payers to stick with Lipitor through the 180-day exclusivity period.

A.20 EARLY OUT-LICENSING BY BIOTECH: TAKE THE MONEY AND RUN

Macugen®

In December 2001, Pfizer announced that it was paying the U.S. start-up company Eyetech Pharmaceuticals US$100 million now and up to US$645 million later for the rights to Macugen, a potential new treatment for age-related macular degeneration (AMD) and diabetic macular edema (DME), two blinding diseases which had been hitherto very difficult to treat. Macugen (pegaptanib) is a pegylated anti-VEGF aptamer, which inhibits the protein that plays a key role in angiogenesis and increased vessel permeability, two of the primary pathological processes responsible for the vision loss associated with neovascular AMD. At this time, Macugen was in Phase III clinical trials for AMD and Phase II for DME, and excitement was high in the ophthalmologist community. In the Phase II AMD clinical program, it had been demonstrated that 26% of patients showed improved vision after treatment with Macugen, whereas the only medical treatment of the disease so far approved— the photodynamic therapy drug Visudyne® (QLT/Novartis)—was only able to stabilize deteriorating vision for a while, but not to improve it.

"We've never seen visual return before like we're seeing in the preliminary studies," said Dr. Steven D. Schwartz, chief of the retina division at the Jules Stein Eye Institute at the University of California at Los Angeles, who had been a consultant to Eyetech. Results of the Phase III trials were expected by the end of 2002, which would mean that the drug could reach the market by 2004 or 2005.

Up to the Pfizer deal, Eyetech had been supported by private financing rounds totaling approximately US$170 million, consisting of a US$157 million initial public offering and a secondary financing.

The future competition for Macugen did not look very strong when Pfizer made their decision to acquire Macugen. Photodynamic therapy, although capable of slowing disease progression, did not seem to hold the promise of improved vision. Genentech was also testing a VEGF inhibitor, Lucentis® (ranibizumab), in AMD, but the development was lagging behind Eyetech, and Lucentis had to be injected into the eye more frequently than Macugen during a course of treatment. Just before the Pfizer announcement, a press release announced that a drug Lilly was developing for DME had failed in Phase III trials.

But as development progressed, reports started to mount up that Lucentis was unexpectedly proving more effective than Macugen. There was a rational basis for this, as Macugen was an aptamer directed against one specific form of VEGF while Lucentis was a monoclonal antibody fragment that inhibited all VEGF isoforms. In June 2003, Genentech gave the development and marketing rights of Lucentis outside of North America to Novartis, while retaining them in the United States and Canada. Novartis was desperate to salvage its AMD franchise, which was based on Visudyne, now that photodynamic therapy was in danger of being rendered obsolete by the new generation of VEGF inhibitors. Efforts were made to accelerate development and close the gap to Macugen.

Macugen was approved by the FDA in December 2004. In August 2005, OSI Pharmaceuticals announced that it had agreed to buy Eyetech for US$1 billion in a stock plus cash deal, a premium of 43% over Eyetech's share price. European approval of Macugen followed in January 2006.

But there were black clouds gathering on the horizon for Macugen. Ophthalmologists were already aware of the fact that there was a potentially superior drug candidate not far behind Macugen, and many physicians were already involved in Lucentis trials. In addition, physicians had noted that the Lucentis antibody fragment was in reality just part of the Avastin® monoclonal antibody, and first experiments indicated that Avastin might be just as effective against AMD as the far more expensive Macugen and Lucentis. Lucentis was duly approved by the FDA in July 2006 and in Europe in January 2007. As a result of all of these factors, Macugen's first full year of sales, 2006, totaled a very disappointing US$100 miliion, and sales were already in decline by the end of the year following the mid-year launch of Lucentis.

In its Annual Report for 2006, OSI stated that "the most noticeable (of OSI's missteps) has been the very disappointing consequences of the 2005 Eyetech acquisition." The report continued "Our decision to acquire Eyetech was based upon three critical assumptions that have proven to be erroneous— that the off-label use of the more promiscuous anti-VEGF agent, Avastin®, would not gain traction due to safety concerns, that the FDA would curtail the unregulated/unapproved reformulation of the Avastin® anti-cancer formulation for injection in the eye, and that Macugen would have a sustainable niche—based on a preferential safety profile—in the market following the launch of Lucentis, another more promiscuous anti-VEGF agent." None of these critical assumptions proved to be correct. OSI decided to completely exit the eyecare business, writing off the US$650 million that it had invested in the acquisition of Eyetech.

Learnings

Eyetech is a great example of a small company managing the life cycle of a new, high-risk development simply by cashing in early and exiting the development. At the price paid, Pfizer did not benefit from Macugen, but the original owners of Eyetech certainly did. And then they did it again by selling the rest of the company to OSI. With the hurdles getting higher for biotechs to themselves evolve into fully integrated drug companies, and the attraction of being a big drug company in any case waning, more and more biotechs are choosing the strategy of cashing in early on their inventions as large drug companies compete for their favors to replenish their failing in-house pipelines.

A.21   CODEVELOPMENT AND COMARKETING DEALS END IN A MEGAMERGER

Merck and Schering-Plough: Zetia®/Vytorin® and Claritin/Singulair®

This case history contains several interesting examples of LCM of different brands, but it is ultimately the tale of a megamerger.

In March 2009, Merck announced that it had agreed to acquire Schering-Plough in a deal worth US$41.1 billion. The combined company would take the Merck name, and Merck CEO Richard Clark would take the reins. In a teleconference Clark said that the merger "makes great strategic sense." He added that the combined strengths of the companies will "create sustainable growth and meaningful value for shareholders." Schering-Plough Chief Executive Fred Hassan called it "the right transaction at the right time." He said the combined pipeline of the two companies would allow them "many, many shots at the goal," meaning greater chances of success in getting new drugs onto the market. The merger was completed at the end of 2009, creating a new company that was the second biggest drugmaker in the world behind Pfizer.

The seeds of the merger were sown some 10 years earlier in the form of collaboration between the two companies on a series of LCM projects.

In May 2000, Merck and Schering-Plough announced the signing of agreements creating two partnerships to develop and market in the United States new prescription medicines in the therapeutic areas of cholesterol management and respiratory disease. The companies stated that they would jointly pursue the development and marketing of Zetia (ezetimibe), Schering-Plough's investigational cholesterol absorption inhibitor, as monotherapy and also as an FDC with Zocor® (simvastatin), Merck's cholesterol-management block-buster. Furthermore, the companies stated that they would also pursue the development and marketing of an FDC of Claritin (loratadine) and Singulair (montelukast sodium) for the treatment of allergic rhinitis and asthma. The activities under these agreements were to be conducted through two partnerships that would be equally owned and managed by Schering-Plough and

Merck. Schering-Plough and Merck would copromote the new medicines resulting from the partnerships.

Let us look separately at these two FDC projects that, 10 years later, formed part of the rationale for the merger between the two companies.

Zetia/Vytorin

At the time that these agreements were being signed, Merck was already marketing Zocor, an HMG-CoA reductase inhibitor that works by blocking an enzyme that is necessary for the body to make cholesterol. It was a highly successful product, with US$4.4 billion annual sales globally in 2000, which left it a close second in the statin class behind Pfizer's Lipitor. Schering-Plough was in the last stages of the development of Zetia/Ezetrol® (ezetimibe), which reduces blood cholesterol by inhibiting absorption of cholesterol in the small intestine. The FDC of these two agents would thus act to reduce blood cholesterol by two different mechanisms of action, giving it an at least theoretical edge over the other statins on the market, especially the market leading Lipitor.

The first job was to get Zetia approved in the United States, and this was achieved in October 2002. The labeled indications covered both monotherapy and free combination therapy—with statins—of primary hypercholesterolemia. In March 2003, Ezetrol (the brand name of ezetimibe in Europe) completed the Mutual Recognition Procedure in Europe. It was widely acknowledged that Zetia was less powerful than current statins like Zocor, but Schering-Plough was banking on Zetia being capable of boosting the effectiveness of statins and thus reducing the dose that had to be given. This was an important consideration, as in 2002, there were growing concerns that statins could cause muscle weakness, and in extreme cases, even fatal rhabdomyolysis. Just one year earlier Bayer's statin Baycol® had been withdrawn from the market for this very reason. Initially, it certainly seemed that Zetia's novel mechanism of action was winning friends. While AstraZeneca's new statin, Crestor®, only had global sales of US$130 million in 2003, Zetia finished its first full year on the market at US$600 million. There was one hiccough in June 2003 when the Zetia label was modified to include angioedema as a side effect, but no black box warning was required so that Zetia's main selling point, its safety profile, was not impacted too dramatically.

In April 2004, Inegy® (the European brand name of Vytorin) was approved in Germany as the first European country, triggering the start of a Mutual Recognition procedure.

Three months later, in July 2004, Vytorin was approved by the FDA with the following labeled indications (virtually the same as those accepted in Germany):

- as adjunctive therapy to diet, to reduce elevated total-C, LDL-C, Apo B, TG, and non-HDL-C, and to increase HDL-C in patients with primary (heterozygous familial and nonfamilial) hypercholesterolemia or mixed hyperlipidemia, and

- for the reduction of elevated total-C and LDL-C in patients with homozygous familial hypercholesterolemia, as an adjunct to other lipid-lowering treatments (e.g., LDL apheresis) or alone, if such treatments are unavailable.

Four dosages were approved, each containing 10 mg of ezetimibe and the simvastatin doses 10 mg, 20 mg, 40 mg, or 80 mg.

Vytorin had met its goal of gaining approval for first-line therapy of patients with high blood cholesterol. Analysts and physicians were split on whether this was a good or a bad thing. For the supporters, who had largely bought into the concept of Zetia reducing the dose of statin required and thus improving safety, Vytorin represented a better way of dosing patients. Moreover, the timing of the Vytorin launch could not have come at a better time in the United States, as its use was supported by new recommendations to lower LDL down to 70 mg/dL in certain patients. The addition of Zetia enabled Zocor to achieve LDL reductions similar to the more potent statins such as Lipitor and Crestor. This particularly played out with primary care physicians who were focused on meeting LDL targets, while cardiologists were focused on the potential value of other lipid markets such as LDL and triglycerides which came with other statin combinations.

Merck also employed an attractive pricing strategy for Vytorin, essentially throwing the Zocor component in for free, making the cost of Vytorin significantly more attractive than the cost of a free combination of Zetia with an alternative statin. This was the first significant time when a branded company had put together two molecules that both still had patent protection into the same FDC, but still threw in one of the components for free.

But critics were concerned that there were no long-term outcome data available for Zetia, and therefore no certainty that the LDL reduction seen with Vytorin would translate into the same reduction in clinical events that was seen when a more potent statin than Zocor was used alone. The critics argued that Vytorin should not be used as a first-line treatment, and should be reserved only for patients who failed to reach target LDL levels with maximum statin doses, or who were intolerant to such high doses.

From the business perspective, the approvals were very timely for Merck in particular. The basic patent on Zocor was due to expire in June 2006, giving the marketing folk two years to convert physicians and patients from Zocor to Vytorin before generic simvastatin flooded the market. Cannibalization of the Zetia sales by Vytorin was not a major concern for Schering-Plough, as they were already sharing sales of this brand with Merck as part of the partnership agreement. The Zetia patent would not expire until 2017.

In 2005, sales of Zetia and Vytorin exceeded US$2.4 billion, with each product contributing over US$1 billion to the total. Cannibalization of Zetia sales by Vytorin was clearly less than many analysts had expected, as Zetia was also being used in free combination with statins other than Zocor. Zocor sales declined to US$4.4 billion, representing a drop in market share of 3%

between 2004 and 2005, but this was due as much to reduced marketing spend by Merck in anticipation of patent expiry in 2006 as to any cannibalization by Vytorin. The newest statin on the market, Crestor, grew sales to US$1.3 billion in the same year. Clearly, both Zetia and Vytorin were competing effectively in the crowded hypercholesterolemia market.

Merck's basic patent on Zocor duly expired in June 2006, and Ranbaxy Laboratories (at the 80 mg strength) and Teva (all other strengths) were cleared by the FDA to launch generic simvastatin with 180-day exclusivity.

In 2006, Vytorin and Zetia each sold for nearly US$2 billion, considerably softening the blow to Merck of US$1 billion lower sales on Zocor following its genericization. Much of this growth was driven by a TV, print, and radio advertising campaign that cost the joint venture US$128 million, according to data from Nielsen Monitor-Plus. The TV ads illustrated how Vytorin targets two different causes of high cholesterol, "food and family." The narrator explained, "Cholesterol can come from fettuccine Alfredo, but also from your Uncle Alfredo." The ads were voted the fifth-most effective prescription drug commercial by IAG Research, a company that rates effectiveness of TV advertising. Obviously, this advertising also encouraged the use of Zetia in free combination in patients receiving statins other than simvastatin, and thus piggy-backed on the marketing spend of the statins that were still patented, including Crestor and Lipitor.

This happy situation continued through 2007, albeit with a slower growth rate, as Vytorin sales grew to US$2.8 billion and Zetia sales to US$2.4 billion. It seemed that Merck had all but compensated for the negative impact of the patent expiry of Zocor, and that the much smaller Schering-Plough also had two blockbusters on its hands.

But then, in January 2008, the first cloud appeared on the horizon. Disappointing results from a long-awaited trial, the ENHANCE study, indicated not only that Vytorin was no more effective than the now genericized simvastatin in reducing plaque formation in the carotid arteries, but also that the patients receiving Vytorin actually had more plaque formation.

In March 2008, a panel convened by the American College of Cardiology concluded that Vytorin and Zetia should be used only after all other cholesterol-lowering drugs fail until such time as research would prove that the medications work. The panel's spokesman, Harlan Krumholz of Yale University, said "Our strongest recommendation is that people need to go back to statins. If you were put on this drug before you were fully treated on a statin, you should go back."

And then, in November 2009, a small study published in the *NEJM* indicated that even niacin, an old standby in the treatment of hypercholesterolemia, was more effective than Zetia in preventing plaque formation when used in conjunction with statins. This study had been sponsored by Abbott, who marketed niacin under the brand name Niaspan®.

As Merck's and Schering-Plough's woes grew, a class-action lawsuit was brought late in 2009, alleging that the companies had violated consumer protection and other laws in claiming efficacy for Zetia and increased efficacy for Vytorin over and above statins, and particularly generic simvastatin, resulting in consumers and insurers paying too much. This litigation was settled with a US$41.5 million payment.

There was a brief cancer scare regarding Vytorin when one clinical trial found a higher rate of cancer among patients taking the drug than among those taking placebo, but the FDA moved quickly to dispel this fear.

As a result of all of these setbacks, the combined sales of Zetia and Vytorin stopped growing and went into decline, dropping by over US$1 billion between 2007 and 2009.

In March 2010, as at least one health insurer moved to discourage the use of Vytorin and Zetia by doubling its co-pay, Merck announced that the Data Safety Monitoring Board (DSMB) of its IMPROVE-IT study, a 17,000 patient outcomes trial comparing Vytorin® and simvastatin with the number of cardiac events as its end point, had performed a prespecified interim analysis of efficacy data, reviewed safety data, and approved continuing the study. While Merck's confidence in continuing this trial may have impressed some stakeholders that there was still optimism that Vytorin and Zetia could be re-established as a breakthrough in the treatment of hypercholesterolemia, results are not expected before 2013, and even then, the predetermined number of cardiac events may not have been reached, delaying the result still further. By 2013, the patent on Lipitor, the statin class leader, will have been expired for 2 years and the availability of cheap generic atorvastatin will make it even harder for Vytorin and Zetia to relive their past glories, even if the results of IMPROVE-IT are positive. And the basic patent on Zetia, and thus the protection of the FDC Vytorin, is due to expire in 2017.

Claritin/Singulair

The second FDC that was the subject of an agreement between Merck and Schering-Plough in 2000 was that of Claritin with Singulair, two oral drugs used in asthma and allergy.

Claritin (loratadine) was Schering-Plough's second-generation antihistamine indicated for the treatment of seasonal allergic rhinitis, or hay fever. It is described in more detail in Case History 7. Claritin had first been approved by the FDA in 1993, and its patent was due to expire in 2002. Singulair (montelukast) was Merck's leukotriene receptor antagonist used for the prophylaxis and chronic treatment of asthma. It had first been approved by the FDA in 1998, and its patent was due to expire in 2012. The target indications for the FDC announced in 2000 were allergic rhinitis and asthma.

So from the business perspective, this FDC was a neat mirror image of the hypercholesterolemia FDC. This time, it was Merck that possessed the component with the longer patent life and Schering-Plough that was looking for a defense against patent expiry. The big difference was, of course, that the asthma/allergy FDC looked like a much lower risk proposition in that both components had already obtained regulatory approval and were already well established on the market. Unlike in the case of the hypercholesterolemia FDC, where the companies agreed to first codevelop Zetia, this second deal only governed the FDC with Schering-Plough and Merck continuing to market their existing products separately.

In December 2002, Merck obtained FDA approval for Singulair tablets (and chewable tablets) for the relief of symptoms of seasonal allergic rhinitis in children and adults. While some physicians welcomed the addition of prescription Singulair to their arsenal of therapies for treating hay fever, others—and health insurers—pointed out that Singulair's high price (US$80 per month) was unacceptable since Claritin had become available earlier in the year as an OTC drug at only US$16 per month. Other effective alternatives were also available more cheaply than Singulair, such as GSK's Flonase®.

Development of the hay fever combination continued through 2001, but then stalled in 2002 when trials failed to show that the combination pill was any better for hay fever patients than the two pills administered separately. However, the project was resurrected in 2007 when Merck and Schering-Plough announced that the FDC not only provided relief from sneezing, runny nose, and watery eyes, but also relieved nasal congestion. The "consistent and clinically relevant effect on congestion was not demonstrated with the individual components," the companies claimed. Many analysts felt that this was not a very convincing argument in view of the highly competitive and lower-priced market environment. Merck may also have had reservations, as Singulair—where they did not have to share profits with Schering-Plough—already had the hay fever indication as monotherapy.

The combination pill was duly submitted to the FDA, but in April 2009, the companies announced that the agency had issued a "nonapprovable" letter, effectively spelling the end for this hay fever remedy.

Events had in any case now taken a different turn, with Merck announcing its intention of acquiring Schering-Plough in the month before this FDA rejection. The acquisition of Schering-Plough was completed at the end of 2009, and in July 2010, Merck announced its intention of cutting 15,000 jobs, or 15% of its workforce, to deliver the US$3.5 billion in annual cost savings promised to shareholders as part of the deal.

Learnings

First and above all, this case history demonstrates an elegant partnership agreement which certainly appeared back in 2000 to offer a real win-win situation to both partners.

Second, although Vytorin and Zetia may be too expensive and their effects on disease outcomes unknown, the global sales of each product in 2010 again exceeded US$2 billion. This represents a very creditable performance compared to a total global market for statins of US$26 billion. The desire for a drug to reduce the required dosage of statins, the demonstrated effect of ezetimibe in reducing LDL levels as the value of other lipid markers still remains under question, and the effect of the high marketing investments and direct-to-consumer (DTC) advertising, all combined together to outweigh the lack of long-term safety and efficacy data. Physicians, patients and—to a somewhat lesser extent payers—were convinced that Zetia and Vytorin were valuable additions to the drugs available for treating hypercholesterolemia. The "food and family" message for justifying the dual mechanism of action of Zetia with statins has been simple to understand and well communicated.

Third, as if we didn't already know it, developing new products is a risky business. The Claritin + Singulair FDC really did look like a no-brainer, but the shift of the Claritin brand to OTC and the failure to demonstrate any unique advantage of the combination weighed heavily against the product.

A.22   A HUGELY SUCCESSFUL LLCM SWITCH STRATEGY: BUSINESS NEEDS AND REPUTATIONAL ISSUES COLLIDE

Prilosec® and Nexium

There are so many different perspectives that can be taken in considering one of the most successful and controversial examples of LLCM of the last decade. We will look at it from different viewpoints. Because of the massive public attention that the switch of AstraZeneca's focus from Prilosec to Nexium has attracted, this case history contains quotes from different industry stakeholders and observers.

The Facts

Nexium is AstraZeneca's proton pump inhibitor (PPI) esomeprazole. It is the S-enantiomer of the racemic mixture Prilosec which AstraZeneca had launched in 1989. The sales of Prilosec peaked at US$6 billion in 2000, making it one of the all-time best-selling pharmaceutical brands.

Although the Prilosec composition-of-matter patent expired in early 2001 and pediatric exclusivity in October of the same year, AstraZeneca was able to maintain the exclusivity of the brand until early 2003. But by mid-2003, the market was fully genericized and the price per pill had dropped to US$0.70.

At just about the same time as the composition-of-matter patent on Prilosec expired, but before exclusivity was lost and generics appeared on the market, AstraZeneca gained approval for the follow-up product to Prilosec, Nexium, in February 2001, and was able to switch so many patients and physicians to the new brand before the Prilosec generics arrived 2 years later that disaster for their PPI franchise could be averted. Nexium sales peaked in the mid-2000's at over US$5 billion. With only a minor change in the chemical structure of their blockbuster brand, AstraZeneca had been able to preserve almost all of its PPI sales revenue.

At the time of Nexium's approval by the FDA, Prilosec was approved for the following indications:

- Short-term treatment of active duodenal ulcer
- Treatment in combination with clarithromycin and amoxicillin of *Helicobacter pylori* infection and duodenal ulcer
- Short-term treatment of active benign gastric ulcer
- Treatment of heartburn and other symptoms associated with GERD
- Short-term treatment of erosive esophagitis which has been diagnosed by endoscopy
- Maintenance of healing of erosive esophagitis
- Long-term treatment of pathological hypersecretory conditions (e.g., Zollinger–Ellison syndrome, multiple endocrine adenomas, and systemic mastocytosis)

Nexium's approval by the FDA was based on several clinical trials:

1. Nexium versus Prilosec evaluating healing rates of erosive esophagitis (four trials)
2. Nexium versus placebo in long-term maintenance of healing of erosive esophagitis (two trials)
3. Nexium versus placebo in symptomatic GERD (two trials)
4. Comparison of Nexium in combination with different antibiotics in the eradication of *H. pylori* (two trials)

The labeled indications accepted by the FDA for Nexium, based on the above clinical studies, were

- Short-term treatment in the healing and symptomatic resolution of diagnostically confirmed erosive esophagitis
- Maintenance of symptom resolution and healing of erosive esophagitis
- Treatment of heartburn and other symptoms associated with GERD
- Treatment of patients with *H. pylori* infection and duodenal ulcer disease in combination with amoxicillin and clarithromycin
- All four of the clinical trial blocks had been successful in gaining a labeled indication for AstraZeneca's new product.

The Public Reaction

The public reaction to the approval of Nexium was extremely negative. It was considered by many that AstraZeneca had manipulated the system firstly to delay the entry of generic Prilosec, and secondly to introduce a patented successor molecule to the market that offered no real advantages over the genericized product that it was designed (designed being very much the right choice of word) to replace. Consequently, Nexium has been used by critics of the branded drug industry as a prime example of what the public increasingly sees as Big Pharma's attempts to artificially prolong brand life cycles and therefore delay public access to cheaper medication.

There now follow chronological extracts of some of the many articles and books about the Nexium case that have appeared in the public domain.

> **Gardiner Harris, *Wall Street Journal*, June 6, 2002, wrote**: "Beginning its work in 1995, the AstraZeneca team came up with a list of nearly 50 possible solutions to the (Prilosec®) patent-expiration disaster facing the company. Among the best would be finding a new heartburn drug that worked significantly better. Among the worst: launching a successor drug that was virtually no better but had several more years of patent exclusivity. The group also constructed an elaborate legal defense of Prilosec®'s patents. . . . (Several executives on the team) say Nexium® was among the poorest of the many drug solutions they pondered back in 1995—a new medicine that isn't any better for ordinary heartburn than the one it will succeed. . . . The Prilosec® pattern, repeated across the pharmaceutical industry, goes a long way to explain why the nation's prescription-drug bill is rising an estimated 17% a year."

> **Tom Scully, administrator of the Federal Centers for Medicare and Medicaid, stated at a 2003 AMA meeting**: "You should be embarrassed if you prescribe Nexium®" because it increases costs with no medical benefits.

> **Malcolm Gladwell, *New York Times*, October 25, 2004, wrote**: "In the political uproar over prescription-drug costs, Nexium® has become a symbol of everything that is wrong with the pharmaceutical industry. The big drug companies justify the high prices they charge—and the extraordinary profits they enjoy—by arguing that the search for innovative, life-saving medicines is risky and expensive. But Nexium® is little more than a repackaged version of an old medicine. And the hundred and twenty dollars a month that AstraZeneca charges isn't to recoup the costs of risky research and development; the costs were for a series of clinical trials that told us nothing we needed to know, and a half-billion-dollar marketing campaign selling the solution to a problem we'd already solved."

> **Marcia Angell, former editor-in-chief of the *New England Journal of Medicine*, wrote in her 2004 book *The Truth About The Drug Companies: How They Deceive Us and What To Do About It*:** ". . . Four trials compared Nexium® head to head with Prilosec® (for esophageal erosions), and these were crucial to the marketing strategy. The company wanted to show that Nexium® was better than Prilosec®—an advance over the older drug. . . . But, note what AstraZeneca did. Instead of comparing

likely equivalent doses (which would have been no more than 20 and possibly as little as 10 milligrams of Nexium®, versus the standard 20-milligram dose of Prilosec®), the company used higher doses of Nexium®. It compared 20 milligrams and 40 milligrams of Nexium® with 20 milligrams of Prilosec®. With the dice loaded in that way, Nexium® looked like an improvement—but still only marginally so."

Alex Berenson, *New York Times,* **wrote in March 5, 2005**: "Call it the case of the disappearing Prilosec®. For a year, supplies of Prilosec® OTC, a popular heartburn drug sold over the counter, have fallen far short of demand. Procter & Gamble, which markets the drug, first promised that more Prilosec® would be available by December, and then by January…. Procter & Gamble and its partner, AstraZeneca, a British drug company that owns the rights to Prilosec® OTC, say they underestimated demand for the drug and are working to increase production and correct the shortage.

But many Wall Street analysts, consumer advocates and academic researchers who study drug costs discount that explanation and say they believe that AstraZeneca could easily meet demand for the drug if it chose.

The shortage of Prilosec® has been very good for AstraZeneca's bottom line because it has increased sales of Nexium®."

Let us round off this case history by quoting one last figure. According to IMS data, Nexium was the second best-selling drug in the United States in 2010, with sales of US$6.3 billion.

Learnings

It would be perfectly possible to write a whole book on the LCM of the PPI franchise at AstraZeneca. This particular case history deals only with one aspect, the switch from prescription Prilosec to prescription Nexium, and even this involved a whole battery of LLCM strategies including secondary patents, patent defense, indication expansion, OTC switching, pediatric exclusivity, and modified chemistry. Many other strategies were employed during the Prilosec and Nexium life cycles. For example, in April 2010, the FDA approval was obtained for Vimovo®, an FDC of esomeprazole and naproxen. It is labeled primarily for naproxen's indications, that is, for the relief of signs and symptoms of osteoarthritis, RA, and ankylosing spondylitis, and the esomeprazole has been added to decrease the risk of developing gastric ulcers in patients at risk of developing nonsteroidal anti-inflammatory drug (NSAID)-associated gastric ulcers.

One learning from AstraZeneca's efforts to maintain its PPI franchise during the early to mid-2000s is that necessity is the mother of invention. AstraZeneca had seen one new drug after another fail in late-stage development, and it just could not afford to lose the PPI franchise without a fight, using every available weapon. Apart from the company's problems with Iressa (which are discussed in Case History 17), AstraZeneca had lost Exanta® (thrombosis), Galida® (diabetes), Cerovive® (stroke), and AGI-1067 (cardiovascular), all in Phase III, so maintaining existing sources of revenue was essential for the health of the company, perhaps even for its survival as an independent entity.

The reader is invited to play FDA reviewer regarding the results of the key head-to-head clinical trials testing Prilosec and Nexium in erosive esophagitis. They are shown in Tables A.1 and A.2.

We, the authors of this book, certainly do not wish to imply that AstraZeneca did anything they should not have done in moving PPI sales from Prilosec to its active anantiomer Nexium, nor in trying to maintain Prilosec exclusivity until Nexium had been approved and was well established among physicians.

TABLE A.1. Nexium versus Prilosec—Erosive Esophagitis Healing Rate

Study	No. of Patients	Treatment Groups	Week 4	Week 8	Significance Level[a]
1	588	Nexium 20 mg	68.7%	90.6%	N.S.
	588	Prilosec 20 mg	69.5%	88.3%	
2	654	Nexium 40 mg	75.9%	94.1%	$P < 0.001$
	656	Nexium 20 mg	70.5%	89.9%	$P < 0.05$
	650	Prilosec 20 mg	64.7%	86.9%	
3	576	Nexium 40 mg	71.5%	92.2%	N.S.
	572	Prilosec 20 mg	68.6%	89.8%	
4	1216	Nexium 40 mg	81.7%	93.7%	$P < 0.001$
	1209	Prilosec 20 mg	68.7%	84.2%	

[a] Log-rank test versus Prilosec 20 mg.
Source: Nexium Prescribing Information.

TABLE A.2. Nexium versus Prilosec—Sustained Resolution of Heartburn

Study	No. of Patients	Treatment Groups	Day 14	Day 28	Significance Level[a]
1	573	Nexium 20 mg	64.3%	72.7%	N.S.
	555	Prilosec 20 mg	64.1%	70.9%	
2	621	Nexium 40 mg	64.8%	74.2%	$P < 0.001$
	620	Nexium 20 mg	62.9%	70.1%	$P < 0.05$
	626	Prilosec 20 mg	56.5%	66.6%	
3	568	Nexium 40 mg	65.4%	73.9%	N.S.
	551	Prilosec 20 mg	65.5%	73.1%	
4	1187	Nexium 40 mg	67.6%	75.1%	$P < 0.001$
	1188	Prilosec 20 mg	62.5%	70.8%	

[a] Log-rank test versus Prilosec 20 mg.
Source: Nexium Prescribing Information.

The company was extremely clever and innovative in utilizing all possible avenues to maintain Prilosec's exclusivity until Nexium arrived, and then in magnifying the advantages of Nexium over Prilosec and its generics. But this case does serve as perhaps the best example of how such LLCM strategies are being interpreted by the media, and how this is detracting from the public image of the branded drug industry. Anybody involved in LLCM must understand the public environment in which he or she is working and weigh up the financial benefits to the company of certain LLCM strategies compared to the potential damage to the company's (and indeed the branded drug industry's) reputation and public image.

A.23 COMBINING PRODUCTION OUTSOURCING WITH SETTLEMENT WITH A GENERIC COMPETITOR

Nexium

AstraZeneca's huge commercial success in shifting their PPI business from Prilosec to Nexium shortly before the patent expiry of the former—and the public reactions to this LLCM strategy—are dealt with in detail in Case History 22.

A decade later, it was Nexium's turn to approach patent expiry, and several generic companies were circling above like vultures waiting for a dying animal to expire. Again, AstraZeneca's approach to maximizing the remaining brand value is worth looking at in some detail.

The overall position of AstraZeneca regarding its existing products and R&D pipeline was not that much different from the situation they were facing back in the 1990s. The basic patent on Nexium was due to expire in 2014, although this time there was no new GI successor in the pipeline, and therefore no option to transition the franchise to a new brand as had been done in the case of Prilosec and Nexium. AstraZeneca's statin, Crestor, was performing well, and its first patent listed in the Orange Book was not due to expire until 2016, but otherwise, the product portfolio had recently faced or was about to face some major challenges. Arimidex®, for breast cancer, lost market exclusivity in the United States in 2010, and other products to see sharp falls in sales during 2010 as a result of patent expiry were Casodex® for prostate cancer and Pulmicort® for asthma. In addition to Nexium, the multibillion antipsychotic Seroquel® was going to lose patent protection shortly. Regulatory delays in the United States to several products, including the platelet aggregation inhibitor, Brilinta®, the thyroid cancer drug vandetanib, and the FDC of Crestor with Abbott's TriLipix® had further impacted AstraZeneca's short-term outlook, and motavizumab, for the treatment of respiratory syncytial virus infection in infants, had failed in late development.

So once again AstraZeneca was heavily dependent on its ability to defend existing revenue streams, particularly in the short term.

In late 2005, AstraZeneca had received a notice from Ranbaxy that they had submitted an ANDA for Nexium, containing Paragraph IV certifications of invalidity and/or noninfringement with respect to certain AstraZeneca U.S. patents listed in the Orange Book with expiry dates between 2014 and 2019, including the basic patent which was due to expire in 2014. At the same time, Ranbaxy certified with respect to certain other AstraZeneca patents expiring in 2007 that it would not launch its generic prior to expiry of those patents. AstraZeneca commenced a patent infringement lawsuit within 45 days, thus triggering a 30-month stay on the FDA approving Ranbaxy's ANDA before May 2008.

In April 2008, one month before expiry of the 30-month stay, AstraZeneca announced that it had settled its legal battle with Ranbaxy over Nexium. At the time of this settlement, Nexium had annual sales of US$5.5 billion, making it the second most successful U.S. drug behind Lipitor. Under the terms of the out-of-court deal, Ranbaxy agreed to scrap plans to market a generic in the United States until six months before basic patent expiry in May 2014, and AstraZeneca agreed not to oppose this generic launch. As part of the settlement, AstraZeneca also agreed to outsource the production of esomeprazole magnesium, the active substance of Nexium, to Ranbaxy from May 2009 and formulations from May 2010. Ranbaxy also got authorized generic status for another AstraZeneca drug, the calcium-channel blocker Plendil® and for Prilosec 40-mg tablets.

AstraZeneca stated that the deal was in line with its strategy to outsource the manufacture of active pharmaceutical ingredients entirely by 2018. Responding to FTC criticism that such deals are "unconscionable," AstraZeneca CEO Brennan stated that the deal was "in compliance with the Medicare Modernization Act of 2003." Certainly, AstraZeneca had found a way around the highly controversial reverse payment deals that other companies had been using and incurring the wrath of FTC.

Investors in both companies welcomed the deal, which analysts said sharply reduced the uncertainty surrounding a large part of AstraZeneca's revenues. Immediately following the announcement, AstraZeneca's shares rose by 11%, although they lost most of this rise a week later on disappointing first-quarter Nexium sales.

Unfortunately for Ranbaxy, they were having significant issues which prompted the FDA to deny approval of their production site. As of writing, the issues have not yet been resolved, and it is unlikely that Ranbaxy will be able to supply product in the United States before the end of 2011.

AstraZeneca continued Nexium litigation with generic companies in several countries, including the United States and Canada, while also defending attempts to invalidate its patents with the European Patent Office. In the United States, further deals were cut with Teva and with Dr. Reddy's. By the end of 2011 Ranbaxy's generic was already available in Germany, Spain, and the United Kingdom.

Learnings

While generic companies often state in public that it is their mission to bring cheaper drugs to patients as early as possible, they are often more than willing to enter into settlement agreements with innovators that keep the original drug's premium pricing for as long as possible, provided that the innovator hands over more of this profit to the generic company than they would make by launching a generic. Straight cash deals have come under increasing pressure, and will continue to do so, and it is therefore prudent to find less blatantly obvious methods than "pay-for-delay" deals to ensure that profits are shared between the innovator and the generic company. This AstraZeneca/Ranbaxy deal was one such option.

The outsourcing element of this deal significantly reduced AstraZeneca's production costs, as it is much cheaper to manufacture in India than in the United States or Europe. This benefited AstraZeneca, while Ranbaxy gained additional Nexium manufacturing know-how and capability from AstraZeneca, and was able to ramp up high volume production ahead of U.S. patent expiry in 2014.

A.24   REFORMULATING FOR SUCCESS IN OSTEOPOROSIS

Osteoporosis Drugs: Fosamax, Actonel®, Boniva®, and Aclasta®

Fosamax is Merck's alendronate, Actonel is P&G's and Sanofi-Aventis's risedronate, Boniva is Roche's ibandronate, and Aclasta is Novartis's zoledronate. All are bisphosphonates.

The osteoporosis market is a classic example of a competitive landscape that has been extensively shaped by the power of reformulation. Merck's Fosamax essentially created the market for osteoporosis, launching as a once-daily tablet in 1993 and establishing itself as the brand to beat. The next major class member to take on Fosamax was P&G's Actonel, sold as Optinate® by Sanofi-Aventis outside of the United States, which was first approved for Paget's disease in 1998, and later approved for osteoporosis as a once-daily tablet in 2000.

By this time, with a 6-year head start, Fosamax was already well placed to maintain a market leadership position despite the challenge from Actonel. However, Merck recognized a key unmet need in the market. Based on the GI tolerability profile of the bisphosphonate class, oral formulations had to be taken first thing in the morning before food, and the patients had to stand for at least 30 min after taking the drug. With many osteoporotic patients finding this dosing regimen difficult to manage, there was a critical need to somehow ease the burden.

Merck's approach to meeting this unmet need was not to reduce the side effects, or to eliminate the troublesome dosing ritual, but simply to make patients have to dose less frequently. Merck had found that by increasing the dose sevenfold, the drug could be dosed once weekly with the same overall efficacy as the once-daily drug. Merck therefore launched Fosamax once weekly in mid 2000, at almost the same time that once-daily Actonel gained its approval for osteoporosis.

Fosamax once weekly was a breakaway success, taking more than 80% of franchise sales within the first 2 years and more than doubling the quarter-on-quarter growth rates in both the United States and Europe in the 12 months following launch. In addition to driving franchise growth, the differentiation provided by the once-weekly formulation firmly positioned Actonel as a second-line therapy.

The launch of Fosamax once weekly was a potential disaster for P&G and Sanofi. As such, the development of a similar formulation was prioritized, with again the same sevenfold dosing approach taken to develop Actonel once weekly, and this formulation finally gained approval in the United States in mid-2002. The launch of once-weekly Actonel provided a strong boost to the franchise, even though the impact on Fosamax's continued dominance of first line was still limited.

For the next couple of years, all was quiet on the competitive front, with once-weekly dosing established as the standard of care. Roche gained approval for once-daily Boniva in mid-2003, but did not even bother to launch the drug, as its competitive profile would not be worth the launch investment. Instead, Roche set about developing a more competitive formulation for the real launch, this time choosing to go beyond the current standard of care, and release a once-monthly oral formulation. Positioned as the most convenient oral option available, Boniva once-monthly hit the market in 2005, and its impact was striking. While Fosamax's sales continued to grow as before, the growth of Actonel was completely stunted. Why would patients want a second-line once-weekly therapy when they could get a second-line once-monthly? Roche had essentially taken a drug with a me-too clinical profile and turned it into an almost US$500 million a year brand, by ensuring that its overall brand profile brought innovation and not just equality to the table.

P&G did respond again for Actonel, developing their "2CD" once-monthly formulation (although actually two doses on two consecutive days, once a month), but again they were more than 3 years behind the competition, this time Boniva. Actonel's strategy throughout its development had been more focused on responding to other competitors than on innovating. This may have been a low-risk strategy, but it was never one destined to drive market leadership. That being said, a low-risk strategy that delivers peak sales of close to US$2 billion cannot really be described as a failure!

While the once-monthly formulations remain to this day the most convenient oral formulations, these were not the end of the formulation story in osteoporosis. Shortly after launching the once-monthly oral formulation, Roche and GSK launched the once quarterly IV push injection formulation of Boniva (a 15-second injection, given once every 3 months). This formulation was targeted to patients who still could not tolerate oral therapies, thus giving Boniva complete coverage of all patients that failed on first-line once-weekly therapy. While most certainly not the dominant part of the franchise (U.S. sales of the intravenous formulation account for less than 15% of total Boniva sales), the launch provided two key advantages to Roche/GSK. First, it gave access to patients currently unavailable to the franchise, the oral intolerants, and second, it allowed the companies to effectively position intravenous therapies as only for oral failures, which would prove very useful in the coming years.

Continuing to stretch the boundaries of dosing, Novartis was next to play in the osteoporosis space. They launched Aclasta, a reformulation of the already successful IV therapy Zometa® which dominates the hypercalcemia market for bisphosphonates, as a once-yearly infusion for the treatment of osteoporosis in 2007. As a once-yearly therapy, Aclasta could provide the guaranteed compliance that was such a key issue with oral therapies, while also offering the best clinical fracture reduction data seen to date. Given these very positive factors, some would say Aclasta should have been an easy win. However, while on paper the proposition sounded good, in the real world, the logistical challenges of a 15-min infusion versus a once-a-week or once-a-month tablet were extremely difficult to overcome. Roche and GSK had already established IV dosing as only relevant to patients who could not tolerate oral therapies, and breakout out of this usage environment continues to be a key challenge for Aclasta.

So what is next? Once every 5 years? A once-in-a-lifetime vaccine? Novartis has already gained approval in the United States for once every-two-year dosing for Aclasta in the prevention of postmenopausal osteoporosis. The question now becomes, in the real world, what is the best combination of dosing schedule and route of administration? Even with all the advancements, the real answer is probably that once weekly is still hard to beat.

Learnings

In the early stages of this case history, Merck took significant investment risks in pushing the boundaries of osteoporosis therapy by moving from daily to weekly dosing. P&G were more cautious, taking the role of a follower. Merck reaped the rewards that their approach deserved, but P&G also showed that being a follower and lowering risk can still prove to be a successful strategy, as annual sales of the Actonel franchise peaked at over US$2 billion. That is a pretty impressive return for a conservative approach! Bonviva's particular success was in bringing the new once monthly formulation to market rather than simply copying the once weekly, and then using the once quarterly IV to strategically position the IV route of administration ahead of Aclasta. With Aclasta, Novartis has further increased the interval between doses, but the jury is out on whether this approach is really meeting an unmet need. Despite all of the advances made, for the majority of patients, once-weekly dosing is still hard to beat.

Other aspects of Fosamax LCM are described in Case History 14.

A.25 ISOMERISM, POLYMORPHISM, AND SETTLEMENTS

Plavix®

Plavix (clopidogrel sulfate) is Sanofi-Aventis/BMS's P2Y12 inhibitor for preventing blood clot formation in coronary artery disease, peripheral vascular disease, and cerebrovascular disease. Global sales in 2010 were US$8.6 billion, making Plavix the second best-selling drug in the world behind Lipitor. Plavix was approved in the United States in 1997, and its composition-of-matter patent was due to expire in 2011, with pediatric exclusivity extending protection until 2012. Sanofi-Aventis markets the drug in Europe and BMS, the inventor, in the United States.

The composition-of-matter patent protects the enantiomer of clopidogrel sulfate, and provides an extra 8 years of protection beyond the expiry of the patent on the original racemic mixture.

Based on obviousness, Apotex attempted to invalidate the patent covering the enantiomer, making a Paragraph IV submission and triggering a 30-month stay in early 2004. A few months before the end of this stay, scheduled for August 2006, Sanofi-Aventis and BMS entered negotiations with Apotex to prevent launch of the Apotex generic. An agreement was proposed which would have resulted in Apotex not launching its generic until shortly before patent expiry in 2011. But the FTC rejected this proposed settlement. At this time, BMS was already operating under the terms of a deferred-prosecution agreement following a 3-year investigation into a US$2.5 billion scandal at the company involving "channel stuffing" to meet quarterly sales targets. A federal judge monitoring BMS under the deferred-prosecution agreement reported that the attempted settlement violated the terms of that agreement and recommended that the BMS CEO, Peter Dolan, be fired or BMS would have to face charges. BMS duly terminated Mr. Dolan.

With the proposed settlement now defunct, Apotex launched generic clopidogrel at risk in August 2006 following expiry of the 30-month stay.

But 1 month after the launch of the Apotex generic, a district court granted BMS a preliminary injunction ordering Apotex to stop sales of its generic; however, it did not order Apotex to recall products already sold or shipped.

In its annual report for 2006, BMS stated that the action by Apotex had caused a reduction in the sales of Plavix in 2006 by between US$1.2 billion and US$1.4 billion, an overall 15% decline in Plavix sales for the year.

The litigation continued, and in December 2008, the Federal Circuit finally determined that, although the racemate was in the prior art, the dextrorotatory enantiomer and bisulfate salt were not described "either explicitly or inherently, in any reference," and that the earlier patent would not have guided a person of ordinary skill in the art to either the dextrorotatory enantiomer or its bisulfate salt. Furthermore, the unexpected and unusual properties of the dextrorotatory enantiomer, and the resulting therapeutic benefits, added to the claim of nonobviousness. Finally, in November 2009, the Supreme Court rejected Apotex's appeal of the Federal Circuit decision. This was an important decision, coming as it did after the KSR versus Teleflex ruling, because it confirmed that a patent can still be granted based on the results of drug testing even if trying the experiment itself was an obvious thing to do.

Interestingly, Kroger Inc. and other drug retailers including Walgreen and CVS filed an antitrust lawsuit against BMS and Sanofi-Aventis in 2006, claiming that the proposed settlement between the drugmakers in 2006 had deprived pharmacies of inexpensive, generic copies of Plavix.

BMS and Sanofi-Aventis countered by pointing out that the proposed settlement never took place, and that Apotex had made generic clopidogrel available in 2006. The district court agreed with the brand companies and finally dismissed the retailers' case in March 2010.

Plavix also had its problems in Europe. In 2008, Cimex, a small Swiss generic company, received German approval to market a generic version of Plavix using the besylate salt instead of the sulfate. Cimex's marketing partners were named as Sandoz and Ratiopharm. Sanofi-Aventis filed legal action against the generic version, emphasizing that its European patent on Plavix did not expire until 2013. Cimex had already announced that it would not be attempting to enter the U.S. market because of differences in the clopidogrel patent on the two continents.

By January 2009, the Cimex generic had captured 25% of the German clopidogrel market.

In May 2009, European approval was granted to the Cimex (since renamed Acino) generic, marketed by Ratiopharm and Hexal (Novartis), and also to further generics. Teva obtained approval for "clopidogrel base," and not a salt such as the sulfate or besylate, stabilized using butylated hydroxyanisole (BHA).

In October 2009, Sanofi-Aventis announced plans to launch its own Plavix generic in Europe, to retain at least some market share in face of the cut-price competition.

In March 2010, the European authorities recommended a recall of all Acino clopidogrel manufactured by the Indian company Glochem after regulatory inspection of one of Glochem's production sites revealed deviations from Good Manufacturing Practice (GMP). Sanofi-Aventis immediately issued a statement that they manufactured all clopidogrel-containing products for the European markets in the EU in full compliance with the relevant rules and regulations in force, including GMP.

Learnings

This case of obviousness in the United States was finally resolved after the landmark KSR versus Teleflex ruling, and was decided in favor of the innovator and against the generic company. The higher obviousness hurdle does make it more difficult to obtain effective patent protection for new molecules which are close in structure to those of existing products, but it is still possible if there is truly an innovative step which was not obvious based on prior art.

The European situation provides an example of a generic company tweaking a molecule to circumvent a patent rather than the innovator using the same strategy to provide new patent protection for an existing therapeutic franchise.

A.26 PAYERS VERSUS BRAND FOR PATIENT SELECTION

Plavix and Brilinta

Following its approval over a decade ago, Plavix has become the gold standard for the treatment of acute coronary syndromes (ACS) and has been the only antiplatelet agent available for this indication until the recent approvals of Eli Lilly/Daiichi Sankyo's Effient® (prasugrel) and AstraZeneca's Brilinta (ticagrelor). Despite the widespread use of Plavix, it suffers from a serious drawback—it is a prodrug that needs to be activated by the cytochrome P450 (CYP) enzymes in the liver (especially the CYP2C19) to its active form. Plavix is believed to be ineffective in up to 14% of patients (depending on the patient's ethnicity), known as "poor metabolizers." Poor metabolizers suffer from genetic variability, leaving them unable to effectively activate Plavix to carry out its antiplatelet effect.

In March 2010, the FDA added a boxed-warning to Plavix to warn these patients, who are unable to receive the full benefits of Plavix.

The FDA has recommended the use of genetic tests to identify poor metabolizers and has advised health-care professionals to consider using other antiplatelet agents or using alternative (higher) doses of Plavix on these patients to mitigate the risk of the reduced antiplatelet effect. Despite the advice by organizations like the FDA, American College of Cardiology (ACC), and American Heart Association (AHA) to carry out the genetic tests for nonresponsiveness to Plavix, they have not been readily available in the United States or in the rest of the world.

The treatment of ACS is expected to dramatically change following the approval of Brilinta and Effient since interventionists and cardiologists will now have a choice of three antiplatelet agents to select from when treating their ACS patients. Beyond reducing the incidence of composite CV death, myocardial infarction (MI), or stroke compared to Plavix, Brilinta does not need to be activated and works on patients regardless of whether they suffer from the genetic variability that makes Plavix ineffective. Brilinta's greater efficacy over Plavix comes at the price of a slight increase in the incidence of major bleeding.

In addition to the launch of new antiplatelet agents, Plavix's impending patent expiry will also change the antiplatelet agent landscape as the introduction of generic clopidogrel will reduce the patient potential for all branded antiplatelet agents due to cost-saving pressures exerted by payers. Medco, a leading pharmacy benefit manager (PBM) in the United States, announced in 2010 that it would launch a program to offer genetic tests and genetic counseling to over 10 million patients enrolled with them following a successful pilot program offering genetic tests to patients prescribed the blood-thinning agent, warfarin. As part of their continuous efforts to improve health and lower the costs of care, Medco announced CYP2C19 testing for Plavix patients whose employer or health plans have enrolled their members in the Medco personalized medicine program, at no cost to eligible members or their physicians. Medco has borne the cost of administering these genetic tests itself in an effort to convince payers (insurers) to enrol their insured members with them instead of other PBMs. Medco's value proposition to the insurers is the potential for cost savings it can help to establish using this patient genotypic selection approach.

By promoting testing, Medco can specifically identify those patients who will not respond to Plavix, creating a market for Effient and Brilinta, but in the process, increasing the value of Plavix in the remaining population. It is this broader target population that will likely form the primary competition between brands moving forward. On the one side, the payers would like all of these patients to use cheaper generic clopidogrel. By contrast, the branded players want to demonstrate that their drugs are better than Plavix even in these patients, thus driving much broader uptake. This is where the greatest clash in patient selection approach will likely occur. AstraZeneca, for example, will want to proactively identify patients where Brilinta performs well and drive use in these populations (irrespective of CYP status), while payers such as Medco will want to identify where older drugs perform badly, and restrict Brilinta use to these patients.

In a rare, but aggressive move, Medco decided in 2009 to take the matter into its own hands. Medco announced that it was planning a comparative effectiveness study of Plavix and Effient to examine whether the 70–75% of patients who are "extensive metabolizers" of Plavix will have "comparable outcomes" with patients taking Effient. The 14,000 patient study was launched as part of Medco's Genetics for Generics project, which has the goal of optimizing savings for payers by dispensing off-patent drugs with the aid of genetic tests. According to Medco's Chief Medical Officer Robert Epstein, the goal of the Genetics for Generics program is to "beef up the profile of a generic drug and make it even smarter." In the case of Plavix, the goal will be to counter claims by other branded players that there is no need to test for poor metabolisers as all patients would benefit from their newer drug.

Learnings

BMS and Sanofi-Aventis have grown the Plavix franchise globally through successful LCM strategies. The latest LCM strategy they adopted was conducting the CURRENT-OASIS 7 trial to support doubling the dose of Plavix on

ACS patients undergoing planned percutaneous coronary intervention (PCI). Despite these successes, the advent of Effient and Brilinta together with Plavix's loss of exclusivity will change the ACS treatment dynamics since interventionists and cardiologists will have a choice in prescribing between brands and generics.

The LCM tactic of patient selection—in this case genotypic—will play a critical role in the success of new antiplatelet agents like Brilinta which will compete against the blockbuster incumbent, Plavix. What this case study illustrates, however, is that the decision of which patient selection approach should be taken is not solely the choice of the branded players. Payer groups and other interested stakeholders have a vested interest in ensuring generics are used where possible, and the Medco study highlights the extents to which they will go in the future to ensure branded companies do not have a monopoly on pharmacoeconomic data. The learnings for the brand drug industry are twofold; first, just because a company itself chooses not to develop a patient selection process does not mean someone else will not. In the end it is better to be proactive rather than reactive. Second, once a selection process has been agreed and studies started, this is not the point to sit back and relax. Understanding how studies will be interpreted and how competitor approaches will be considered is critical to ensure stakeholder opinion can be proactively shaped to drive positive uptake.

A.27   LITIGATION CAN DELAY GENERIC ENTRY IN THE OTC FIELD TOO

Prilosec OTC

The switch of AstraZeneca's Prilosec (omeprazole) from prescription to OTC status was approved by the FDA in June 2003. This was just one additional component of the overall LCM of Prilosec/Nexium as described in Case History 22. Prilosec OTC was the first PPI and the first treatment of frequent heartburn to be made available without prescription in the United States. P&G acquired the rights to market the drug from AstraZeneca, agreeing to pay the company a royalty on sales. Because of the safety studies performed by the manufacturer, the product was granted 3 years of exclusivity. Prilosec OTC was protected by two patents listed in the Orange Book, the so-called "960" and "424" patents, which are due to expire in 2014 and 2016, respectively.

In March, 2007, Dr. Reddy's filed an ANDA with Paragraph IV certification, and AstraZeneca filed suit alleging infringement of both patents. The patents claim omeprazole formulations comprising a magnesium salt "having more than 70% crystallinity," and related processes of manufacture. In reply, Dr. Reddy's claimed that their product did not infringe either patent, and produced test results supporting the claim. The district court ordered Dr. Reddy's to provide test samples of their product to AstraZeneca, and ordered AstraZeneca to test them. The results confirmed Dr. Reddy's claims; the samples were less than 1% crystalline; in other words, they were to all intents and purposes amorphous and therefore did not infringe the patents. Accordingly, Dr. Reddy's moved for summary judgment on the grounds of noninfringement.

But AstraZeneca refused to give up. They argued that further evidence would be necessary to persuade them to drop the suit against Dr. Reddy's. Specifically, they alleged that Dr. Reddy's might be manufacturing a crystalline form and then converting it into an amorphous form, which would infringe the patents. The court allowed limited discovery, ordering Dr. Reddy's to produce sections of their ANDA and Drug Master File (DMF), plus a witness with experience of Dr. Reddy's manufacturing process. Based on this documentation and the evidence provided, AstraZeneca was still unable to provide any evidence to the court that would persuade them that Dr. Reddy's process infringed their patents. Still AstraZeneca pressed on, requesting a decision by the district court judge as to the meaning of a phrase "by the addition of water" used in Dr. Reddy's manufacturing process.

In March 2009, the district court finally ruled that there was "no evidence whatever that Dr. Reddy's makes use of a salt with the requisite degree of crystallinity." Later in the year, the Federal Circuit affirmed the district court ruling.

In March 2010, the district court granted Dr. Reddy's motion that AstraZeneca should pay their attorney's fees. The court concluded that "an inference of bad faith exists when a patentee is manifestly unreasonable in assessing infringement, while continuing to assert infringement in court." It therefore ruled that AstraZeneca had an obligation not to file a lawsuit unless it had evidence that Dr. Reddy's was infringing their patents.

AstraZeneca had argued that their behavior was acceptable as a lot of money was at risk. The court reacted very negatively to this assertion. It concluded that this was a ridiculous claim to make, and that AstraZeneca was not free to throw up roadblocks or to assert a claim construction in bad faith—to abuse the court system—just because it was to AstraZeneca's economic advantage to keep a potential competitor off the market. The court found AstraZeneca's behavior to have been "unreasonable, frivolous, anti-competitive and anti-consumer." Accordingly, in April 2010, the court ordered AstraZeneca to pay the attorney's fees.

Learnings

While frivolous litigation can still delay the entry of generics to the market, courts everywhere are losing patience with what is increasingly perceived as a manipulation of the legal system. Brand companies are going to have to become a lot more sophisticated going forward if they want to continue to pursue this dubious LLCM strategy.

A.28 INCONSISTENT COURT DECISIONS CAN HURT BOTH BRAND AND GENERIC COMPANIES

Protonix®

Protonix is Pfizer's (formerly Wyeth's and originally Altana's) PPI pantoprazole sodium indicated for the short-term treatment of erosion and ulceration of the esophagus caused by GERD. It was first approved by the FDA in 2000 as a delayed-release tablet, and then as an injectable in 2001. Protonix sales in the United States for the 12-month period from Q3/2006 to Q3/2007 amounted to US$2.5 billion.

The Protonix story started in the research labs of the German company Altana. Following the success of AstraZeneca's Prilosec, Altana had filed a patent on 18 PPIs (No. 4,555,518, the "518" patent). Although the "518" patent did not disclose pantoprazole itself, one of the claimed compounds was very similar to pantoprazole. Altana subsequently filed a new patent application claiming pantoprazole, and this application was issued in February 1988 (No. 4,758,579, the "579" patent). The Patent Office also granted a 5-year term extension pursuant to the Hatch–Waxman Act, and thus the "579" patent, the composition-of-matter patent on pantoprazole, was due to expire in July 2010 (without pediatric exclusivity).

In early 2004, Teva filed an ANDA with the FDA requesting approval to market a generic version of Protonix. Sun followed with its own ANDA application in 2005. Both generic companies filed Paragraph IV certifications in conjunction with their respective ANDAs, and Altana accordingly filed suit against both parties. As the end of the 30-month stay approached, in mid-2007, Altana filed a motion for preliminary injunction. In response, Teva and Sun both agreed that they had infringed the "579" patent, which Wyeth had licensed exclusively from Nycomed (the new owners of Altana), but claimed that it was invalid because of obviousness. The district court found that a person skilled in the art would have selected the compound similar to pantoprazole in the "518" patent as a lead compound for modification, and also determined that additional references that Teva and Sun had made available to the court provided both the motivation to modify this compound, and the teaching that such a substitution was feasible. Moreover, the district court rejected Altana's position that allowing generic entry into the market would cause irreparable harm. Based on all of this reasoning, the district court accordingly denied Altana's motion for preliminary injunction.

Following the denial of the preliminary injunction, Teva accelerated launch preparations for its generic product, which had already been granted final approval and 180-day coexclusivity with Sun in August 2007, and announced its launch in December of the same year. At the same time, however, Teva also announced that it had entered into settlement discussions with Wyeth/Altana and as part of these negotiations agreed to a standstill agreement pursuant to which Teva agreed not to ship additional product for a period of 30 days. Negotiations evidently broke down, and in January 2008, Wyeth announced that it was launching its own authorized generic through a distribution agreement with Prasco Laboratories, just after Sun announced the launch of its generic. The relaunch of Teva's generic quickly followed, with Teva claiming that Wyeth had broken the truce by launching its own generic.

In their 2008 Annual Report, Wyeth announced that they had "initiated Project Impact, a company-wide program designed to initially address short-term fiscal challenges, particularly the significant loss of sales and profits resulting from the launch of generic versions of Protonix®." The impact of these generic launches on Wyeth was indeed immense, with 80% of branded Protonix sales lost in 2008.

One year after the launch of the Protonix generics, in January 2009, Pfizer announced its takeover of Wyeth. A little over a year on, in April 2010, the jury in the U.S. District Court of New Jersey ruled that the U.S. patent of Protonix held by Nycomed (who had in the meantime acquired Altana) is valid. In July, Judge Jose L. Linares confirmed the jury verdict.

Nycomed immediately stated that together with Pfizer it would seek for damage claims. "Of course, the verdict can be potentially appealed, but this is a great breakthrough for us," said a Nycomed spokeswoman, declining to say how much the company would ask for damage claims. Teva said it planned to pursue all available legal remedies in the case, including appeals. Sun also stated that it still believed the Protonix patent to be invalid and unenforceable, and that it would pursue all available legal action.

The potential damage claims could amount to as much as US$1–2 billion as a result of this verdict and the steep sales decline in brand sales after generic entry to the market. Coming shortly after Teva lost another composition-of-matter patent suit to Novartis over Famvir, this might persuade Teva and other generic companies to reconsider their strategy regarding the at-risk launch of generics of patented drugs, and this would be of huge benefit to the branded drug industry in general.

Finally, in July 2010, New Jersey District Court confirmed the jury verdict in favor of Nycomed, confirming the patent validity and rejecting allegations that the patent was invalid either as obvious or for reasons of double patenting.

Learnings

This case is a good example of how the unpredictable and fluctuating court interpretations of obviousness of patent claims can hurt both innovator and generic company. Following the initial court decision not to block the Teva generic, the at-risk launch of this product and of Wyeth's authorized generic marked the end of Protonix as a significant brand. The later reversal of the decision by a higher court could ultimately cost Teva as much as US$2 billion in damages.

The positive outcome of the litigation from the perspective of the innovator does not help either of the brand companies initially involved in the case,

Wyeth and Altana. During the 6 years that the case dragged on, both companies ceased to exist as independent entities.

A.29 HOLDING ON TO AN ANTIPSYCHOTIC FRANCHISE

Risperdal®/Invega®

Risperdal (risperidone) is J&J's second-generation atypical antipsychotic, indicated for the treatment of the manifestations of psychic disorders, including schizophrenia. It was first approved by the FDA in 1993, and its basic patent expired in December 2007 (2005 in Spain). Initially, Risperdal was made available as color-coded oral tablets ranging in strength from 0.5 mg to 4 mg, and as a 1 mg/mL oral solution. In April 2003, the FDA granted approval for oral disintegrating tablets, Risperdal M-tabs, of 0.5, 1, and 2 mg. Then, in August 2002 (Europe) and October 2003 (United States), approval was granted for Risperdal Consta, a long-acting intramuscular injection with strengths of 25 mg–50 mg supplied in a prefilled syringe and injected every 2 weeks (a 12.5-mg strength was added in 2007). Risperdal Consta was developed using Alkermes's proprietary Medisorb® technology and had the strong advantage of overcoming patient compliance issues inherent in daily oral dosing of patients with psychic disorders.

But already now the battle lines were being drawn for the upcoming patent expiries. In December 2003, Mylan and Dr. Reddy's submitted ANDAs with Paragraph IV certification against the Risperdal patents, triggering a 30-month stay until May 2006, 18 months before basic patent expiry. In October 2006, the District Court of New Jersey ruled that the Risperdal patent was valid, enforceable, and infringed by the Mylan and Dr. Reddy's generics and entered an injunction prohibiting the sale of generic risperidone until after patent expiry. And in 2006, J&J gained approval for the indication of irritability in children with autism, which gave them 6 months of pediatric exclusivity and extended protection against generics of Risperdal until May 2008.

Generic oral risperidone duly entered the U.S. market in mid-2008, reducing 2008 sales of oral Risperdal by 38% compared to 2007. Sales of Risperdal Consta, without generic competition, grew by 16% during the same period. Total sales of the Risperdal franchise dropped from US$4.2 billion in 2006 to US$3.4 billion in 2008. A year later, sales of oral Risperdal had dropped another 60% while Risperdal Consta grew by 9%. But the total vaue of the franchise had fallen to US$2.3 million, over half of which was now Risperdal Consta for which there was no generic competition.

While it had been extending and defending its Risperdal franchise, J&J had also been developing a successor. Invega (paliperidone) extended-release (once-daily) tablets were approved by the FDA in April 2006. Invega utilized the Oros® extended-release technology of Alza, a J&J subsidiary. Invega Sustenna, a long-acting intramuscular injection, was approved in July 2009.

Paliperidone is the active metabolite of risperidone rather than a truly new active substance.

Invega's once-daily oral formulation was expected to improve compliance over twice-daily Risperdal/generic risperidone, and it possesses a slightly better side-effect profile, but risperidone has a faster onset of action and comparable efficacy, and the generic is much, much cheaper. Recognizing the modest advantage of their new drug over the old, J&J priced Invega slightly lower than Risperdal in order to encourage psychiatrists to switch patients to the new drug. Invega Sustenna has a bigger advantage over Risperdal Consta, as it only needs to be injected every 4 weeks instead of 2, and there are no Risperdal Consta generics available. Invega Sustenna has the additional selling points of a ready-to-use formulation, no refrigerated storage, and the use of standard needles.

In light of these factors, J&J is actively switching patients from Risperdal Consta, resulting in a decline in revenues of the older product as Invega Sustenna gains market share. Although Risperdal Consta has market exclusivity in the United States until mid-2012, and 25 patents are listed in the Orange Book with expiry dates from 2013–2020, J&J has clearly transferred its loyalties to Invega Sustenna. In August 2009, J&J stopped a project with Alkermes to develop a monthly Risperdal injection, a move that sent Alkermes's shares down by 9%. So while J&J seems to have lost the oral market to generic risperidone, it may well be successful in switching injections from a dependency on risperidone to Invega Sustenna.

Learnings

Was J&J's management of its schizophrenia franchise a success or not? There were good and bad elements. The move from oral Risperdal to intramuscular Risperdal Consta was managed well, and around half of the franchise sales survived the expiry of the basic risperidone patent, thanks to J&J's success in switching physicians and patients to the patented intramuscular formulation. Invega oral was not a success, but Invega Sustenna was.

Oral Invega was just not differentiated enough from oral Risperdal to stand a realistic chance of success once generic resperidone became available. The attraction of once-daily dosing instead of twice-daily could not compensate for the huge price differential between brand and generic, a message that we have repeated several times in this book.

Invega Sustenna's superior dosing schedule and the fact that no intramuscular generics were available should enable J&J to move a large part of their Risperdal Consta sales to Invega Sustenna, which also has a longer patent life and where J&J does not have to share its profits with Alkermes. The bottom line? J&J's schizophrenia franchise was worth US$4.7 million in 2007. They will have done well if they can hang on to a third of these sales in the mid-term.

A.30   LCM CREATES AN ALMOST IMMORTAL BRAND

Voltaren®

Novartis gained the first approval for its NSAID, diclofenac, in 1974, under the brand name Voltaren. The basic patent expired in 1985, yet in 2010, annual global brand sales of the Voltaren franchise, including the OTC range, is still believed to have exceeded US$1 billion.

This success was made possible by a broadly based LCM strategy which has been sustained for more than 30 years. Many different LCM measures were implemented at different points during this long life cycle.

Voltaren is marketed in a wide range of oral formulations, including enteric-coated tablets, slow-release tablets and capsules, film-coated tablets, hard-gelatin capsules, suspensions, granules, dispersible tablets, and powder. While the active substance of Voltaren is diclofenac sodium, some of the administration forms are branded as Cataflam® and contain the potassium salt instead. Cataflam was claimed to have a faster onset of action, and is positioned for acute disease in markets where both brands are available.

In addition to these oral administration forms, Voltaren is also available as injectable solutions, topical gels, suppositories, and eye drops. In India it is marketed in a base containing capsaicin as Voveran® Thermagel. (Voveran is the Indian brand name for Voltaren, and it is called Voltarol® in the United Kingdom).

In some markets, it is sold as an FDC with cholestyramine (Flotac®, available in various South American countries), with a broad range of pain indications, or with codeine (Combaren®, available in some European countries), for the treatment of cancer pain.

Voltaren is marketed in more than 120 countries, but no two markets have exactly the same product range, and the individual formulations are often positioned differently according to local needs and regulatory factors.

Different dosage strengths are offered depending on indication and disease severity. Tablets, for example, are available at 25 mg, 37.5 mg, 50 mg, 75 mg, and 100 mg, while suppositories are available at 12.5 mg, 25 mg, and 100 mg.

Voltaren is also available OTC in some markets, for example, as topical Voltaren Emugel globally, and as Voltaren Thermagel in India, and as a low-dose (12.5 mg) tablet.

Voltaren is indicated for the treatment of pain, and depending on the market and presentation form has labeling for osteoarthritis, RA, ankylosing spondylitis, menstrual pain, gout, muscle and tendon pain, sprains, rheumatism, tumor pain, postoperative pain, pain after cataract surgery, and even "pain due to other causes."

Today, Voltaren sales are particularly strong in self-pay markets, because brand loyalty is a far more important factor there than in countries where third-party payers are likely to insist on generic diclofenac. Thus, India, Brazil, and Mexico are among the biggest markets for Voltaren. In 2009, Voveran was still the largest selling domestic drug in India. Japan is another major Voltaren market, although this is likely to change as the pressure to prescribe and dispense generics increases. But despite the availability of numerous generics, Voltaren still enjoys significant sales in Europe, including in France and Germany.

In addition to all of this, Novartis's generics arm, Sandoz, also markets generic diclofenac in oral forms, as an injectable and as suppositories.

Voltaren sales were expected to suffer because of the introduction of COX-2 inhibitors in the same indications, but the spectacular failure of Vioxx®, following the appearance of serious cardiovascular side effects and its withdrawal from world markets, effectively eliminated competition from this new drug family and allowed Voltaren to continue to flourish.

Learnings

One of the main learnings from the LCM of Voltaren, and the reason for including it in this book, is that it is dangerous to try to extrapolate all aspects of past successes one-on-one into the future. Many of the strategies which contributed to the success of Voltaren during the 1970s, 1980s, and 1990s would not work as well today. Premium pricing of line extensions and the use of a different salt, for example, would be highly unlikely to meet with the same success today, and it is unlikely that Novartis would today undertake the wide spectrum of clinical trials that health authorities would now demand for a product to achieve such broad indications in its labeling.

However, the Voltaren case does also contain elements which are still very applicable today to the LCM of mature, patent-expired brands. These include

- Switch (part of) the franchise to OTC
- Focus on self-pay markets, where the patient and not the third-party payer makes the buying decision
- Create local line extensions, including reformulations and FDCs, where regulatory hurdles are low and/or price premiums are feasible.

In the COX-2 crisis, Voltaren undoubtedly benefited from the fact that is was an old, well-established drug. It was not tested for cardiovascular safety as extensively as the new drug class, although recent research suggests that traditional NSAIDs may carry a similar degree of cardiovascular risk as do the withdrawn COX-2 inhibitors.

It is also worth asking just how big the Voltaren brand might be today if diclofenac was still patented. Following the demise of the COX-2 inhibitors and in view of the persisting unmet need for effective painkillers, a figure of US$5 million annual sales might be considered reasonable. Looked at this way, patent-expired Voltaren may only be realizing 15% or so of the potential it could aspire to were there to be no generics on the market.

A.31 LCM OF A WOMEN'S HEALTH FRANCHISE

The Yasmin® Family

Yasmin is Bayer's FDC oral contraceptive containing drospirenone and ethinyl estradiol. It was introduced in the United States in mid-2001. Drospirenone was a known substance, and the product was protected by three secondary patents listed in the Orange Book, but primarily by the "531" patent which was due to expire in 2020.

In late 2005, Bayer launched an FDC of drospirenone and estradiol under the trade name Angeliq® for the treatment of menopausal symptoms such as hot flashes and vaginal dryness. Angeliq is protected solely by the "395" patent (which is also listed for both Yasmin and Yaz®).

Bayer launched Yaz in early 2006. Yaz combines drospirenone and ethinyl estradiol, but the latter is dosed one-third lower than in Yasmin. The initial approval was for oral contraception, and then in early 2007, the indication of acne treatment in women aged over 14 years was added. It is protected by 10 secondary patents listed in the Orange Book, of which the "531" patent is again of key importance.

In January 2005, Barr filed its ANDA for a generic Yasmin product with Paragraph IV certification against the three patents listed in the Orange Book. Bayer filed a patent infringement suit, triggering a 30-month stay which expired in September 2007, as the FDA accepted Barr's filing in March 2005.

In January 2007, Barr submitted an ANDA for a Yaz generic with Paragraph IV certification against all 10 Bayer patents listed in the Orange Book. Again, Bayer filed a suit triggering a 30-month stay.

In October 2007, Watson filed for a Yaz generic, again with Paragraph IV certification.

In March 2008 a U.S. District Court invalidated Bayer's "531" patent on grounds of obviousness, relying heavily on the KSR versus Teleflex judgment. The "531" patent claims pharmaceutical formulations of micronized drospirenone and ethinyl estradiol. The two key issues in the case were whether it would have been obvious to

- micronize drospirenone so as to increase its bioavailability
- not protect the drospirenone from the gastric environment with an enteric coating.

Drospirenone is a relatively difficult molecule to formulate due to its poor water solubility and sensitivity to acid.

Bayer argued that prior art taught away from micronizing acid-sensitive drugs like drospirenone, but the court concluded: "Undoubtedly, there would be some concern about dissolution of a poorly water soluble acid sensitive drug, but the person of ordinary skill in the art could conclude that micronization is a viable option." Similarly, while Bayer asserted that the prior art taught that acid-sensitive drugs must be enteric coated, the court agreed with Barr's argument, finding that "inter- and intra-subject variability is a major disadvantage" of enteric coating, and concluding therefore that one "could not rule out formulating a micronized drospirenone without enteric coating." Furthermore, the court concluded that a prior art reference teaching that drospirenone isomerzies when exposed to hydrochloric acid *in vitro* should be discounted because its results were not corroborated by *in vivo* studies. In addition to concluding that the invention claimed in the "531" patent would have been obvious, the court felt that the invention was obvious to try. As in KSR versus Teleflex, the court concluded that "there are a finite number of identified predictable solutions." In this case, based on the prior art as a whole, micronizing and immediately releasing drospirenone was obvious to try. Bayer appealed the decision.

In June 2008, Bayer and Barr signed supply and licensing agreements for both Yasmin and Yaz for the United States. Under the terms of this agreement, Bayer supplied Barr with a generic version of Yasmin, which Barr marketed only in the United States. Barr paid Bayer a fixed percentage of the revenues from the product sold by Barr. The agreement stipulated that Bayer could continue to pursue its appeal of the court decision invalidating Bayer's "531" patent for Yasmin. Were Bayer to prevail in its appeal, Bayer would receive a larger share of Barr's revenues from the product. Furthermore, it was agreed that Bayer would grant Barr a license to market a generic version of Yaz in the United States starting in July 2011. Bayer would supply Barr with product. Should Bayer lose patent lawsuits in the United States against other companies concerning Yaz before that date, at that time Bayer would begin supplying the product to Barr, and Barr would begin marketing the generic. Barr would pay Bayer a fixed percentage of the revenues from the product sold by Barr.

Accordingly, Barr launched its branded generic version of Yasmin, Ocella®, in July 2008.

Also in 2008, Watson and Sandoz both submitted ANDAs with Paragraph IV certification for Yasmin generics. Bayer duly filed suit against both companies, alleging patent infringement. In reply, Watson and Sandoz filed counterclaims alleging, among other things, the invalidity of various Bayer patents. Sandoz further alleged that the agreement between Bayer and Barr was anticompetitive and violated antitrust and unfair competition laws.

And another 2008 development that was to have a major impact on the future of Bayer's Yasmin/Yaz franchise was the announcement by Teva in July that it intended to acquire Barr. The acquisition was approved by the U.S. FTC in December 2008.

In August 2009, a three-judge panel affirmed the lower court ruling invalidating the "531" patent covering Yasmin due to obviousness.

In June 2010, Teva announced that it had commercially launched Gianvi®, the company's branded generic version of Yaz, and had been awarded 180-day exclusivity as the first filer. This move came as a surprise to many analysts who had expected Teva to wait with its launch until July 2011, in accordance with the agreement of June 2008 between Bayer and Barr. A Bayer spokesman promptly announced that Bayer would sue Teva for patent infringement.

Teva's decision to launch Gianvi at risk was partly motivated by the fact that the 30-month stay on Watson's ANDA for its Yaz generic expired in May 2010.

In June 2010, Bayer sued Teva for false advertising and for patent infringement. Bayer claimed that Teva was marketing Gianvi using Physician Prescribing Information that falsely claimed that Gianvi's ethinyl estradiol is "stabilised by betadex as a clathrate," but that based on Bayer's testing of the product this was not true. Bayer sought a temporary restraining order and a preliminary injunction to stop Teva from making false claims about Gianvi, and from infringing Bayer's "338" patent which covers ethinyl estradiol drugs stabilized by betadex as a clathrate. Teva admitted before a federal court that it had indeed misrepresented the usage of betadex as a clathrate.

In the meantime, several other branded generics of Yaz and Yasmin have entered the U.S. market, including Sandoz's Loryna® and Syeda® and Watson's Zarah®.

As of June 2011, Bayer was still pursuing patent infringement cases against Teva, Sandoz, and Mylan. In Europe, Bayer's fortunes for Yasmin took a further blow in July 2011. Bayer commented in a press release that the European Patent Office had revoked the key patent protecting Yasmin following an appeal from generics company Hexal, part of the Sandoz group, against an earlier decision in 2006 that confirmed the patent. The Bayer spokeswoman commented that the decision would take immediate effect, but declined to comment on how soon rivals could bring copycat versions to market.

The prospects for the Yasmin family of products had taken another dramatic turn for the worse in late 2010 when class action lawsuits alleging serious health side effects to some of the users of Yasmin and Yaz were initiated. At this point, there had already been about 4000 individual cases against the two drugs in the United States, claiming that they caused strokes, pulmonary embolisms, and various heart problems. Moreover, many young women taking these drugs had to have their gall bladders removed.

Bayer's ideas for protecting the Yasmin franchise do seem to be running out. FDCs of both Yasmin and Yaz with folic acid look like nonstarters against low-priced Yasmin and Yaz generics, and Bayer's new contraceptive Natazia® (Qlaira® in Europe) is forecast to replace only a small fraction of the lost Yasmin/Yaz sales.

Learnings

Bayer had done a good job of maximizing the potential of drospirenone during the lifetime of the Yasmin and Yaz secondary patents by introducing a variety of formulations with different estrogen content and a different number of active days in the cycle to counteract the side effects of hormonal therapy. The battery of secondary patents and the active defense of these patents succeeded in delaying generic entry. When these defenses were finally destined to fail, a "win-win" settlement was agreed with a generic company, and this strategy may only have fallen apart because of the acquisition of Barr by Teva. Bayer's defense of the Yasmin family of products would have been successful for even longer had it not fallen foul of the tougher interpretation of obviousness following the KSR versus Teleflex ruling.

A.32 INDICATION EXPANSION/NEW DOSAGE STRENGTH

Zometa/Reclast® (Aclasta)

Novartis's bisphosphonate Zometa (zoledronic acid) was first launched in 2000 and made its debut on the U.S. market in 2001, approved for the treatment of hypercalcemia of malignancy. The first indication expansion in the United States was achieved in 2002, with the addition of the indications multiple myeloma and bone metastases of solid tumors. It is available as a 4-mg dosage (in a 5-mL vial) administered by 15-min intravenous infusion repeated after a week in the case of hypercalcemia, or every 3–4 weeks in the case of multiple myeloma and bone metastases. Zometa quickly became the gold-standard treatment for hypercalcemia associated with malignancy.

Novartis then pursued an indication expansion strategy that took the drug into a completely new physician and patient population. It was also given a new brand name, Aclasta (EU) resp. Reclast (United States). In early 2007, the FDA approved Reclast for the treatment of the niche indication Paget's disease, and in late 2007 for the much larger indication osteoporosis. Novartis demonstrated to the FDA's satisfaction that the optimal dosage of zoledronic acid in these indications was 5 mg rather than the 4 mg used for the cancer indications, and formulated it as a 100-mL ready-to-give infusion in place of the 5-mL vial used in cancer. Aclasta's strongest selling point in osteoporosis was that it only has to be dosed once yearly.

The composition-of-matter patent on zoledronic acid is due to expire in September 2012, but the product has been awarded pediatric exclusivity which extends exclusivity until March 2013. The pediatric trial indicated that the drug should not be used in children, but to gain pediatric exclusivity, it is not necessary to prove utility of a drug in children, just to conduct pediatric trials according to the Pediatric Written Request (PWR) (United States) or Pediatric Investigation Plan (PIP) (EU). In addition to its basic patent, Aclasta/Reclast is protected by additional formulation patents until 2022, but these are not listed in the FDA's Orange Book.

With the separate physician and patient populations and slightly different dosage strength (4 mg versus 5 mg), Novartis has been able to clearly separate the identity of its two brands. However, early off-label prescribing of Zometa for osteoporosis (reported in Datamonitor, "Pipeline Insight 2007: Osteoporosis") suggests that Aclasta/Reclast sales may suffer significantly once the zoledronic acid composition-of-matter patent expires in early 2013. Teva holds 180-day exclusivity, and once this expires in late 2013 and other generic agents enter the market, there is likely to be a considerable price discrepancy between generic zoledronic acid and Aclasta/Reclast.

Even so, with 6 years of exclusivity remaining between approval in 2007 and primary patent expiry in 2013, the decision to develop the osteoporosis indication would seem to have been a good one for Novartis. The key question remains whether their chosen clinical strategy was the best in the circumstances. Novartis chose to conduct one of the largest clinical programs in the history of osteoporosis, banking on the strong clinical data to drive uptake and overcome the barriers to entry of once-yearly infusion. By contrast, rival Boniva from Roche was supported by a very limited clinical program, relying on a simple "one tablet, once a month" ease of use story. In the end, Boniva has been more successful in terms of sales, and most likely even better still in terms of profit. Again, right concept, but potentially not the optimum approach.

Learnings

We shall have to wait until 2013 to see whether Novartis has succeeded in maintaining a significant market share with premium-priced Aclasta/Reclast once the composition-of-matter patent on zoledronic acid expires in the major markets. But thanks to its indication expansion strategy, Novartis has already been successful in getting zoledronic acid prescribed by a new group of physicians to a whole new patient population. Will the 4-mg and 5-mg dosages for the two indications be too close to ward off generic erosion once Zometa generics appear on the market? Time will tell.

Note: Page numbers in *italics* refer to figures, those in **bold** to tables.

Pharmaceutical Lifecycle Management: Making the Most of Each and Every Brand, First Edition. Tony Ellery and Neal Hansen.
© 2012 John Wiley & Sons, Inc. Published 2012 by John Wiley & Sons, Inc.

384 INDEX

Printed and bound by CPI Group (UK) Ltd, Croydon, CR0 4YY

27/10/2024

14580134-0001